Black Health in the South

EDITED BY

Steven S. Coughlin
Lovoria B. Williams
Tabia Henry Akintobi

JOHNS HOPKINS UNIVERSITY PRESS   BALTIMORE

© 2023 Johns Hopkins University Press
All rights reserved. Published 2023
Printed in the United States of America on acid-free paper
9 8 7 6 5 4 3 2 1

Johns Hopkins University Press
2715 North Charles Street
Baltimore, Maryland 21218
www.press.jhu.edu

Cataloging-in-Publication Data is available from the Library of Congress.
A catalog record for this book is available from the British Library.

ISBN: 978-1-4214-4546-5 (hardcover)
ISBN: 978-1-4214-4547-2 (ebook)

Special discounts are available for bulk purchases of this book. For more information, please contact Special Sales at specialsales@jh.edu.

Contents

Part Four: Future Directions

Contributors

TABIA HENRY AKINTOBI, PhD, MPH

Professor and Chair of Community Health and Preventive Medicine
Principal Investigator and Director, Prevention Research Center
Associate Dean, Community Engagement
Morehouse School of Medicine
Atlanta, GA

BRITTNEY T. ANDERSON, MD

Assistant Professor, Family, Internal, and Rural Medicine
College of Community Health Sciences
The University of Alabama
Tuscaloosa, AL

CANDACE BEST, PhD

Associate Professor, Department of Psychological Sciences
Augusta University
Augusta, GA

CAMILLE BURNETT, MPA, APHN-BC, RN, BSCN, DSW, CGNC, FAAN

Associate Vice President, Education and Health Equity
Executive Associate Director, Institute for Inclusion, Inquiry and
    Innovation (iCubed)
Office of Institutional Equity, Effectiveness and Success
Virginia Commonwealth University
Richmond, VA

TIFFANY E. BYRD, MPH, CHES

Doctoral Candidate, Department of Health Promotion, Education,
    and Behavior
Arnold School of Public Health
University of South Carolina
Columbia, SC

KERRI L. CAVANAUGH, MD, MHS
Associate Professor of Medicine
Vanderbilt University School of Medicine
Nashville, TN

CHARLTON COLES, PhD
Consultant, Center for Research on Health Disparities
Clemson University
Clemson, SC

STEVEN S. COUGHLIN, PhD, MPH
Professor and Interim Head, Division of Epidemiology
Department of Population Health Sciences
Augusta University
Augusta, GA

MARTHA R. CROWTHER, PhD, MPH
Associate Dean for Research & Health Policy
Professor, Community Medicine & Population Health
Professor, Family, Internal, & Rural Medicine
Investigator, Institute for Rural Health Research
The University of Alabama
Tuscaloosa, AL

YENDELELA L. CUFFEE, PhD, MPH
Assistant Professor, Program in Epidemiology
College of Health Science
University of Delaware
Newark, DE

CASEY L. DANIEL, PhD, MPH
Director of Epidemiology and Public Health and Assistant Professor
University of South Alabama College of Medicine
University of South Alabama Mitchell Cancer Institute
Chair, Alabama Comprehensive Cancer Coalition
Mobile, AL

STACY N. DAVIS, PhD, MPH

Assistant Professor, Department of Health Behavior, Society and Policy

School of Public Health

Rutgers University

Piscataway, NJ

RACHEL FISSELL, MD

Assistant Professor of Medicine

Division of Nephrology and Hypertension

Department of Medicine

Vanderbilt University Medical Center

Nashville, TN

FAITH E. FLETCHER, PhD, MA

Assistant Professor, Center for Medical Ethics and Health Policy

Baylor College of Medicine

Houston, TX

LYNN E. GLENN, PhD, APRN-C

Assistant Professor, Department of Biobehavioral Nursing

College of Nursing

Augusta University

Augusta, GA

CLEMENT K. GWEDE, PhD, MPH, RN, FAAN

Senior Member/Professor, Moffitt Cancer Center

Morsani College of Medicine

University of South Florida

Tampa, FL

RYAN A. HARRIS, PhD, CEP, FACSM

Professor of Medicine, Pediatrics, Physiology & Graduate Studies

Augusta University

Augusta, GA

KATHIE L. HERMAYER, MD, MS

Professor of Medicine and Endocrinology, College of Medicine

Medical University of South Carolina

Charleston, SC

LUCY A. INGRAM, PhD, MPH

Associate Professor, Department of Health Promotion, Education, and Behavior

Associate Dean for Academic Affairs and Online Education

Arnold School of Public Health

University of South Carolina

Columbia, SC

CAROLYN JENKINS, DRPH, MSN, MS, RN, RD, LD, FAAN

Professor Emerita, College of Nursing

Medical University of South Carolina

Mount Pleasant, SC

ANTONIKA KADIRI, MPH

Doctoral Candidate, Department of Health Promotion, Education, and Behavior

Arnold School of Public Health

University of South Carolina

Columbia, SC

ERNEST KANINJING, DRPH, MPH, MBA, CHES

Assistant Professor of Public Health, School of Health & Human Performance

Georgia College

Milledgeville, GA

GASTON KAPUKU, MD

Associate Professor, Department of Medicine

Augusta University

Augusta, GA

ANNA KUCHARSKA-NEWTON, PhD, MPH

Assistant Professor, Department of Epidemiology
Cardiovascular Epidemiology Program
The Gillings School of Global Public Health
University of North Carolina at Chapel Hill
Chapel Hill, NC

DANIEL LACKLAND, DRPH

Professor, College of Medicine
Medical University of South Carolina
Charleston, SC

AUNDREA E. LOFTLEY, MD

Assistant Professor, Department of Medicine
College of Medicine
Medical University of South Carolina
Charleston, SC

GEORGIANA LOGAN, PhD, MS

Assistant Professor, Department of Health Science
Minority Health Institute
Marshall University
Huntington, WV

JOHN S. LUQUE, PhD, MPH

Professor, Institute of Public Health
Florida Agricultural and Mechanical University
Tallahassee, FL

PAUL C. MANN, MD

Associate Professor of Pediatrics
Acting Division Head, Neonatology
Director, Center for Bioethics and Health Policy
Augusta University
Augusta, GA

DANIELLE L. McDUFFIE, MA
The University of Alabama
Tuscaloosa, AL

FOLAKEMI T. ODEDINA, PhD
Professor and Associate Director, Center for Health Equity and
    Community Engagement Research
Director, CHCR Global Health Disparities Initiatives
Mayo Clinic
Jacksonville, FL

BRUCE OVBIAGELE, MD, FRCP
Chief of Staff and Associate Dean
Professor, Department of Neurology
University of California San Francisco
San Francisco Veterans Affairs Health Care System
San Francisco, CA

VERONICA G. PARKER, PhD
Director, Center for Research on Health Disparities
Professor/Biostatistician
School of Nursing
Clemson University
Clemson, SC

SIDDHARTHA ROY, DRPH, MPH
Assistant Professor, Department of Family and Community
    Medicine
Pennsylvania State University College of Medicine
Hershey, PA

SAMANTHA SOJOURNER, PhD
Assistant Professor, Department of Medicine
Augusta University
Augusta, GA

EBELE M. UMEUKEJE, MD, MPH
Assistant Professor, Division of Nephrology and Hypertension
Department of Medicine
Vanderbilt University Medical Center
Nashville, TN

MARLO VERNON, PhD
Assistant Professor, Department of Medicine
Augusta University
Augusta, GA

COLLEEN WALTERS, DNP, MSN
Assistant Professor, College of Nursing
Augusta University
Augusta, GA

JASMINE WASHINGTON, MD
Nephrology Fellow
Division of Nephrology and Hypertension
Department of Medicine
Vanderbilt University Medical Center
Nashville, TN

LOVORIA B. WILLIAMS, PhD, APRN-BC, FAAN
Associate Professor, College of Nursing
University of Kentucky
Lexington, KY

MARIANNE K. WILSON, MD
Assistant Professor, Department of Medicine
College of Medicine
Medical University of South Carolina
Charleston, SC

CLAYTON C. YATES, PhD
Professor and Director, Center for Biomedical Research
Tuskegee University
Tuskegee, Alabama

LUFEI YOUNG, PhD, APRN
Associate Professor, College of Nursing
Augusta University
Augusta, GA

Preface

This volume was written by outstanding contributors who are nationally and internationally recognized for their work. It provides important information about the health and well-being of African Americans in the southern United States. The audience for the book includes graduate students, health professionals, members of health advocacy organizations, and researchers from many different disciplines, including epidemiology, behavioral science, medicine, nursing, sociology, health disparities, policy studies, and African American studies. This book will likely also be of interest to members of nonprofit organizations, government agencies, and health advocacy organizations. Practitioners at local, state, and federal agencies and departments will also find it relevant.

The book is organized in four parts. The first part, Foundations, provides an overview of the health of African Americans in the southern United States and information about several foundational topics: the social determinants of health and disease; race, racism, and health disparities; poverty, income, and health equity; and access to quality, culturally appropriate health care. The second part of the book, Methods, discusses research approaches that are important for addressing health disparities among African Americans in the South. These include health intervention studies, faith-based interventions, and clinical/community based research networks. The third part, Health Disparities, discusses disparities in cardiovascular disease, diabetes, kidney disease and end-stage renal disease, interpersonal violence, mental health, major forms of cancer, maternal health, and infant mortality. The last part of the book, Future Directions, examines approaches to ameliorating and eliminating health disparities among African Americans in the southern United States.

Our hope is that this unique volume will provide a pivotal discussion of the prevalence of, determinants of, and potential solutions to health disparities that affect African Americans in the South and elsewhere in the United States. We anticipate that it will stimulate efforts to prevent and control these disparities for the benefit of at-risk communities and future generations of African Americans.

I   FOUNDATIONS

1

Overview

STEVEN S. COUGHLIN, PhD, MPH,

LOVORIA B. WILLIAMS, PhD, FNP-BC, FAAN,

and TABIA HENRY AKINTOBI, PhD, MPH

The southern United States is a geographic and cultural region of the United States located between the western United States and the Atlantic Ocean. It is south of the midwestern United States and northeastern United States and north of the Gulf of Mexico and Mexico. The region is known for its culture and history. As defined by the US census, the region includes 16 states (Delaware, Florida, Georgia, Maryland, North Carolina, South Carolina, Virginia, West Virginia, Alabama, Kentucky, Mississippi, Tennessee, Arkansas, Louisiana, Oklahoma, and Texas).[1] However, Delaware, Maryland, and the District of Columbia remained with the Union during the Civil War. As of 2020, an estimated 114,555,744 people, or 37% of all US residents, lived in the South, the nation's most populous region.[2]

The historical and cultural development of the South have been influenced by the institution of slave labor on plantations in the Deep South, the legacy of racism magnified by the Civil War and Reconstruction, the segregated system of separate schools and public facilities known as Jim Crow laws that remained in effect until the 1960s, and the presence of a large proportion of African Americans in the population.[3] After the Civil War, the South's population, infrastructure, and economy were devastated.[4] Thousands of people were on the move as African Americans strove to reunite with families separated by slave sales. Other freed people moved from plantation areas to cities or towns. African Americans in the South were made free citizens and were given the right to vote with the passage of the Thirteenth, Fourteenth, and Fifteenth Amendments to the Constitution of the United States. Secret vigilante organizations such as the Ku Klux Klan arose quickly after the war's end that used lynching, physical attacks, house burnings, and intimidation to keep African Americans from exercising their political rights. Jim Crow laws were passed to segregate public facilities and services, including transportation. In the late 19th and early 20th centuries, thousands of African Americans left the South for cities in the Northeast and Midwest in the movement known as the Great Migration.[5] In their pursuit of justice and voting rights, African Americans participated in large-scale activism during the Civil Rights Movement of the 1950s and 1960s. Most of the major events in the movement occurred in the South.

Historically, the South relied heavily on agriculture and was highly rural until after 1945; it has since become more industrialized and urban.[6] The expansion of cotton cultivation after 1800 required more slave labor, and the institution became an integral part of the South's economy.[7] In the early 20th century, invasion of the boll weevil devastated cotton crops in the South, prompting more African Americans to leave the South for northern and western cities. World War II was a time of dramatic change in the poor, heavily rural South as the federal government developed new industries and military bases. Farming shifted from cotton and tobacco to include cattle, rice, soybeans, corn, and other foods. Industrial growth increased in the 1960s and greatly accelerated into the 1980s and 1990s. Several large urban areas in Texas, Georgia, and Florida grew to over four million people. In the late 20th century, the South's service economy, manufacturing base, high-technology industries, and financial sector experienced a boom. However, the ten poorest big cities in the United States include Memphis, Tennessee, and Miami, Florida. In 2011, nine of the ten poorest states were in the South.[8] The South has lower percentages of high school graduates, lower household incomes, and a lower cost of living than the rest of the United States.

African American descendants of the slaves who were brought into the South compose the second largest racial minority in the United States; according to the 2000 federal census, they account for 12.1% of the total population. The majority of the African American population remains concentrated in the South. This group has contributed heavily to elements (Christianity and the Bible Belt, foodways, art, and music) of southern culture today.[9]

Health Disparities among African Americans

Compared to other racial groups, African Americans have a higher risk of adverse health outcomes and premature mortality. Life expectancy in the United States in 2015 was 75.7 years for African Americans compared to 87.7 years for Asian / Pacific Islanders and 79.2 years for whites.[10] The disparity in life expectancy, which is particularly pronounced for African American men, is driven by marked racial disparities in leading causes of death such as heart disease, diabetes, and homicide.[10] African Americans also experience pronounced disparities in cancer mortality.[11–15]

African Americans have poorer cardiovascular health and higher cardiovascular disease (CVD) mortality than non-Hispanic whites. The high burden of CVD among African Americans is a primary cause of disparities in life expectancy between African Americans and whites.[16] The higher prevalence of CVD risk factors (e.g., hypertension, diabetes mellitus, and obesity) underlies the relatively earlier age of onset of CVDs among African Americans. Hypertension is highly prevalent among African Americans and contributes to disparities in stroke, heart failure, and peripheral artery disease.[16] The prevalence of diagnosed and undiagnosed hypertension among African American men (42.4%) and women (44%) $\geq$ 20 years of age is among the highest in the world.[16]

The excess in stroke mortality for African Americans is substantially larger in southern states than in nonsouthern states.[17] The Stroke Belt is a region of the southeastern United States that has 50% higher stroke mortality rates.[17] African Americans living in southern states are at higher risk of death from stroke than are whites.[17] At age 55 years, the risk of dying from stroke is about three times greater for African Americans than whites.[17] The reasons for the Stroke Belt are unknown but may include regional differences in stroke risk factors such as hypertension, obesity, and diabetes.

African American men develop diabetes mellitus 1.52 times more often than white men, and African American women are 2.14 times more likely to develop diabetes than white women.[16] The combined prevalence of diagnosed and undiagnosed type 2 diabetes mellitus is 21.8% in African Americans and 11.3% in non-Hispanic whites.[18] African Americans are twice as likely to die from diabetes than non-Hispanic whites.[19] In a study of racial disparities in diabetes mortality in the 50 most populous US cities, African Americans had statistically significantly higher mortality rates than whites in 39 of the 41 cities included in analyses.[19] The prevalence of diagnosed diabetes is higher in southern states than in nonsouthern states.[20]

Obesity rates are higher among African Americans than whites. Among adults $\geq$ 20 years of age, African American women had the highest rates of obesity at 58%, followed by African American men (38%), white men (34%), and white women (33%).[21] Nine southern states (Mississippi, Louisiana, West Virginia, Alabama, Oklahoma, Arkansas, South Carolina, Kentucky, and Texas) have obesity rates that are among the highest in the nation.[22,23] Rates for hypertension and diabetes for these states are also the highest in the nation.[23] The southern United States also has the largest number of people who die from stroke.

Although reduced obesity, a healthy diet, increased physical activity, and the use of health care services can improve population health and health equity, these factors are influenced by social determinants such as income, employment, and education.[10,11] Neighborhood socioeconomic status (SES) is inversely related to diabetes and hypertension. African Americans are four times more likely than whites to live in the lowest SES neighborhoods.[11] Poverty rates are two times higher among African Americans (25.4%) than among non-Hispanic whites (10.4%).[10] Unemployment rates are more than two times higher among African Americans than among non-Hispanic whites.[10] There are also substantial disparities in educational attainment. Fewer African Americans graduate from high school (72.5%) than non-Hispanic whites (87.2%).[11]

The health disparities that are seen among African Americans, particularly those who live in southern States, are not limited to cardiovascular disease, diabetes, and obesity. African Americans who live in the South also have increased risks of sexually transmitted diseases, HIV/AIDS, infant mortality, and mental health conditions.[24-27] The HIV epidemic is most pronounced in the South, which has the highest rates of HIV infection.[26] In the United States, approximately 46% of people living with HIV reside in the South. African Americans are disproportionately affected: the HIV diagnosis rate among African Americans is eight times that of whites.[27] In 2016, African Americans accounted for 54% of all new HIV diagnoses in the South.[27] African American women account for 69% of all HIV diagnoses among women in the South.[28] African American men who have sex with other men account for 59% of all HIV diagnoses among African Americans in the South.[28]

The Causes of Health Disparities

African Americans who live in the southern United States have a unique history that includes hundreds of years of slavery, injustices experienced during the Jim Crow era, the Great Migration, the Civil Rights Movement, and contemporary experiences that include reverse migration from cities in the Midwest and Northeast to the South, the Black Lives Matter movement, and continued efforts to address inequities and structural problems that affect the lives and health of African Americans. The legacy of slavery and the limitations on civil rights until the middle of the 20th century have had an important effect on the social, economic, cultural, and political experiences of African Americans in this region. These factors have resulted in significant racial and socioeconomic health disparities.[29]

The work of Michael Marmot and others has highlighted the importance of social gradients in the relative deprivation that is a driving force in health disparities.[30] Socioeconomic factors such as unemployment, lack of education, poverty, and income inequality are among the most important social determinants of health. Economists use the Gini coefficient to measure income inequality. From 1990 to 2018, the Gini coefficient in the United States rose from 0.43 to 0.49, reflecting a nationwide increase in income inequality. Income disparities frequently coexist with other sociopolitical determinants of health, which include access to health insurance, rates of employment, quality of education, support for public assistance programs, and access to quality health care. Unequal access to these social resources for marginalized racial/ethnic groups, particularly African Americans, leads to increased hospitalization, illness, and death across many chronic diseases.[31,32] In 2018, all 17 states in the South were among the top 20 with respect to highest income inequality.[33]

It is well established that low-income people are at increased risk of an array of adverse health outcomes and are more likely to die prematurely. Numerous studies have documented a socioeconomic gradient: people on each step of the socioeconomic ladder exhibit improved health outcomes over the people on the rung below.[34,35] Compared to whites, African Americans receive less income at the same education levels and have markedly less wealth at equivalent income levels. These disparities in income are reflected in racial differences in life expectancy. A 1998 study found that for each mile of the twelve-mile Metro route from downtown Washington, DC, to Montgomery County, Maryland, the life expectancy of the resident population increased by approximately a year and a half.[36]

Social determinants of health play an important role in creating and sustaining health disparities among African Americans. Frameworks of social determinants build on the social gradient concept, the ideas that individuals with lower social status have greater health risks and lower life expectancy than those with higher status and that the impact of social position can accumulate over time.[37] Social determinants of poor health include inadequate food and nutrition, lack of education, unemployment, inadequate housing, and lack of access to affordable, quality health care; social support; and social connections (social networks). The social context in which people live and work influences their health. For example, social connections between neighbors and greater social cohesion and social capital have been found to be protective against depression.[38] Conversely, exposure to interpersonal violence has been associated with increased depression, depressive symptoms, and posttraumatic stress disorder.[38] Racial discrimination, food insecurity, poor family relationships, and a history of abuse and neglect have also been associated with negative mental health outcomes.[37] In contrast, living with family, satisfaction with family relationships, and family connectedness have been associated with fewer depressive symptoms.[37]

The World Health Organization defines the social determinants of health as the "conditions in which people are born, grow, work, live and age, and the wider set of forces and systems shaping the conditions of daily life."[39] Adverse childhood experiences, including exposure to domestic violence, parental incarceration, and parental mental illness, are strongly associated with adverse health consequences later in life. The Institute of Medicine notes that the social environment may influence health behavior by "shaping norms, enforcing patterns of social control, providing or not providing environmental opportunities to engage in particular behaviors, reducing or producing stress, and placing constraints on individual choice."[40] The environmental context of living in an area of low or underemployment, high crime, residential crowding, and poorer living conditions contributes to a state of chronic psychosocial stress.[41-44] Accordingly, behavioral and metabolic risk factors are increased disproportionately among those with high psychosocial chronic stress, leading to a strain on the coping abilities of individuals.[45-47] Chronic stress due to a disadvantaged social environment may independently affect health outcomes negatively. One hypothesized mechanism for the relationship between chronic stress and poor health outcomes lies within the hypothalamus-pituitary-adrenal (HPA) pathway. Increased HPA dysfunction has been associated with lower socioeconomic status, higher cortisol variability, and increased measurements of central adiposity.[46,48] Chronic stress due to a disadvantaged social environment may independently impact health outcomes negatively.

Some consider racism to be a social determinant of health for people of color. Structural racism refers to the ways societies foster racial discrimination through mutually reinforcing and unequal systems of housing, education, employment, earnings, credit, health care, and criminal justice.[49] These patterns and practices reinforce discriminatory beliefs, values, and distribution of resources.[49] Structural racism is reflected in the residential segregation of African Americans, which is associated with adverse birth outcomes, decreased longevity, increased risk of chronic disease, and increased rates of homicide.[49,50] As Williams et al. note, "Racial residential segregation refers to the occupancy of different neighborhood environments by race that was developed in the U.S. to ensure that whites resided in separate communities from blacks. Segregation was created by federal policies as well as explicit governmental support of private policies such as discriminatory zoning, mortgage discrimination, red-lining and restrictive covenants."[50]

The pathways through which structural racism and residential segregation harm health include exposure to dilapidated housing, the substandard quality of the social and built environments, limited opportunities for high-quality education and desirable employment, and restricted access to quality health care.[49] Residential segregation systematically shapes access to, use of, and quality of health care, at the individual, neighborhood, provider, and health care system levels.[49-51]

In addition to substandard housing and residence in high crime areas, examples of structural or systemic problems that adversely affect health include poverty, lack of health insurance, inadequate access to health care, lack of education, health illiteracy, lack of transportation, and food insecurity. For example, as the result of redlining and other historical and contemporary injustices, African Americans are less likely to own a home or to have built up home equity, which places them at risk of financial distress if they experience an illness such as heart attack, stroke, or cancer. Although redlining is no longer legal, discrimination in the rental and housing markets against communities of color is still pervasive.[49] Another example of a structural problem that contributes to health disparities is the War on Drugs and the tough-on-crime policies enacted in the 1970s and 1980s that stereotyped African Americans as drug addicts and disproportionately targeted them for incarceration.[49]

Racism harms health through multiple pathways. It exposes people to adverse physical, social, and economic systems and can lead to maladaptive coping behaviors.[49] These exposures can accumulate over the life course and across generations. Interpersonal racism has been shown to have adverse effects on psychological well-being, mental health, and the consumption of alcohol, cigarettes, and illicit drugs.[49]

Phelan and Link argue that the combination of our expanded capacity to control death and disease and the presence of social and economic inequalities creates health disparities by race and SES: "When we develop the ability to control disease and death, the benefits of this new-found ability are distributed according to resources of knowledge, power, prestige, and beneficial social connections. Those who are advantaged with respect to such resources benefit more from new health-enhancing capabilities and consequently experience lower mortality rates. Disparities are the result. This explanation for health disparities is a core component of the theory of fundamental social causes."[52]

The determinants of health disparities are complex and multifactorial. They include biologic and behavioral individual factors, barriers to providers and health care systems that include differences in income, education, and health insurance coverage. Racial disparities may be due to differences in biology, increased comorbid conditions, suboptimal patient-physician interactions, and structural problems such as lack of transportation and decreased access to quality care. The use of community coalitions is a valuable approach for addressing health disparities in African American communities.[53,54] Improving the cultural competence of health care providers and the health care system are examples of evidence-based approaches to reducing health disparities.

A life course perspective, which recognizes the influence of historical changes on human behavior, is useful for understanding health disparities.[55,56] This perspective recognizes the linkages between early life experiences and later experiences in adulthood. For example, behavioral risk factors (e.g., cigarette smoking and alcohol consumption) over the life course may contribute more to adverse birth outcomes than current behavioral risk factors during pregnancy.[57] The early programming model of health disparities posits that exposures in early life could influence future risk of adverse health outcomes such as adverse birth outcomes and adult-onset chronic diseases.[57] Early life socioeconomic disadvantage has been associated with risk of adolescent and adult diseases independent of adolescent or adult SES.[58] The cumulative pathways model conceptualizes declining health as cumulative wear and tear to the body's allostatic systems.[57] Allostatic load reflects physiological changes across different biological regulatory systems in response to chronic social and environmental stress.[58] The life course perspective also emphasizes the ways that humans are interdependent and gives special attention to the family as the primary arena for experiencing and interpreting the wider social world. This perspective sees humans as capable of making choices and constructing their own life journeys within systems of opportunities and constraints.

Despite the importance of social determinants of health, genetic and epigenetic factors also contribute to adverse health outcomes and health disparities among African Americans. For example, adverse birth outcomes, which are rooted in institutionalized social disadvantage and structural racism, are mediated through complex interactions with genetic predisposition and expression.[59] Asthma prevalence and mortality in the United States are higher for African American children and adults than for their white counterparts.[60] Socioeconomic factors, racial discrimination, differential access to medical care, differential access to housing, patterns of medical care use, and biologic factors such as genetic variation in vulnerability to effects of exposures may contribute to these disparities.[60]

Recent advances in exposomics are also contributing to our understanding of health disparities. The exposome consists of all of the exposures an individual incurs over a lifetime (as an embryo, as a fetus, as a newborn, in early childhood, in preadolescence, in adolescence, in young adulthood, in middle age, in older adulthood, and in old age) and how those exposures are related to human health.[61] The exposome is dynamic and evolves throughout the lifetime of an individual. It includes internal and external environmental exposures to things such as microorganisms, alcohol, and tobacco and social, economic, and psychological exposures to factors such as social capital, education, and mental stress.[61] The exposome concept takes into account the full spectrum of possible exposures (diet, dietary supplements, food additives, pesticide residues, microbial organisms and infections, geophysical exposures, environmental pollution, smoking, alcohol consumption, exercise, infections, vaccinations, occupational exposures, consumer products, therapeutic drugs, severe stress, etc.), the timing of exposures, and acute and chronic responses to exposures.[62] In contrast to the genome, the exposome is highly variable and dynamic and evolves throughout the lifetime of an individual.

Diet is an important example of a culturally influenced environmental determinant of health that likely contributes to health disparities in the southern United States. Traditional African American food, colloquially called soul food, includes a variety of leafy greens, corn, starchy vegetables, grains, fried meats, whole milk, and buttermilk. Many of these ingredients contain high levels of fat, cholesterol, and sodium. Soul food has its roots in slavery when slaves received undesirable cuts of meats. African slaves used their knowledge of their West African heritage and food preparation techniques to develop a new, flavorful cuisine in the New World. The knowledge of West African food preparation, recipes, and crops that slaves brought to the continent are cultural traditions that have affected food practices in the southern United States.[63,64] Examples of soul food include sweet potato casserole, hot water cornbread, and grits flavored with salt and fat. In contemporary epidemiological studies, the southern dietary pattern characterized by added fats, fried food, eggs, organ and processed meats, and sugar-sweetened beverages has been associated with acute coronary heart disease and overall mortality.[65,66] African American men in the Stroke Belt were found to have lower intakes of sodium, potassium, magnesium, and calcium, and higher intake of cholesterol than white men.[67]

Addressing Health Disparities among African Americans in the South

Efforts to address health disparities among African Americans, including those who reside in the southern United States, are furthered by evidence-based interventions to improve the health of diverse communities. This includes information provided by the Centers for Disease Control and Prevention's Community Guide[68] and by leading health advocacy organizations and professional associations. Interventions that the Community Guide has identified as having sufficient evidence of effectiveness, based on systematic literature reviews, can be recommended to local and state health departments and other stakeholders for routine use in public health. Instances where the Community Guide has concluded that there is insufficient evidence that an intervention is effective in improving health suggest opportunities for further research.

Efforts to address health disparities often occur at the local level. Health needs assessments, Geographic Information Systems analyses, geospatial analyses, and qualitative research such as focus groups are often helpful for prioritizing health concerns and planning health interventions at the local level. Including members of the affected community in the planning process facilitates input from a diverse range of residents and provides more insight into the needs of the local community.[29] There is a need for interventions that incorporate the engagement of patients and stakeholders in developing, testing, and disseminating interventions.[69]

One promising approach to addressing health disparities is community-based participatory research (CBPR), a collaborative approach to research that equitably involves all partners, including community members affected by the health topic being addressed, representatives of organizations, and academic researchers in the research process.[70] This approach includes partnerships between academic and community organizations with the goal of increasing the value of the research product for all partners. CBPR addresses health disparities and inequities in diverse communities, including groups that are socially disadvantaged, marginalized, or stigmatized or that have suffered historical injustices. CBPR takes into account the strengths and insights that community and academic partners bring to framing health problems and developing solutions. Instead of focusing solely on health problems or other concerns, CBPR highlights community resilience, resources, and opportunities for positive growth.[70,71] It emphasizes shared decision-making, co-learning, reciprocal transfer of expertise between community members and academic partners, and mutual ownership of research products. The combination of experiences of community members with public health science provides a deeper understanding of complex social phenomena, thereby providing more relevant interventions and increasing the likelihood that the interventions will be successful. The CBPR research paradigm represents a fundamental shift in how academic researchers view community residents, from patients and research subjects who may benefit from medical advances to essential partners who can energize their communities to develop effective, sustainable interventions to improve health and eliminate health disparities.[72]

Eliminating or reducing health disparities likely requires multilevel interventions that are directed at more than one level of influence (e.g., individual, neighborhood, health care provider, health care system, policy).[73] In selecting interventions, it may be important to address an individual's social and physical environment, the health care system he or she accesses, and individual-level factors such as smoking cessation, weight management, or the use of cancer screening tests.[73] As Plescia and Emmanuel have noted, interventions can address multiple levels of the socioecological model, including changes at the policy level: "Many interventions designed to address health disparities emphasize reaching individuals or small groups with the greatest needs and a visible burden of suffering. However, interventions designed using a socioecological model have far greater impact. Changes in policy, systems, and the environment can have further reach and greater capacity to address the underlying causes of poor health and health disparity."[29]

African American communities have resources and strengths to draw upon that can address health disparities and improve quality of life. Examples include the importance of the church in the daily lives of many African Americans, the social support provided by family and friends, and resources provided by community-based organizations. Eliminating and reducing health disparities among African Americans in the southern United States requires collaboration among members of the target population and key stakeholders, including community partners; local, state, and federal governments; academic researchers; members of health advocacy organizations; private foundations; and policy makers. Cross-sectoral efforts that include representatives from health care, education, housing, employment, and financial services may be required to address structural problems that contribute to health disparities.

REFERENCES

1. United States Census Bureau. "Census Regions and Divisions of the United States." N.d. https://www2.census.gov/geo/pdfs/maps-data/maps/reference/us_regdiv.pdf.

2. Mackun, Paul, and Steven Wilson. Population Distribution and Change: 2000 to 2010. 2010 Census Briefs, March 2011. https://www.census.gov/content/dam/Census/library/publications/2011/dec/c2010br-01.pdf.

3. Allen, John O., and Clayton E. Jewett. *Slavery in the South: A State-by-State History.* Westport, CT: Greenwood Press, 2004.

4. McPherson, James M. *Battle Cry of Freedom: The Civil War Era.* New York: Oxford University Press, 1998.

5. Mickey, Robert. *Paths Out of Dixie.* Princeton, NJ: Princeton University Press, 2015.

6. Grantham, Dewey W. *The South in Modern America.* New York: HarperCollins, 1994.

7. Rodriguez, Junius P., ed. *Slavery in the United States: A Social, Political, and Historical Encyclopedia.* 2 vols. Santa Barbara, CA: ABC-CLIO, 2007.

8. 24/7 editors. "America's Poorest States." 24/7 Wall Street. September 20, 2012. Last

updated March 26, 2020. https://247wallst.com/investing/2012/09/20/americas-poorest -states-2/.

9. Wilson, Charles R., and William Ferris, eds. *Encyclopedia of Southern Culture*. Chapel Hill: University of North Carolina Press, 1989.

10. Singh, G. K., G. P. Daus, M. Allender, C. T. Ramey, E. K. Martin, C. Perry, A. A. De Los Reyes, and I. P. Vedamuthu. "Social Determinants of Health in the United States: Addressing Major Health Inequality Trends for the Nation, 1935–2016." *International Journal of Maternal and Child Health and AIDS* 6 (2017): 139–164.

11. Noonan, A. S., H. E. Velasco-Mondragon, and F. A. Wagner. "Improving the Health of African Americans in the USA: An Overdue Opportunity for Social Justice." *Public Health Reviews* 37 (2016): article 12.

12. Coughlin, S. S., D. S. Blumenthal, S. J. Seay, and S. A. Smith. "Toward the Elimination of Colorectal Cancer Disparities among African Americans." *Journal of Racial and Ethnic Health Disparities* 3 (2016): 555–564.

13. Coughlin, S. S., W. Yoo, M. S. Whitehead, M. S., and S. A. Smith. "Advancing Breast Cancer Survivorship among African-American Women." *Breast Cancer Research and Treatment* 153 (2015): 253–261.

14. Coughlin, S. S., P. Matthews-Juarez, P. D. Juarez, C. E. Melton, and M. King. "Opportunities to Address Lung Cancer Disparities among African Americans." *Cancer Medicine* 3 (2014): 1467–1476.

15. Smith, Z. L., S. E. Eggener, and A. B. Murphy. "African American Prostate Cancer Disparities." *Current Urology Reports* 18 (2017): 81.

16. Carnethon, M. R., J. Pu, G. Howard, M. A. Albert, C. A. M. Anderson, A. G. Bertoni, M. S. Mujahid, L. Palaniappan, H. A. Taylor Jr., et al. "Cardiovascular Health in African Americans. A Scientific Statement from the American Heart Association." *Circulation* 136 (2017): e393–e423.

17. Howard, G., D. R. Labarthe, J. Hu, S. Yoon, and V. J. Howard. "Regional Differences in African Americans' High Risk for Stroke: The Remarkable Burden of Stroke for Southern African Americans." *Annals of Epidemiology* 17 (2007): 689–696.

18. Menke, A., S. Casagrande, L. Geiss, and C. C. Cowie. "Prevalence of and Trends in Diabetes among Adults in the United States, 1988–2012." *Journal of the American Medical Association* 314 (2015): 1021–1029.

19. Rosenstock, S., S. Whitman, J. F. West, and M. Balkin. "Racial Disparities in Diabetes Mortality in the 50 Most Populous US Cities." *Journal of Urban Health* 91 (2014): 873–885.

20. Barker, L. E., K. A. Kirtland, E. W. Gregg, L. S. Geiss, and T. J. Thompson. "Geographic Distribution of Diagnosed Diabetes in the U.S.: A Diabetes Belt." *American Journal of Preventive Medicine* 40 (2011): 434–439.

21. Benjamin, E., M. J. Blaha, S. E. Chiuve, M. Cushman, S. R. Das, R. Deo, S. D. de Ferranti, J. Floyd, M. Fornage, et al. "Heart Disease and Stroke Statistics—2017 Update: A Report from the American Heart Association." *Circulation* 135 (2017): e146–e603.

22. Centers for Disease Control and Prevention. "Adult Obesity Facts." 2021. https://www.cdc.gov/obesity/data/adult.html.

23. Karp, D. N., C. S. Wolff, D. J. Wiebe, C. C. Branas, B. G. Carr, and M. T. Mullen. "Re-

assessing the Stroke Belt: Using Small Area Spatial Statistics to Identify Clusters of High Stroke Mortality in the United States." *Stroke* 47 (2016): 1939–1942.

24. Reif, S., K. L. Geonnotti, and K. Whetten. "HIV Infection and AIDS in the Deep South." *American Journal of Public Health* 96 (2006): 970–973.

25. Prejan, J., T. Tang, and H. I. Hall. "HIV Diagnoses and Prevalence in the Southern Region of the United States, 2007–2010." *Journal of Community Health* 38 (2013): 414–416.

26. Natural Center for HIV/AIDS, Viral Hepatitis, STD, and TB Prevention (U.S.), Division of HIV/AIDS Prevention. "HIV in the United States by Geography." https://stacks.cdc .gov/view/cdc/50232.

27. Nunn, A., W. L. Jeffries IV, P. Foster, K. McCoy, C. Sutten-Coats, T. C. Willie, Y. Ransome, R. G. Lanzi, E. Jackson, et al. "Reducing the African American HIV Disease Burden in the Deep South: Addressing the Role of Faith and Spirituality." *AIDS and Behavior* 23 (2019): 5318–5330.

28. Centers for Disease Control and Prevention. "HIV in the Southern United States." Issue Brief, September 2019. https://www.cdc.gov/hiv/pdf/policies/cdc-hiv-in-the-south -issue-brief.pdf.

29. Plescia, M., and C. Emmanuel. "Reducing Health Disparities by Addressing Social Determinants of Health: The Mecklenburg County Experience." *North Carolina Medical Journal* 75 (2014): 417–421.

30. Marmot, M. "Social Justice, Epidemiology and Health Disparities." *European Journal of Epidemiology* 32 (2017): 537–546.

31. Kearney, M. S., and P. B. Levine. "Income Inequality, Social Mobility, and the Decision to Drop Out of High School." *Brookings Papers on Economic Activity* (Spring 2016): 333–380.

32. Henry Akintobi, T. Jacobs, D. Sabbs, K. Holden, R. Braithwaite, L. N. Johnson, D. Dawes, and L. Hoffman. "Community Engagement of African Americans in the Era of COVID-19: Considerations, Challenges, Implications, and Recommendations for Public Health." *Preventing Chronic Disease* 17 (August 13, 2020). https://www.cdc.gov/pcd/issues /2020/20_0255.htm.

33. Semega, J., M. Kollar, E. A. Shrider, and J. F. Creamer *Income and Poverty in the United States: 2019.* U.S. Census Bureau, Current Population Reports, P60-270. September 15, 2020. Washington, DC: U.S. Government Publishing Office, 2020.

34. Kawachi, I., B. Kennedy, and R. G. Wilkinson. *Income Inequality and Health: A Reader.* New York: New Press, 1999.

35. Daniels, N., B. Kennedy, and I. Kawachi. "Justice Is Good for Our Health: How Greater Economic Equality Would Promote Public Health." *Boston Review* 25 (2000): 4–19.

36. Murray, C. J. L., C. M. Michaud, M. T. McKenna, and J. S. Marks. *US Patterns of Mortality by County and Race: 1965–94.* Cambridge, MA: Harvard Center for Population and Development Studies, 1998.

37. Alegria, M., A. NeMoyer, I. Falgas, I., Y. Wang, and K. Alvarez. "Social Determinants of Mental Health: Where We Are and Where We Need to Go." *Current Psychiatry Reports* 20 (2019): 95.

38. Diez Roux, A., and C. Mair. "Neighborhoods and Health." *Annals of New York Academy of Sciences* 1186 (2010): 125–145.

39. World Health Organization. *World Conference on Social Determinants of Health: Meeting Report, Rio de Janeiro, Brazil, 19–21 October 2011*. https://www.who.int/publications /i/item/9789241503617.

40. Institute of Medicine (US) Committee on Assuring the Health of the Public in the 21st Century. *The Future of the Public's Health in the 21st Century*. Washington, DC: National Academies Press, 2003.

41. Rogers, R. G., R. A. Hummer, C. B. Nam, and K. Peters. "Demographic, Socioeconomic, and Behavioral Factors Affecting Ethnic Mortality by Cause." *Social Forces* 74: (1996): 1419–1438.

42. Dana, R. H. *Multicultural Assessment Perspectives for Professional Psychology*. Boston: Simon & Schuster, 1993.

43. Baum, A., J. P. Garofalo, and A. M. Yali. "Socioeconomic Status and Chronic Stress: Does Stress Account for SES Effects on Health?" *Annals of the New York Academy of Sciences* 896 (1999): 131–144.

44. Anderson, N. B., and C. A. Armstead. "Toward Understanding the Association of Socioeconomic Status and Health: A New Challenge for the Biopsychosocial Approach." *Psychosomatic Medicine* 57 (1995): 213–225.

45. Lantz, P. M., J. S. House, J. M. Lepkowski, D. R. Williams, R. P. Mero, and J. Chen. "Socioeconomic Factors, Health Behaviors, and Mortality: Results from a Nationally Representative Prospective Study of US Adults." *Journal of the American Medical Association* 279 (1998): 1703–1708.

46. Rozanski, A., J. A. Blumenthal, K. W. Davidson, P. C. Saab, and L. Kubzansky. "The Epidemiology, Pathophysiology, and Management of Psychosocial Risk Factors in Cardiac Practice: The Emerging Field of Behavioral Cardiology." *Journal of the American College of Cardiology* 45 (2005): 637–651.

47. Pampel, F. C., P. M. Krueger, and J. T. Denney. "Socioeconomic Disparities in Health Behaviors." *Annual Review of Sociology* 36 (2010): 349–370.

48. García-León, M. Á., J. M. Pérez-Mármol, R. Gonzalez-Perez, M. Garcia-Rios, and M. I. Peralta-Ramírez. "Relationship between Resilience and Stress: Perceived Stress, Stressful Life Events, HPA Axis Response during a Stressful Task and Hair Cortisol." *Physiology & Behavior* 202 (2019): 87–93.

49. Bailey, Z. D., N. Krieger, M. Agenor, J. Graves, N. Linos, and M. T. Bassett. "Structural Racism and Health Inequities in the USA: Evidence and Interventions." *Lancet* 389 (2017): 1453–1463.

50. Williams, D. R., J. Lawrence, and B. David. "Racism and Health: Evidence and Needed Research." *Annual Review of Public Health* 40 (2019): 105–125.

52. Phelan, J. C., and B. G. Link. "Controlling Disease and Creating Disparities: A Fundamental Cause Perspective." *Journal of Gerontology* 60B (2005): 27–33.

53. Anderson, L. M., K. L. Adeney, C. Shinn, S. Safranek, J. Buckner-Brown, and L. K. Krause. "Community Coalition-Driven Interventions to Reduce Health Disparities among Racial and Ethnic Minority Populations." *Cochrane Database of Systematic Reviews* 6 (June 15, 2015): CD009905.

54. Akintobi, T. H., L. Goodin, E. Trammel, D. Collins, and D. S. Blumenthal. "How Do You Set Up and Maintain a Community Advisory Board?" Chapter 5, 136–138, in Clinical

and Translational Science Awards Consortium, Community Engagement Key Function Committee, and Task Force on the Principles of Community Engagement, *Principles of Community Engagement*, 2nd ed. Washington, DC: United States Department of Health and Human Services, 2011.

55. Lynch, J., and G. D. Smith. "A Life Course Approach to Chronic Disease Epidemiology." *Annual Review of Public Health* 26 (2005): 1–35.

56. D. A. Lawlor and G. D. Mishra, eds. *Family Matters: Designing, Analyzing, and Understanding Family-Based Studies in Life Course Epidemiology*. New York: Oxford University Press, 2009.

57. Lu, M. C. and N. Halfon. "Racial and Ethnic Disparities in Birth Outcomes: A Life-Course Perspective." *Maternal and Child Health Journal* 7 (2003): 13–30.

58. Braveman, P. and L. Gottlieb. "The Social Determinants of Health: It's Time to Consider the Causes of the Causes." *Public Health Reports* 129 (suppl. 2) (2014): 19–31.

59. Stevenson, D. K., R. J. Wong, N. Aghaeepour, M. S. Angst, G. L. Darmstadt, D. B. DiGiulio, M. L. Druzin, B. Gaudilliere, R. S. Gibbs, et al. "Understanding Health Disparities." *Journal of Perinatology* 39 (2019): 354–358.

60. Gold, D. R. and R. Wright. "Population Disparities in Asthma." *Annual Review of Public Health* 26 (2005): 89–113.

61. Wild, C. P. "Complementing the Genome with an 'Exposome': The Outstanding Challenge of Environmental Exposure Measurement in Molecular Epidemiology." *Cancer Epidemiology Biomarkers & Prevention* 14 (2005): 1847–1850.

62. Coughlin, S. S. "Toward a Road Map for Global -Omics: A Primer on -Omic Technologies." *American Journal of Epidemiology* 180 (2014): 1188–1195.

63. Bower, A. L., ed. *African American Foodways: Explorations of History and Culture*. Urbana: University of Illinois Press, 2007.

64. Vance, K. E. "Culture, Food, and Racism: The Effects on African American Health." Honors thesis. University of Tennessee at Chattanooga, 2018.

65. Shikany, J. M., M. M. Safford, P. K. Newby, R. W. Durant, T. M. Brown, and S. E. Judd. "Southern Dietary Pattern Is Associated with Hazard of Acute Coronary Heart Disease in the Reasons for Geographic and Racial Differences in Stroke (REGARDS) Study." *Circulation* 132 (2015): 804–814.

66. Shikany, J. M., M. M. Safford, J. Bryan, P. K. Newby, J. S. Richman, R. W. Durant, T. M. Brown, and S. E. Judd. "Dietary Patterns and Mediterranean Diet Score and Hazard of Recurrent Coronary Heart Disease Events and All-Cause Mortality in the REGARDS Study." *Journal of the American Heart Association* 7 (2018): e008078.

67. Newby, P. K., S. E. Noel, R. Grant, S. Judd, J. M. Shikany, and J. Ard. "Race and Region Are Associated with Nutrient Intakes among Black and White Men in the United States." *Journal of Nutrition* 141 (2) (2011): 296–303.

68. Centers for Disease Control and Prevention. "The Community Guide." http://www thecommunityguide.org.

69. Purnell, T. S., E. A. Calhoun, S. H. Golden, J. R. Halladay, J. L. Krok-Schoen, B. M. Appelhans, and L. A. Cooper. "Achieving Health Equity: Closing the Gaps in Health Care Disparities, Interventions, and Research." *Health Affairs* 35 (2016): 1410–1415.

70. Coughlin, S. S., S. A. Smith, and M. E. Fernandez, eds. *Handbook of Community-Based Participatory Research*. New York: Oxford University Press, 2017.

71. Braithwaite, R., T. Akintobi, D. Blumenthal, and M. Langley. *Morehouse Model: How One School of Medicine Revolutionized Community Engagement and Health Equity*. Baltimore, MD: Johns Hopkins University Press, 2020.

72. Oetzel, J. G., N. Wallerstein, B. Duran, S. Sanchez-Youngman, T. Nguyen, K. Woo, J. Wang, A. Schultz, J. Keawe'aimoku Kaholokula, et al. "Impact of Participatory Health Research: A Test of the Community-Based Participatory Research Conceptual Model." *BioMed Research International* (2018): 7281405.

73. Paskett, E., B. Thompson, A. S. Ammerman, A. N. Ortega, J. Marsteller, and D. Richardson. "Multilevel Interventions to Address Health Disparities Show Promise in Improving Population Health." *Health Affairs* 35 (2016): 1429–1434.

2

Racism and Health

Implications for Health Disparities

STEVEN S. COUGHLIN, PhD, MPH,

LOVORIA B. WILLIAMS, PhD, FNP-BC, FAAN,

RYAN A. HARRIS, PhD, CEP, FACSM,

and GASTON KAPUKU, MD

In recent decades, a burgeoning literature has examined the many ways that racism and discrimination continue to adversely affect the health of African Americans and other people of color. The term racism includes an ideology of superiority that categorizes and ranks various groups and includes negative attitudes and beliefs about groups seen as different and differential treatment of those groups by individuals and social institutions.[1] Race is a socially constructed category that emerged in the context of social and economic oppression and has been used to promote and sustain economic, cultural, political and legal systems of inequality.[1,2] Racism devalues and disempowers groups defined as inferior and allocates social resources and opportunities such as education, employment, housing, and health care differentially. The most profound impact of racism is at the level of social institutions that shape the socioeconomic opportunities and life chances of racialized groups.[1] Given the body of research regarding race and health, the Centers for Disease Control and Prevention recently joined the American Medical Association, the American Nurses Association, and other health organizations to declare that racism is a critical threat to public health.[3-5] These recent acknowledgements of the negative health effects of racism underscore what several researchers have emphasized: that racism is a neglected but important social force that adversely affects the health of racial and ethnic populations.[6-8]

This chapter provides a summary of the adverse physical and mental health outcomes that have been associated with racism and discrimination with a particular focus on the health of African Americans in the United

States. Definitions of key concepts appear below, including structural racism, cultural racism, and individual-level discrimination.

Structural Racism, Cultural Racism, and Individual-Level Discrimination

A growing body of literature shows that centuries of pervasive racism in the United States has had a profoundly negative effect on the health of African Americans and on the ways they engage with the health care system. Slavery, the Jim Crow era, and persistent biased health care has contributed to the fact that African Americans experience the worst health care and health outcomes across many illnesses of any racial/ethnic group in the United States and partly accounts for the fact that the life expectancy of African Americans is four years lower than that of whites.[9] Through its educational system and practices, the health care institution in the United States has perpetuated racialized theories of inferiority, such as the idea that race is a biological variable. This has contributed to the fact that some African Americans do not trust the health care system.[10,11]

As Williams et al. have noted, structural racism—which has also been referred to as institutional racism—exists within multiple social systems, including the housing, labor, and credit markets and the education, criminal justice, and health care systems.[12] For example, the Social Security Act of 1935 created a system of old age insurance and unemployment insurance that is based on employment. However, the act's exclusion of agricultural workers and domestic servants disproportionately affected African American men and women.[13]

In the public health literature, racial residential segregation is one of the most widely studied mechanisms of institutional racism. The practice of redlining that the Federal Housing Administration initiated in 1934 resulted in segregated neighborhoods. This government body promoted segregation by making it legal for banks to deny mortgages to African Americans who wanted to buy property in predominantly white neighborhoods. In addition, the federal government subsidized builders who mass produced suburban neighborhoods for whites.[13] Although racial residential segregation has been illegal since the Fair Housing Act of 1968, its pervasive and basic structures, including the concentration of urban poverty, remain largely intact.[12] Residential segregation harms health in both direct and indirect ways, including the high concentration of dilapidated housing in distressed neighborhoods, exposure to toxins and pollutants, limited opportunities for high-quality education and employment, and decreased access to quality health care.[13] Racial residential segregation shapes access to and the quality of health care at the neighborhood, provider, and individual levels.[14]

Moreover, the socioeconomic disadvantage resulting from public and private disinvestment in predominately African American neighborhoods makes it difficult for health care facilities in those neighborhoods to attract primary care providers and specialists.[13] Although health disparities exist in many chronic diseases, racial residential segregation has been generally associated with poorer health and a higher risk of low birth weight and pre-term birth among African Americans.[12,15] In addition, segregation has been positively associated with cancer diagnoses at late stages and with lower survival rates for African Americans with breast and lung cancer.[16]

The housing policies of the 1950s have had lasting effects on the health of African Americans by restricting them to urban settings that limit opportunities for upward mobility, such as quality education and access to adequate health care. Moreover, neighborhoods of color are more likely than white neighborhoods to lack grocery stores, healthy environments and safe, well-lit places to walk, all of which are social determinants of good health.

Structural racism is an ongoing concern. For example, the criminal justice system in the United States (which includes police departments, courts, prosecutors, and parole and probation agencies) disproportionately criminalizes African Americans.[13,17] Structural racism refers to the ways societies foster racial discrimination through mutually reinforcing systems of unequal access to housing, education, employment, earnings, credit, health care, and criminal justice.[13] These patterns and practices reinforce discriminatory beliefs and values and how resources are distributed.[13] As Bailey et al. note, institutional racism in one sector reinforces it in others, forming a large interconnected system of structural racism.[13] Racism interacts with other social institutions, shaping and being shaped by them, to reinforce, justify, and perpetuate a racial hierarchy.[12] Structural racism is likely the most important way that racism affects health.

Williams et al. define cultural racism as the "instillation of the ideology of inferiority in the values, language, imagery, symbols, and unstated assumptions of the larger society."[12] It creates an environment in which the system of racism can flourish. Cultural racism, which can underlie both institutional- and individual-level discrimination, is manifested through media, stereotyping, and norms within society. It can lead to social policies that create and maintain structures that provide differential access to opportunities. Additionally, cultural racism can lead to individual-level bias that can perpetuate discrimination against group members.[12]

Discrimination is the most frequently studied form of racism in the health literature.[12] It includes self-reported discrimination and inequitable access to opportunities and resources by race and ethnicity because individuals and institutions treat racial groups differently. Self-reports of discrimination can lead to altered physiological reactions and changes in health behaviors (e.g., smoking and drinking) that can lead to adverse health outcomes. Examples of physiological reactions to perceived discrimination include increased allostatic load, inflammation, greater oxidative stress, and dysregulation in cortisol.[12,18,19] Importantly, environmental stressors in general can exacerbate a pro-inflammatory/pro-oxidant state. In fact, epidemiological studies in humans have established a relationship between adversity early in life, such as low parental socioeconomic status (SES) and cardiovascular disease (CVD) in adulthood by altering disease progression.[20–23] Packard et al. reported positive associations with low parental SES (status of the childhood home, father's occupation) and biomarkers of chronic inflammation and vascular dysfunction in adults.[24] Taken together, these data provide insight into the link between inflammation and how adversity during childhood predisposes a person to poor adult health.

Associations between Racial Discrimination and Physical Health Outcomes

Self-reported racial discrimination has been associated with adverse physical health outcomes in several recent reviews. Studies indicate positive associations between perceived discrimination and adverse cardiovascular outcomes, obesity, hypertension, poor sleep, high-risk behaviors, cigarette smoking, and alcohol use and abuse.[12,19,25–30] Although some systematic reviews have found weak associations between racism and hypertension and blood pressure,[27] racial disparities in health outcomes persist and further research into the contributing mechanisms is warranted. The adverse effects of hypertension and exposures such as alcohol use and smoking can accumulate over the life course and contribute to poor outcomes.[13] Paradise et al., who systematically reviewed the literature on racism as a determinant of health, found that racism is associated with poorer general health and poorer physical health.[19]

African Americans not only have a greater incidence of the CVD, their all-cause mortality is significantly greater than that of their white counterparts.[31] According to a review by Lewis et al. of perceived discrimination and CVD, large-scale epidemiological and community-based investigations of the association between self-reported experiences of discrimination and objective indices of CVD have not been done until recently.[26] Most of this research has examined associations between self-reported discrimination and indices of CVD among African Americans.[26] Among the traditional risk factors for CVD, measures of clinical hypertension, resting blood pressure as a continuous measure, and ambulatory blood pressure monitoring have been the most frequently studied. Lewis et al. found that studies to date have provided mixed evidence for an association of CVD with self-reported experiences of discrimination.[26] However, findings from the reviewed studies suggest that associations may be sex-specific and may depend on psychosocial processes (e.g., the ways those who experience discrimination interpret and express their own racial or social identity and coping style).

Racism has both physiological and social impacts. African Americans experience heightened psychological stress due to discrimination.[32] Some,[32-35] but not all[36-38] studies reported that compared to European Americans, African Americans experience increased cardiovascular responsivity both to laboratory stressors and in the real world. In addition, African Americans are prone to show biobehavioral stress-induced biological perturbations that include a derangement of the hypothalamic-pituitary-adrenal axis, overexpression of the renin-angiotensin system, increased endothelin-1, higher oxidative stress, enhanced inflammation, and mishandling of salt. Various behavioral coping styles are developed to counter environmental stress. The imbalance between stress and coping mechanisms culminate in early manifestations of cardiovascular disease owing to heart and vessel dysfunction.

Bernardo et al. conducted a systematic review of the literature on interpersonal discrimination and markers of adiposity.[25] The review focused on longitudinal studies. Results from the ten studies they included support a positive association between self-reported discrimination and body mass index among women. Waist circumference showed a similar pattern of association with discrimination, but an inverted U-shaped association was also found.[25] Overall, markers of adiposity were consistently associated with discrimination.

Black et al. reviewed the literature on perceived racism/discrimination and health among African American women.[39] Nineteen studies met the inclusion criteria. They found consistent evidence for the relationship between perceived racism/discrimination and breast cancer risk and adverse birth outcomes (low birth weight and preterm birth). Five of the six studies on adverse birth outcomes showed a significant negative association between perceived racism/discrimination and infant birth weight and gestational age. The results of these studies also suggest a dose-response relationship; more frequent or lifetime exposure to discrimination had a larger effect on birth outcomes. Findings were inconsistent for the relationship between perceived racism/discrimination and heart disease risk factors.[39]

Associations between Racial Discrimination and Mental Health Outcomes

In the health sciences literature, racism has been primarily conceptualized as a psychosocial stressor. The strongest evidence in the scientific literature is for adverse effects of perceived racial discrimination on psychological well-being, mental health, and related health practices such as eating patterns and the consumption of cigarettes, alcohol, and drugs.[13,30,40,41] The most consistent evidence of its adverse health effects is for mental health (e.g., anxiety, depression, psychological distress, and posttraumatic stress).[13,30]

Gilbert and Zemore, who systematically reviewed the literature on discrimination and alcohol consumption, found that articles generally supported a positive association between discrimination and drinking alcohol.[28] Although the included studies were conducted in various countries, the largest number of studies related to racial discrimination among African Americans in the United States, followed by discrimination due to sexual orientation and gender. Studies of racial/ethnic discrimination focused almost exclusively on interpersonal discrimination.[28]

In a review of racial/ethnic discrimination and health observed in community studies, Williams et al. found that mental health was the most common outcome examined.[42] Of the 25 associations examined for psychological distress, 20 studies reported a positive association between discrimination and distress.[42] Of the four studies that examined the relationship between perceived discrimination and a diagnosis of major depression, three found a positive association. Other studies focused on generalized anxiety disorder, psychosis, anger, and early initiation of substance use. All reported a positive association with discrimination.

Interventions to Address Racism

There is a critical need to identify interventions that can ameliorate and eliminate the negative effects of racism on health. Interventions aimed at structural racism must be addressed in the context of the interrelated social mechanisms and leverage points though which racism operates.[13] For example, racial residential segregation is a key leverage point by which institutional racism creates and sustains racial economic inequities.[13] As Williams et al. note, dismantling the institutional mechanisms of segregation will require a scaling up of interventions that address its underlying mechanisms.[12] Multilevel interventions that address multiple processes of racism simultaneously are more likely to be effective than single interventions. The civil rights policies of the 1960s are important examples of race-targeted policies that improved socioeconomic opportunities and living conditions and reduced health disparities.[12] Interventions to improve household income, education, and employment opportunities have also been linked to health benefits.[43] In additions, interventions are needed to diversify the health professions and adequately train all staff on culturally sensitive care. However, there is a paucity of evidence that indicates that these interventions affect health outcomes.[12,44] Lastly, routine data analysis and reporting of medical encounters by race and social vulnerability index will provide the opportunity to elucidate disparate health care outcomes and to develop effective strategies to address them.[45]

Summary and Conclusions

Achieving health equity requires that all individuals and populations be valued equally, that historical injustices be recognized, and that resources be provided according to need.[46] The United States is experiencing a resurgence of racism, xenophobia, and other forms of intolerance.[47] These trends have clear deleterious consequences for the health and well-being of many racial and ethnic groups, including African Americans in the South. Leadership is necessary to challenge the racism that operates at structural, institutional, and individual levels in the United States. Comprehensive approaches are more likely to reshape policy and practice and to change individual attitudes and behaviors in ways that ameliorate and eliminate racism.[47]

To date, the body of scientific research on racial discrimination and health has primarily focused on the stress of perceived unfair treatment—that is, individual-level or interpersonal racism. A focus on structural racism is also needed to advance health equity and improve population health.[1] Structural racism has had an important role in shaping the distribution of the social determinants of health and the health of African Americans, including those who live in the southern United States.

REFERENCES

1. Williams, D. R., Y. Yu, and J. S. Jackson. "Racial Differences in Physical and Mental Health. Socio-Economic Status, Stress and Discrimination." *Journal of Health Psychology* 2 (1997): 335–351.

2. Omi, M., and H. Winant. *Racial Formation in the United States: From the 1960s to the 1980s.* New York: Routledge, 1986.

3. American Medical Association. "AMA Board of Trustees Pledges Action Against Racism, Police Brutality." Press release, June 7, 2020. https://www.ama-assn.org/press-center/ama-statements/ama-board-trustees-pledges-action-against-racism-police-brutality.

4. American Nurses Association. "The American Academy of Nursing and the American Nurses Association Call for Social Justice to Address Racism and Health Equity in Communities of Color." Press release, August 4, 2020. https://www.nursingworld.org/news/news-releases/2020/the-american-academy-of-nursing-and-the-american-nurses-association-call-for-social-justice-to-address-racism-and-health-equity-in-communities-of-color/.

5. Centers for Disease Control and Prevention. "Racism and Health." Last reviewed November 24, 2021. https://www.cdc.gov/healthequity/racism-disparities/index.html.

6. Williams, D. R., R. Lavizzo-Mourey, and R. C. Warren. "The Concept of Race and Health Status in America." *Public Health Reports* 109 (1994): 26–41.

7. King, G., and D. R. Williams. "Race and Health: A Multidimensional Approach to African American Health." In *Society and Health*, ed. B. C. Amick, S. Levine, D. C. Walsh, and A. Tarlov, 93–130. New York: Oxford University Press, 1996.

8. Krieger, N., D. L. Rowley, A. A. Herman, B. Avery, and M. T. Phillips. "Racism, Sexism, and Social Class: Implications for Studies of Health, Disease, and Well-Being." *American Journal of Preventive Medicine* 9 (suppl. 6) (1993): 82–122.

9. Freedman, V. A., and B. C. Spillman. "Active Life Expectancy in the Older US Population, 1982–2011: Differences between Blacks And Whites Persisted." *Health Affairs* 35 (2016): 1351–1358.

10. Byrd, W. M., and L. A. Clayton. "An American Health Dilemma: A History of Blacks in the Health System." *Journal of the National Medical Association* 84 (1992):189–200.

11. Fofana, M. O. "The Spectre of Race in American Medicine." *Medical Humanities* 39 (2013): 137–141.

12. Williams, D. R., J. A. Lawrence, and B. A. Davis. "Racism and Health: Evidence and Needed Research." *Annual Review of Public Health* 40 (2019): 105–125.

13. Bailey, Z. D., N. Krieger, M. Agénor, J. Graves, N. Linos, and M. T. Bassett. "Structural Racism and Health Inequities in the USA: Evidence and Interventions." *Lancet* 389 (2017):1453–1463.

14. White, K., J. S. Haas, and D. R. Williams. "Elucidating the Role of Place in Health Care Disparities: The Example of Racial/Ethnic Residential Segregation." *Health Services Research* 47 (2012): 1278–1299.

15. Williams, A. D., M. Wallace, C. Nobles, and P. Mendola. "Racial Residential Segregation and Racial Disparities in Stillbirth in the United States." *Health & Place* 51 (2018): 208–216.

16. Landrine, H., I. Corral, J. G. L. Lee, J. T. Efird, M. B. Hall, and J. K. Bess. "Residential Segregation and Racial Cancer Disparities: A Systematic Review." *Journal of Racial and Ethnic Health Disparities* 4 (2017): 1195–11205.

17. Pager, D., and H. Shepherd. "The Sociology of Discrimination: Racial Discrimination in Employment, Housing, Credit, and Consumer Markets." *Annual Review of Sociology* 34 (2008): 181–209.

18. Lewis, T. T., C. D. Cognurn, and D. R. Williams. "Self-Reported Experiences of Discrimination and Health: Scientific Advances, Ongoing Controversies, and Emerging Issues." *Annual Review of Clinical Psychology* 11 (2015): 407–440.

19. Paradise, Y., J. Ben, N. Denson, A. Elias, N. Priest, A. Pieterse, A. Gupta, M. Kelaher, and G. Gee. "Racism as a Determinant of Health: A Systematic Review and Meta-Analysis." *PLOS ONE* 10 (2015): e0138511.

20. Johnson, R. C., and R. F. Schoeni. "Early-Life Origins of Adult Disease: National Longitudinal Population-Based Study of the United States." *American Journal of Public Health* 101 (2011): 2317–2324.

21. Dong, M., W. H. Giles, V. J. Felitti, S. R. Dube, J. E. Williams, D. P. Chapman, and R. F. Anda. "Insights into Causal Pathways for Ischemic Heart Disease: Adverse Childhood Experiences Study." *Circulation* 110 (2004):1761–1766.

22. National Scientific Council on the Developing Child. "Early Experiences Can Alter Gene Expression and Affect Long-Term Development." Working Paper No. 10. 2010. https://developingchild.harvard.edu/resources/early-experiences-can-alter-gene-expression-and-affect-long-term-development/.

23. Danese, A., T. E. Moffitt, H. Harrington, B. J. Milne, G. Polanczyk, C. M. Pariante, R. Poulton, and A. Caspi. "Adverse Childhood Experiences and Adult Risk Factors for Age-Related Disease: Depression, Inflammation, and Clustering of Metabolic Risk Markers." *Archives of Pediatric and Adolescent Medicine* 163 (2009): 1135–1143.

24. Packard, C. J., V. Bezlyak, J. S. McLean, G. D. Batty, I. Ford, H. Burns, J. Cavanagh, K. A. Deans, M. Henderson, et al. "Early Life Socioeconomic Adversity Is Associated in Adult Life with Chronic Inflammation, Carotid Atherosclerosis, Poorer Lung Function and Decreased Cognitive Performance: A Cross-Sectional, Population-Based Study." *BMC Public Health* 11 (2011). https://doi.org/10.1186/1471-2458-11-42.

25. Bernardo, C. de O., J. L. Bastos, D. A. Gonzales-Chica, M. A. Peres, and Y. C. Paradies.

"Interpersonal Discrimination and Markers of Adiposity in Longitudinal Studies: A Systematic Review." *Obesity Reviews* 18 (2017): 1040–1049.

26. Lewis, T. T., D. R. Williams, M. Tamene, and C. R. Clark. "Self-Reported Experiences of Discrimination and Cardiovascular Disease." *Current Cardiovascular Risk Report* 8 (2014): 365.

27. Dolezsar, C. M., J. J. McGrath, A. J. M. Herzig, and S. B. Miller. "Perceived Racial Discrimination and Hypertension: A Comprehensive Systematic Review." *Health Psychology* 33 (2014): 20–34.

28. Gilbert, P. A., and S. E. Zemore. "Discrimination and Drinking: A Systematic Review of the Evidence." *Social Science & Medicine* 161 (2016): 178–194.

29. Slopen, N., T. T. Lewis, and D. R. Williams. "Discrimination and Sleep: A Systematic Review." *Sleep Medicine* 18 (2018): 88–95.

30. Pascoe, E. A., and L. S. Richman. "Perceived Discrimination and Health: A Meta-Analytic Review." *Psychology Bulletin* 135 (2009): 531–554.

31. Beydoun, M. A., H. A. Beydoun, N. Mode, G. A. Dore, J. A. Canas, S. M. Eid, and A. B. Zonderman. "Racial Disparities in Adult All-Cause and Cause-Specific Mortality among US Adults: Mediating and Moderating Factors." *BMC Public Health* 16 (2016): 1113.

32. Chung, B., M. Meldrum, F. Jones, A. Brown, R. Daaood, and L. Jones. "Perceived Sources of Stress and Resilience in Men in an African-American Community." *Progress in Community Health Partnerships: Research, Education, and Action.* 8 (2014): 441–451.

33. Treiber, F. A., L. Musante, G. Kapuku, C. Davis, M. Litaker, and H. Davis. "Cardiovascular (CV) Responsivity and Recovery to Acute Stress and Future CV Functioning in Youth with Family Histories of CV disease: A 4-Year Longitudinal Study." *International Journal of Psychophysiology.* 41 (2001): 65–74.

34. Anderson, N. B., J. D. Lane, H. Monou, R. B. Williams Jr., and S. J. Houseworth. "Racial Differences in Cardiovascular Reactivity to Mental Arithmetic." *International Journal of Psychophysiology* 6 (1988):161–164.

35. Light, K. C., and A. Sherwood. "Race, Borderline Hypertension, and Hemodynamic Responses to Behavioral Stress before and after the Beta-Adrenergic Blockade." *Health Psychology* 8 (1989): 577.

36. Goldstein, I. B., and D. Shapiro. "The Cardiovascular Response to Postural Change as a Function of Race." *Biological Psychology* 39, nos. 2–3 (1995): 173–186.

37. Falkner, B., and H. Kushner. "Race Differences in Stress-Induced Reactivity in Young Adults." *Health Psychology* 8, no. 5 (1989): 613.

38. Saab, P. G., M. M. Llabre, N. Schneiderman, B. E. Hurwitz, P. G. McDonald, J. Evans, W. Wohlgemuth, P. Hayashi, and B. Klein. "Influence of Ethnicity and Gender on Cardiovascular Responses to Active Coping and Inhibitory-Passive Coping Challenges." *Psychosomatic Medicine* 59, no. 4 (1997): 434–446.

39. Black, L. L., R. Johnson, and L. VanHoose. "The Relationship between Perceived Racism/Discrimination and Health among Black American Women: A Review of the Literature from 2003–2013." *Journal of Racial and Ethnic Health Disparities* 2 (2015): 11–20.

40. Krieger, N. "Discrimination and Health Inequities." *International Journal of Health Services* 44 (2014): 643–710.

41. Ge, G. C., and C. L. Ford. "Structural Racism and Health Inequities." *Du Bois Review* 8 (2011): 115–132.

42. Williams, D. R., H. W. Neighbors, and J. S. Jackson. "Racial/Ethnic Discrimination and Health: Findings from Community Studies." *American Journal of Public Health* 93 (2003): 200–208.

43. Williams, D. R., and S. A. Mohammed. "Racism and Health I: Pathways and Scientific Evidence." *American Behavioral Scientist* 57 (2013): 1152–1173.

44. Truong, M., Y. Paradies, and N. Priest. "Interventions to Improve Cultural Competency in Healthcare: A Systematic Review of Reviews." *BMC Health Services Research* 14 (2014). https://bmchealthservres.biomedcentral.com/articles/10.1186/1472-6963-14-99.

45. Ogojiaku, C. N., J. C. Allen, R. Anson-Dwamena, K. S. Barnett, O. Adetona, W. Im, and D. B. Hood. "The Health Opportunity Index: Understanding the Input to Disparate Health Outcomes in Vulnerable and High-Risk Census Tracts." *International Journal of Environmental Research and Public Health* 17 (2020): 5767.

46. Jones, C. P. "Toward the Science and Practice of Anti-Racism: Launching a National Campaign against Racism." *Ethnicity & Disease* 28 (suppl. 1) (2018): 231–234.

47. Smedley, B. D. "Multilevel Interventions to Undo the Health Consequences of Racism: The Need for Comprehensive Approaches." *Cultural Diversity & Ethnic Minority Psychology* 25 (2019): 123–125.

3

Access to Quality, Culturally Appropriate Health Care

BRITTNEY T. ANDERSON, MD

Black people in the South need access to quality health care that is culturally appropriate in order to improve their overall health. Barriers to this access include racism and race bias in medicine, a low number of practicing Black physicians who disproportionally assume the care of Black patients, and other institutional and systemic barriers that negatively impact the health of Black Americans living in the South. Efforts to directly address these issues include incorporating cultural competency training in medical education and in the health care workforce, developing processes to recruit Black students into medicine to increase the number of practicing Black physicians, and recognizing attributes that Black patients seek in health care providers that may lead to more trusting relationships and better health outcomes.

Racism and Race Bias in Health Care

The concern is great that racism and race bias may contribute to poor health outcomes for Black people, particularly in the South, which has longstanding ties to slavery, segregation, and institutional racism. Black people in the South do not readily forget stories of maltreatment of Black patients. These stories include (but are not limited to) those of the men enrolled in The Tuskegee Study of Untreated Syphilis in the Negro Male in Alabama and the countless Black women throughout the South who were sterilized without their consent. Antebellum southern medical journals extensively document how white physicians treated Black slaves, giving credibility to the oral tradition that Blacks were objects of learning and experimentation for physicians and medical schools (Fisher 1968). In 1860, an editorial in the *Savannah Journal of Medicine* noted abundant clinical opportunities in southern medical schools for the study of disease in the large Negro population in the region (Savannah Journal of Medicine 1859–1860). These stories and others created a deep mistrust of medicine and science in some Black people that is reflected in patients' hesitation to participate in clinical trials, receive preventive health services, seek medical attention, and follow prescribed regimens. This history of maltreatment means that some Black patients have a general distrust of white health care providers. They prefer to be cared for by Black providers. Unfortunately, the low number of Black physicians in the United States is not enough to meet this demand.

In addition to this historical context, there is also a current and very real issue of race bias among some white providers that perpetuates Black patients' mistrust of the health care industry. While medical professionals should seek to provide appropriate treatment to all patients regardless of their race, this is not always the case. Health care workers may exhibit both implicit bias (the unintentional and unacknowledged preference for one group over another) and explicit biases that negatively affect both the patient experience and overall health outcomes. While it is difficult to obtain a true determination of physicians' explicit race bias using traditional research methods because social norms may prevent study participants from sharing their true opinions, implicit bias among physicians has been widely studied. Implicit bias in physicians correlates with unequal care of patients (Chapman, Kaatz, and Carnes 2013, 1504–1510). This bias can lead to assumptions based on stereotypes and to different treatment plans among patients based on their race. Some ways that implicit race bias and discrimination may manifest in patient care include longer times in waiting rooms for Black patients, less time spent with Black patients, approaching Black patients in a condescending manner, less thorough clinical workup of Black patients, and fewer special privileges to Black patients than those afforded to others (Hall et al. 2015, e61). Oliver and colleagues evaluated whether or not white physicians' implicit views of Blacks affected their clinical decision making and found that even though physicians reported that they gave similar care to Black and white patients, they demonstrated implicit pro-white bias, reported an explicit preference for white people, and had beliefs that Blacks were less medically cooperative than whites (Oliver et al. 2014, 184). In contrast, Black physicians have been shown to exhibit significantly less implicit race bias, regardless of the patient's race (Chapman, Kaatz, and Carnes 2013, 1508).

Bias on the part of physicians, whether it is implicit or explicit, may make them less likely to offer treatment regimens to a Black patient that they would offer to a white patient. It may also cause them not to recommend and perform certain screening and treatments that are the universal standard of care. Racial disparities are well documented in health care settings, particularly in the emergency department setting, where research shows that physicians are less likely to order diagnostic tests, such as EKGs, cardiac monitoring, oxygen saturation measurement, and chest X-rays for Black patients who report chest pain (Pezzin, Keyl, and Green 2007). Black patients being treated for pain in emergency rooms are less likely to receive appropriate and timely analgesic management, more likely to have a prolonged emergency department stay, and less likely to be admitted to the hospital (Shah et al. 2015, 1005). Both Blacks and Hispanics in emergency rooms have been shown to be significantly less likely to receive any antidote for acute drug overdose (Wilder et al. 2018).

Both real and perceived discriminations are barriers to health for Black patients. This is perhaps felt most acutely in the South, where centuries of systemic racism have been pervasive and normalized and have great potential to be translated into the health care setting.

Cultural Competence in Medical Education

Ensuring that medical practitioners provide culturally sensitive and unbiased care is a major step toward decreasing the health disparities Black patients face. As the United States continues to become more culturally diverse, it is imperative that health care providers are aware of the cultural views their patients have that may affect their health outcomes. The medical professional workforce continues to be dominated by white practitioners and it is reasonable to assume that most of them will care for Black patients, who have different cultural backgrounds than their own, at some point in their careers. It is important that non-Black health care professionals caring for Black patients understand the complexity of the role culture plays in the lives of these patients. Moreover, it is important for health care providers to understand the culture of Black patients in the South (i.e., their customs, values, and beliefs) in order to understand factors that may lead to disease processes and to make realistic and feasible health care plans. Culture can directly affect patients' perceptions about diet, exercise, and medication. When providers fail to take social and cultural factors into account, they may resort to stereotyping that influences their behavior toward patients and the decisions they make about patient care that could affect the overall health of the patient (Van Ryn and Burke 2000). Alternatively, when providers recognize the effect of cultural influences on patients and incorporate this knowledge into patient care, they are better able to build relationships and trust with Black patients. It is important for physicians to be both culturally aware and culturally competent.

Culturally competent care acknowledges and incorporates the importance of culture, assesses cross-cultural relations, is vigilant about the dynamics that result from cultural differences, seeks to expand cultural knowledge, and adapts services to meet culturally unique needs (Betancourt et al. 2003). Several models have described cultural competence; most describe it as a continuum. The widely used Cross model defines cultural competence as a six-stage developmental process in which the individual progresses from cultural destructiveness (i.e., the individual has attitudes and participates in policies and practices that are destructive to cultures and individuals within a culture) to a level of advanced cultural competence or proficiency (i.e., the individual holds culture in high esteem and pays careful attention to the dynamics of difference, continuously works to expand their cultural knowledge and resources, and uses a variety of adaptations to better meet the needs of minority populations) (Cross et al. 1989, 13–17).

A review of health care provider education interventions yielded evidence that cultural competence training improves the knowledge, attitudes, and skills of health professionals and impacts patient satisfaction (Beach et al. 2005, 366). Therefore, teaching cultural competence to medical students is essential. Health care professionals do not necessarily start out being culturally competent; they develop cultural competence over time through training, experience, guidance, and self-evaluation (Cross et al. 1989, 25). Recently, there has been a necessary shift in medical education to incorporate cultural competency training in the curricula for medical students and residents. The standards of the Liaison Committee on Medical Education state that medical students must be self-aware of personal biases in their approach to health care delivery, must demonstrate an understanding of the effects that social and cultural systems have on their patients' health, and must know how to recognize and address cultural, racial, and ethnic biases and disparities in the diagnosis and treatment of disease (International Association of Medical Colleges 2020). Similarly, the Accreditation Council on Graduate Medical

Education requires that physicians in training demonstrate respect and responsiveness to a patient's culture as part of its professionalism competency (Accreditation Council of Graduate Medical Education 2020). These are positive steps that at least acknowledge the need to train the physician workforce to be culturally competent.

Currently, there is no uniform model for conducting the cultural competence training of health professionals. Training occurs using several curricular methods that include case scenarios, cultural immersion, group discussions, lectures, and clinical experiences. Contact time for such training can be a one-time session or multiple sessions over a period of time (Beach et al. 2005, 360–362). The effectiveness of cultural competency education can be measured by determining whether the training changes clinicians' behaviors, improves the patient-provider relationship, and improves health outcomes (Agency for Healthcare Research and Quality 2014).

It is important to recognize that even within one minority group different cultures can exist. Thus, it is vital that cultural training does not lead to stereotyping. This is particularly important in the case of Black people. Not only can various cultures be seen among those living in different regions, but cultures may also differ among those living in the same region. For example, in the South, the culture of certain Blacks living in Charleston, South Carolina, may differ from those in New Orleans, Louisiana, whose culture may also be different from those in Selma, Alabama. True cultural competence views minority groups as distinctly different from one another and as having numerous subgroups, each with important cultural characteristics (Cross et al. 1989, 17). The goal of introducing the idea of cultural competency in medical education is not to strive to teach future practitioners everything they will need to know about a minority group but instead to make them aware that different cultures exist and that their attention to these varying cultures, especially those that are different from their own, is essential to achieving both patient satisfaction and best health outcomes.

Given the documented effectiveness of cultural competency training and the overwhelming proportion of non-minorities in the health care industry, similar training should be conducted among practicing physicians, nurses, and other members of the health care team and staff. Specifically, targeting non-Black physicians could result in more culturally competent care for Black patients in the midst of a deficiency in the numbers of Black physicians.

Shortage of Black Physicians

Currently, only 5% of physicians in the United States identify as Black or African American (Association of American Medical Colleges 2019c). There has been only minimal change in this percentage in several decades, certainly not enough that the percentage of Black physicians matches that of the general population; Black people account for roughly 13.2% of the country's inhabitants. It is widely realized that Black physicians disproportionately provide medical care for Black patients and communities, elevating the need to address this scarcity of Black physicians. Historical context contributes to the lack of Black physicians, but modern-day barriers also exist and perpetuate the shortage of Black students who matriculate into and graduate from medical school. Chief among the concerns about the shortage of Black physicians is the disparity in the number of Black male physicians, which is less than 3% of all active physicians and has been declining in recent decades (Association of American Medical Colleges 2018a).

Black physicians have historically experienced rejection and racism in the field of medicine and in organized medicine. This history exposes the systemic and institutional bias in the field of medicine and the negative impact this bias continues to have on the number of Black physicians and consequently on the health of Black patients. In the 18th century, scientific racism falsely labeled Blacks as inferior based on supposed biological racial differences (Garrod 2006, 55). This idea carried into the 19th century and beyond. It led white physicians to assume that Black people were mentally inferior and to the disqualification of Blacks from many medical institutions in the United States, particularly in the South, although few northern medical schools and medical societies accepted Blacks. At their inception in the mid-19th century, medical societies afforded physicians professional contacts and relationships, information about the latest medical advancements, training opportunities, access to hospital and licensing privileges, and the general ability to have a successful practice. Exclusion from these societies based on race led to significant barriers and practice constraints for Black physicians (Baker et al. 2009, 502).

Although the American Medical Association, which was founded in 1847, never formally adopted exclusion criteria for Blacks, it developed a state-based structure that effectively excluded most Black physicians from membership (Baker 2009, 501). This exclusion was particularly notable in the

South, where Black physicians formed their own local societies. In 1895, leading Black physicians formed the National Medical Association, which supported Black physicians who were graduating in small numbers from northern white medical schools, international medical schools, and the growing number of medical schools established in the South. From 1868 to 1907, 15 medical colleges were established with the intent of educating Black physicians, including twelve schools in Kentucky, Louisiana, Mississippi, North Carolina, and Tennessee. These schools were small and financially constrained, but they produced Black physicians who would provide exclusive care for Black patients.

In 1908, Alexander Flexner, a white educator from Kentucky, was commissioned to lead a review of medical schools in the United States and Canada. The purpose of this study was to raise the standards of medical education. Flexner's report led to the closure of over half of the 150 medical schools in the country, including all but two of the institutions devoted to training Black physicians (Johnston 1984). The closure of these Black medical schools significantly inhibited the production of Black physicians to care for the nine million Blacks, 90% of the country's Black population, who were living in the segregated South at that time (Baker 2009, 509). The AMA accepted this damning report and sealed the fate of these Black medical colleges and prospective Black physicians and the fate of citizens who relied on their care. The subsequent integration of African Americans into white medical colleges was gradual and slow over the next several decades. The Flexner Report has long-reaching consequences even today, more than 100 years after its publication.

Presently, there are four medical schools whose primary focus is training Black physicians: Howard University College of Medicine in Washington, DC; Meharry Medical College in Nashville, Tennessee; Charles R. Drew Medical School in Los Angeles, California;, and Morehouse School of Medicine in Atlanta, Georgia. While these institutions matriculate a large percentage of Black students annually, there is still a disparity in the number of Black students entering medical training. *Diversity in Medicine: Facts and Figures 2019*, a publication of the Association of American Medical Colleges, reports that only 7.1% of students who matriculated into US medical schools in 2019 were Black (Association of American Medical Colleges 2019b). Not only are acceptance rates of Black students into medical school low; the number of applications submitted are also low in relation to other groups. In 2018, only

8.4% of applicants identified as Black or African American (Association of American Medical Colleges 2019d). This suggests that systemic factors are real and perceived barriers to a career as a physician for Black students. Black high school students cited financial challenges related to attending college and postgraduate education, the time commitment required to become a physician, the stress related to the difficulty of coursework, limited opportunities in and exposure to medicine, lack of family and peer support, perceptions of physicians as largely white males, lack of knowledge about the field of medicine, and perceived racism in the medical field and health care institutions as barriers to a career in medicine (Rao and Flores 2007, 998–990). The cost of postgraduate training can be a significant challenge for many Black students and is often cited as a deterrent to pursuing a medical degree. Black students, on average, enter medical school with higher debt than their white counterparts. It is reported that 22.9% of Black students entering medical school complete their premedical education with $50,000 or more of debt, higher than any other racial/ethnic group of students. Only 8.1% of white students have this amount of debt as they enter medical school (Association of American Medical Colleges 2019a). Financial and other challenges must be addressed if the number of Black medical school applicants and matriculants is to increase.

Although overall the numbers remain low, the proportions of Black medical school graduates have changed, leading to a concerning decline in the number of Black male physicians in this country. Since 1986, the proportion of Black female medical school graduates has increased 53% and the proportion of Black male graduates has declined 39%. In 2015, the gender gap among Black or African American graduates was 31% (Association of American Medical Colleges 2017). While rates for both Black male and female physicians remain low, Black men face unique challenges, including society's general mistrust of Black men, stereotypes and social biases against Black men, unpreparedness for college admission, and lack of mentorship (Oliver et al. 2020, S77–S79). Black males have significantly poorer educational outcomes compared to other major demographic groups in the United States. The trajectory of these outcomes begins in elementary education and continues through higher education (Palmer et al. 2010, 105). Research shows that early academic problems that disparage Black males include the fact that educators are less likely to impart positive expectations that they will attend college compared to whites, lower representation in gifted education programs or coursework, disproportionate disciplinary action, and the fact that Black males are labeled with behavior problems or learning disabilities at much higher rates than their white counterparts (Palmer et al. 2010, 109).

There is also a pronounced gender disparity among Black men and women related to higher education in other fields. African American males lag behind their female and white male counterparts in college admission and completion, largely due to lack of preparedness. As few as 1 in 15 are adequately prepared for college-level work (Palmer et al. 2010, 109). Black men account for 4.3% of the total enrollment at four-year higher education institutions in the United States. Many of them experience significant challenges as they work to complete their degree; more than two-thirds of Black men who start college do not graduate within six years (Harper 2006, 14). All of these constructs present Black men with specific challenges to becoming successful applicants to and graduates of medical school. The decrease in Black male graduates is discouraging, as is the overall low number of Black physicians, which is not growing at the same rate as that of other underrepresented minorities.

Barriers to Recruiting and Retaining Physicians in Predominantly Black Communities

There is a devastating gap in the overall health of Black communities compared to that of white communities. This is particularly noteworthy in the South, where obesity, diabetes, and metabolic syndrome are prevalent (Gurka, Flipp, and DeBoar 2018). Nationally, Blacks have a lower life expectancy at birth compared to whites and experience death from hypertension, diabetes, chronic lung disease, and preterm delivery at rates significantly higher than whites (U.S. Department of Health and Human Services Office of Minority Health 2019). Lack of access to care is chief among the reasons for these disparities and includes factors such as fewer primary care physicians in Black communities to address preventive care and chronic disease, even fewer specialty physicians to treat the most serious of these cases, and fewer physician-staffed health care facilities in predominantly Black and low-income communities. This highlights the need to recruit and retain physicians in predominantly Black areas.

At the turn of the 20th century, the proportion of Black physicians practicing in the South was similar to the proportion of Black people living in the region. But by the 1970s, only 32% of active physicians were in the South, even though 53% of the Black population resided there (Gray 1977, 520). Most recent data from the Office of Minority Health shows that 58% of the US Black population lives in the South (U.S. Department of Health and Human Services Office of Minority Health 2019). There is scant data on the current distribution of Black physicians, although trends show that the proportion of Black physicians practicing in the South is unlikely to be similar to the population. As was the case for Black physicians a century ago, Black physicians today tend to care for a large percentage of Black, underserved, and uninsured patients. In 2018–2019, when medical school matriculants were asked, "Do you plan to work primarily in an underserved area?" an overwhelming 60.5% of Black or African American matriculants answered yes, the highest of any race/ethnicity (Association of American Medical Colleges 2019e). The need to increase the number of Black students entering the medical field is urgent in order to increase the overall care of Black communities. It is especially important to disperse new Black medical graduates to geographic areas that would result in better access to care for Black Americans.

Blacks in the South suffer from chronic and preventable diseases at an alarming rate. Primary care physicians are essential for providing the necessary screening of these diseases and providing education that will prevent them. Black physicians often choose primary care fields. In 2018, 41.4% of Black physicians in the United States were primary care physicians, a proportion that was second only to that of American Indian or Alaska Native physicians practicing primary care (41.5%) (Association of American Medical Colleges 2018b). Increasing the number of Black physicians would undoubtedly increase the number of physicians practicing primary care among Black patients.

The factors physicians consider when choosing a location to practice vary, but broadly speaking, they include well-studied factors such as personal characteristics, financial dynamics, medical school programs, and location characteristics. Multiple studies show that physicians who self-identified as belonging to an underrepresented minority group were more likely than their colleagues to locate in high-need practice areas (Goodfellow et al. 2016, 1316). Specifically, Black physicians are significantly more likely than white physicians to practice in a lower-income neighborhood and more likely to treat Black patients (Bach et al. 2004, 579). The amount of education debt seems to have direct inverse relationship to physicians' choice of practice location. Those with little educational debt may be more likely to accept lower-reimbursed positions treating underserved patients. Conversely, those with higher debt may be more likely to accept scholarships, loan repayment programs, or other incentives in return for their service to an underserved area and population. Incentive programs have been widely used to recruit physicians to underserved areas to practice, largely through Title VII of the Public Health Service Act. Physicians who received Title VII funding during medical school and residency were more likely to locate their practice in underserved areas than those who did not (Krist et al. 2005). Medical training curricula and programs that focus on underserved areas were also more likely to graduate physicians who would practice in underserved communities (Goodfellow et al. 2016, 1316).

The makeup of the community is also a factor when physicians choose where they will practice. Location characteristics include physician wages, the number of other physicians providing care in the area, the area's unemployment rate and per capita income, proportion of population by age, and proportion of population by race (Chou and Lo Sasso 2009). According to the American Communities Project, the predominantly Black counties in the South, which stretch from Virginia to Texas, are home to 16.4 million people. Only 20.5% of the residents of these counties have a college degree, 7% are unemployed, and the median household income is $37,500 (American Communities Project 2020). According to Census Bureau data, the national Black median household income in 2017 was $40,165, compared to $65,845 for white households. In this same year, 55.5% of Blacks used private health insurance (compared to 75.4% of whites) and 43.9% of Blacks relied on Medicaid or public health insurance (compared to 33.7% of whites) (U.S. Department of Health and Human Services Office of Minority Health 2019).

Medicaid, which was enacted in 1965 to finance health care for the poor, has provided health care of large numbers of low-income Black and white Americans. Similarly, the Medicare program was established in 1965 to reduce the financial burden of the elderly and disabled seeking medical care. The creation of Medicare and Medicaid accelerated the process of desegregation in health care facilities in the South, as institutions that receive these federal funds are prohibited from discriminating on the basis of race (Davis et al. 1987, 227). However, many people who would benefit from access to Medicaid, particularly poor Blacks in the South, are not afforded this opportunity by their state. As of 2020, twelve states, including Tennessee, North Carolina, South Carolina, Georgia, Florida, Alabama, Mississippi, and Texas, have not formally adopted an expansion of Medicaid, thereby preventing many in these southern states from access to health care and better health outcomes.

Komaromy et al. found that communities with high proportions of Black and Hispanic residents were four times as likely as others to have a shortage of physicians (Komaromy et al. 1996, 1306). The introduction of community health centers in 1965 has had a positive impact on the provision of affordable, accessible, quality, and value-based primary health care, regardless of ability to pay, to otherwise underserved groups, including low-income Black communities across the South. But such centers must be staffed by health care providers who will commit to practicing with this population and in these communities, preferably over the long term in order to build relationships within the community. Retaining physicians in underserved areas is a point of concern, especially when considering that many physicians who enter underserved areas to practice do so with a debt of loan repayment or a scholarship obligation or in order to obtain US residency status. In some cases, a pattern evolves whereby physicians leave these communities at the end of their obligatory commitments, thereby creating a revolving door of care for patients. This disrupts the continuity that is needed to build trusting relationships and effect change to the health of the population within the community.

There is an obvious need to increase access to health care in Black communities, particular in the South. In order to increase access, it will be necessary to increase the number of providers, decrease the distance people need to travel to receive medical care, and increase the ability of patients to pay for visits and prescribed treatments. However, even when services are more accessible, Blacks may face racial discrimination from non-Black physicians that makes it difficult for them to obtain adequate care (Jones and Rice 1987).

Black Patient Responsiveness to Black Physicians

Medical segregation, a system whereby Black patients were cared for solely by Black physicians, was particularly prominent in the South after the Civil War. Black physicians were limited where they could practice and the number of physicians and institutions who would treat Black patients was very small. Today, after the civil rights legislation of the 1960s and population migration, these restrictions are less harsh. However, an interesting link remains between Black patients and Black physicians that is important to understand in order to address some of the health outcomes of Black patients.

Research finds that patients tend to choose physicians and determine their satisfaction based on the physician's interpersonal skills and communication, perceived level of knowledge, time spent with patients, and interest in patients' concerns (Hill and Carter 1991, 491–496). Shared experiences and cultural beliefs may drive some patients' preferences. To that end, race concordance, or matching, among patients and their health care providers has been widely studied and is important to consider in the discussion of Black patients. A study that evaluated doctor-patient race concordance and association with greater satisfaction with care found that Black patients who could choose their physician were more likely to choose a Black physician and were more likely to report greater satisfaction with their physician than those who were not race concordant (Laveist and Nuru-Jeter, 2002, 302). The hypotheses about patients' preference for physician concordance include that patients may have more trust and a greater level of comfort with physicians of their same race group (Laveist and Nuru-Jeter, 2002, 303). Trust is an essential component to a good relationship between a patient and physician and is an important factor that leads to shared treatment goals and best outcomes. Higher patient trust is significantly associated with positive physician affect; patients are more trusting of their physicians if they show interest in their needs, are friendly and responsive, are not assertive, show empathy, and are not hurried (Martin et al. 2013, 153–156). Black Americans are significantly less likely to trust health care professionals and the health care system than white Americans (Halbert et al. 2006, 899). This medical mistrust has serious negative consequences for the health of Black patients. Medical mistrust has been shown to delay preventive health care in Black men who report experiencing everyday racism and perceive racism in health care at significantly high rates (Powell et al. 2019, 110).

Black patients' beliefs about racial discrimination in health care is a large component of mistrust and has been found to be associated with choosing a Black physician (Chen et al. 2005, 142). Generally, physician-patient race concordance should lead to better-quality care and greater patient satisfaction. While it is difficult to objectively measure the care that Black patients receive from Black physicians, patients seem to perceive better care, which likely contributes to their positive responsiveness to Black physicians. The chronic medical conditions that predispose the Black community to death at higher rates require regular and close follow-up. Research shows that patients tend to use more health care and are less likely to postpone care when they have physicians who are of their own race or ethnicity (Laveist, Nuru-Jeter, and Jones 2003, 319)

Despite the apparent preference among Black patients for Black physicians and research that supports Black patients' responsiveness to Black physicians, most Black patients in America have a white physician, largely due to the fact that there is a significantly higher number of white physicians in the country. The goal is not to return to racial segregation in health care; instead, the goal is to increase the number of Black physicians and provide patients with more choices that might align with their preferences in order to obtain the best health outcomes.

Black communities, particularly in the South, have a great need for physicians and health care providers who are accessible, well trained, compassionate, and can provide culturally competent care. In order to improve the health of Black people living in the South, and reduce the current health disparities, it is imperative to recognize this need and adjust accordingly. This can be done by acknowledging the presence of systemic racism and physician race bias and working toward preparing physicians and other health care workers to be culturally competent and better prepared to care for Black patients. Another means of improving care and physician access for Black patients would be to increase the number of practicing Black physicians. Action must be taken to reverse the unfortunate trend in the numbers of Black physicians, particularly Black male physicians, being produced. The first step to doing so is addressing the personal and institutional barriers that Black students face when they apply to medical schools. The second step is programs and policies that ensure that Black medical students complete their degree.

Increasing the data specifically related to the provision of health care to Blacks in the South would fill gaps in the literature and would offer information needed in order to provide better and more culturally appropriate access to health care for Black people in the South. Specifically, gathering more information from patients and health care providers regarding race bias in the South and its effect on patient health would be beneficial. There is also need for updated information on the distribution of Black physicians and the numbers of those currently practicing in the South. This could help with identifying current deficits and forecasting future needs in southern Black communities. Research involving Black physicians who practice in the South and factors that contribute to their remaining in the South would also be valuable and would perhaps aid in recruiting Black physicians to the South.

America's South is widely known for its long history of maltreatment of Blacks, from slavery to sharecropping to Jim Crow to the present day. The result of this racism is a large population of Blacks living in the South who still harbor a mistrust of what they believe is an unfair health care system that will have a negative impact on their health. Because of this negative history, the provision of quality, culturally appropriate care to Black patients in the South must be a goal that we view as necessary, impactful, and attainable.

REFERENCES

Accreditation Council of Graduate Medical Education. 2020. "Common Program Requirements." December 1, 2020. https://www.acgme.org/what-we-do/accreditation/common-program-requirements/.

Agency for Healthcare Research and Quality. 2014. "Improving Cultural Competence to Reduce Health Care Disparities for Priority Populations." Accessed December 1, 2020. http://effectivehealthcare.ahrq.gov/products/cultural-competence/research-protocol.

American Communities Project. 2020. "African American South." Accessed December 1, 2020. http://www.americancommunities.org/community-type/african-american-south/.

Association of American Medical Colleges. 2017. "At a Glance: Black and African American Physicians in the Workforce." Accessed December 1, 2020. http://www.aamc.org/news-insights/glance-black-and-african-american-physicians-workforce.

———. 2018a. "Percentage of Physicians by Sex and Race/Ethnicity, 2018." Diversity in Medicine: Facts and Figures, 2019. Accessed December 1, 2020. https://www.aamc.org/data-reports/workforce/interactive-data/figure-20-percentage-physicians-sex-and-race/ethnicity-2018.

———. 2018b. "Primary Care Versus Nonprimary Care Physicians by Race/Ethnicity, 2018." Diversity in Medicine: Facts and Figures, 2019. Accessed December 1, 2020. https://www.aamc.org/data-reports/workforce/interactive-data/figure-26-primary-care-versus-nonprimary-care-physicians-race/ethnicity-2018.

———. 2019a. "Amount of Premedical Education Debt for U.S. Medical School Matriculants by Race/Ethnicity, Academic Year 2018–2019." Diversity in Medicine: Facts and Figures, 2019. Accessed December 1, 2020. https://www.aamc.org/data-reports/workforce/interactive-data/figure-10-amount-premedical-education-debt-us-medical-school-matriculants-race/ethnicity-academic.

———. 2019b. "Percentage of Acceptees to U.S. Medical Schools by Race/Ethnicity (Alone),

Academic Year 2018–2019." Diversity in Medicine: Facts and Figures, 2019. Accessed December 1, 2020. https://www.aamc.org/data-reports/workforce/interactive-data/figure -6-percentage-acceptees-us-medical-schools-race/ethnicity-alone-academic-year-2018 -2019#:~:text=Diversity%20in%20Medicine%3A%20Facts%20and%20Figures%202019, -New%20section&text=Of%20accepted%20applicants%2C%20nearly%20half,Latino %2C%20or%20of%20Spanish%20Origin.

———. 2019c. "Percentage of All Active Physicians by Race/Ethnicity, 2018." Diversity in Medicine: Facts and Figures, 2019. Accessed December 1, 2020. https://www.aamc.org /data-reports/workforce/interactive-data/figure-18-percentage-all-active-physicians -race/ethnicity-2018#:~:text=Among%20active%20physicians%2C%2056.2%25%20 identified,as%20Black%20or%20African%20American.

———. 2019d. "Percentage of Applicants to U.S. Medical Schools by Race/Ethnicity (Alone), Academic Year 2018–2019." Diversity in Medicine: Facts and Figures, 2019. Accessed December 1, 2020. https://www.aamc.org/data-reports/workforce/interactive-data/figure -2-percentage-applicants-us-medical-schools-race/ethnicity-alone-academic-year -2018-2019#:~:text=Diversity%20in%20Medicine%3A%20Facts%20and%20Figures %202019,-New%20section&text=Apart%20from%20White%20applicants%20(46.8 ,were%206.2%25%20of%20the%20pool.

———. 2019e. "Percentage of U.S. Medical School Matriculants Planning to Practice in an Underserved Area by Race/Ethnicity, Academic Year 2018–2019." Diversity in Medicine: Facts and Figures, 2019. Accessed December 1, 2020. https://www.aamc.org/data -reports/workforce/interactive-data/figure-11-percentage-us-medical-school -matriculants-planning-practice-underserved-area-race.

Bach, Peter, Hoangmai Pham, Deborah Schrag, Ramsey Tate, and Lee Hargraves. 2004. "Primary Care Physicians Who Treat Blacks and Whites." New England Journal of Medicine 351 (6): 575–584.

Baker, Robert, Harriet Washington, Oloade Olakanmi, Todd Savitt, Elizabeth Jacobs, Eddie Hoover, and Matthew Wynia. 2009. "Creating a Segregated Medical Profession: African American Physicians and Organized Medicine, 1846–1910." Journal of the National Medical Association 101 (6): 501–512.

Beach, Mary, Eboni Price, Tiffany Gary, Karen Robinson, Aysegul Gozu, Ana Palacio, Carole Smarth, et al. 2005. "Cultural Competence: A Systematic Review of Health Care Provider Educational Interventions." Medical Care 43 (4): 356–373.

Betancourt, Joseph, Alexander Green, J. Emilio Carrillo, and Owusu Ananeh-Firempong. 2003. "Defining Cultural Competence: A Practical Framework for Addressing Racial/ Ethnic Disparities in Health and Health Care." Public Health Reports 118 (4): 293–302.

Chapman, Elizabeth, Anna Kaatz, and Molly Carnes. 2013. "Physicians and Implicit Bias: How Doctors May Unwittingly Perpetuate Health Care Disparities." Journal of General Internal Medicine 28 (11): 1504–1510.

Chen, Frederick, George Fryer, Robert Phillips, Elisabeth Wilson, and Donald Pathman. 2005. "Patients' Beliefs About Racism, Preferences for Physician Race, and Satisfaction with Care." Annals of Family Medicine 3 (2): 138–143.

Chou, Chiu-Fang, and Anthony Lo Sasso. 2009. "Practice Location Choice by New Physicians: The Importance of Malpractice Premiums, Damage Caps, and Health Profession

Shortage Area Designation." *Health Services Research* 44: 1271–1289. https://www.ncbi
.nlm.nih.gov/pmc/articles/PMC2739028/.

Cross, Terry, Barbara Bazron, Karl Dennis, and Mareasa Isaacs. 1989. *Towards a Culturally
Competent System of Care: A Monograph of Effective Services for Minority Children Who
Are Severely Emotionally Disturbed*. Washington, DC: CASSP Technical Assistance Cen-
ter, Georgetown University Child Development Center.

Davis, Karen, Marsha Lillie-Blanton, Barbara Lyons, Fitzhugh Mullan, Neil Powe, and Diane
Rowland. 1987. "Health Care for Black Americans: The Public Sector Role." *Milbank
Quarterly* 65 (suppl. 1): 213–247.

Fisher, W. 1968. "Physicians and Slavery in the Antebellum Southern Medical Journal."
Journal of the History of Medicine and Allied Sciences 23 (1): 36–49.

Garrod, Joel. 2006. "A Brave Old World: An Analysis of Scientific Racism and BiDil®." *McGill
Journal of Medicine* 9 (1): 54–60.

Goodfellow, Amelia, Jesus Ulloa, Patrick Dowling, Efrain Talamantes, Somi Chheda, Curtis
Bone, and Gerardo Moreno. 2016. "Predictors of Primary Care Physician Practice Loca-
tion in Underserved Urban or Rural Areas in the United States: A Systemic Literature
Review." *Academic Medicine* 91 (9): 1313–1321.

Gray, Lois. 1977. "The Geographic and Functional Distribution of Black Physicians: Some
Research and Policy Considerations." *American Journal of Public Health* 67 (6): 519–526.

Gurka, Matthew, Stephanie Flipp, and Mark DeBoar. 2018. "Geographical Variation in the
Prevalence of Obesity, Metabolic Syndrome, and Diabetes Among U.S. Adults." *Nutrition and Diabetes* 8: article 14. Accessed December 1, 2020. https://doi.org/10.1038
/s41387-018-0024-2.

Halbert, Chanita, Katrina Armstrong, Oscar Gandy, and Lee Shaker. 2006. "Racial Differences in Trust in Health Care Providers." *Archives of Internal Medicine* 166 (8): 896–901.

Hall, William, Mimi Chapman, Kent Lee, Yesenia Merino, Tainayah Thomas, Keith Payne,
Eugenia Eng, Steven Day, and Tamera Coyne-Beasley. 2015. "Implicit Racial/Ethnic Bias
among Health Care Professionals and Its Influence on Health Care Outcomes: A Systematic Review." *American Journal of Public Health* 105 (12): e60–e76.

Harper, Shaun. 2006. "Reconceptualizing Reactive Policy Responses to Black Male College
Achievement: Implications from a National Study." *Focus: Magazine of the Joint Center
for Political and Economic Studies* 14.

Hill, C. Jeanne, and S. J. Carter. 1991. "Factors Influencing Physician Choice." *Hospital and
Health Services Administration*. 36 (4): 491–503. http://link.gale.com/apps/doc/A11556953
/ITOF?u=tusc49521&sid=ITOF&xid=34d73574.

International Association of Medical Colleges. 2020. "LCME Accreditation Standards." Accessed December 1, 2020. https://www.iaomc.org/lcme.htm.

Johnston, George. 1984. "The Flexner Report and Black Medical Schools." *Journal of the
National Medical Association* 76 (3): 223–225.

Jones, Woodrow, and Mitchell Rice. 1987. "Black Health Care: An Overview." In *Health Care
Issues in Black America*, ed. Woodrow Jones and Mitchell Rice, 1–20. New York: Greenwood Press.

Komaromy, Miriam, Kevin Grumbach, Michael Drake, Karen Vranizan, Nicole Lurie, Dennis Keane, and Andrew Bindman. 1996. "The Role of Black and Hispanic Physicians in

Providing Health Care for Underserved Populations." *New England Journal of Medicine* 33 (20): 1305–1310.

Krist, Alex, Robert Johnson, David Callahan, Steven Woolf, and David Marsland. 2005. "Title VII Funding and Physician Practice in Rural or Low-Income Areas." *Journal of Rural Health* 21 (1): 3–11.

Laveist, Thomas, and Amani Nuru-Jeter. 2002. "Is Doctor-Patient Race Concordance Associated with Greater Satisfaction of Care?" *Journal of Health and Social Behavior* 43 (3): 296–306.

Laveist, Thomas, Amani Nuru-Jeter, and Kiesha Jones. 2003. "The Association of Doctor-Patient Race Concordance with Health Services Utilization." *Journal of Public Health Policy* 24 (3): 312–323.

Martin, Kimberly, Debra Roter, Mary Beach, Kathryn Carson, and Lisa Cooper. 2013. "Physician Communication Behaviors and Trust Among Black and White Patients with Hypertension." *Medical Care* 51 (2): 151–157.

Oliver, Kelvin, Mridula Nadamuni, Christina Ahn, Marc Nivet, Byron Cryer, and Dale Okorodudu. 2020. "Mentoring Black Men in Medicine." *Academic Medicine* 95 (12). S77–S81.

Oliver, M. Norman, Kristen Wells, Jennifer Joy-Gaba, Carlee Hawkins, and Brian Nosek. 2014. "Do Physicians' Implicit Views of African Americans Affect Clinical Decision Making?" *Journal of American Board of Family Medicine* 27 (2): 177–188. https://www.jabfm .org/content/27/2/177.

Palmer, Robert, Ryan Davis, James Moore, III, and Adriel Hilton. 2010. "A Nation at Risk: Increasing College Participation and Persistence Among African American Males to Stimulate U.S. Global Competitiveness." *Journal of African American Males in Education* 1 (2): 105–124.

Pezzin, Liliana, Penelope Keyl, and Gary Green. 2007. "Disparities in the Emergency Department Evaluation of Chest Pain Patients." *Academic Emergency Medicine* 14 (2): 149–156.

Powell, Wizdom, Jennifer Richmond, Dinushika Mohottige, Irene Yen, Allison Joslyn, and Giselle Corbie-Smith. 2019. "Medical Mistrust, Racism, and Delays in Preventative Health Screening among African-American Men." *Behavioral Medicine* 45 (2): 102–117. Accessed December 1, 2020. https://doi.org/10.1080/08964289.2019.1585327.

Rao, Vijaya, and Glenn Flores. 2007. "Why Aren't There More African American Physicians? A Qualitative Study and Exploratory Inquiry of African American Students' Perspectives on Careers in Medicine." *Journal of the National Medical Association* 99 (9): 986–993.

Savannah Journal of Medicine. "Southern Institutions." 1859–1860. *Savannah Journal of Medicine* 2: 352–354.

Shah, Adil, Cheryl Zogg, Syed Zafar, Eric Schneider, Lisa Cooper, Alyssa Chapital, Susan Peterson, R. J. Thorpe Jr., et al. 2015. "Analgesic Access for Acute Abdominal Pain in the Emergency Department among Racial/Ethnic Minority Patients: A Nationwide Examination." *Medical Care* 53 (12): 1000–1009.

U.S. Department of Health and Human Services Office of Minority Health. 2019. "Profile: Black/African Americans." Accessed December 1, 2020. http:www.minorityhealth.hhs .gov/omh/browse.aspx?lvl=3&lvlID=61.

Van Ryn, Michelle, and Jane Burke. 2000. "The Effect of Patient Race and Socio-Economic

Status on Physicians' Perceptions of Patients." *Social Science and Medicine* 50 (6): 813–828.

Wilder, Marcee, Lynne Richardson, Robert Hoffman, Gary Winkel, and Alex Manini. 2018. "Racial Disparities in the Treatment of Acute Overdose in the Emergency Department." *Clinical Toxicology* 56 (12): 1173–1178. https://www.ncbi.nlm.nih.gov/pmc/articles/PMC6318059/.

II METHODS

4

Health Intervention Studies

CASEY L. DANIEL, PhD, MPH,

and YENDELELA L. CUFFEE, PhD, MPH

Reducing health disparities and achieving health equity is a primary goal in the field of public health. Social determinants of health such as poverty, educational attainment, and environmental conditions as well as social and cultural issues such as discrimination and medical mistrust are major contributors to racial health disparities. These inequities have persisted for centuries in the United States, although efforts to narrow and one day eliminate these gaps have increased over time. But how can this be accomplished? One of the most effective methods of reducing health disparities is implementing health interventions, particularly those designed to meet the unique needs of the population. Many types of health interventions have been utilized to improve African American health, with varying success. This chapter explores the history of health interventions for African Americans in the United States, modern-day initiatives, and the various types of interventions that have been employed and their effectiveness.

Brief Historical Background on Health Interventions to Address Health of African Americans in the United States

Some of the earliest formal intervention efforts focused on African American populations began at the start of the 20th century. African Americans at that time had significantly poorer health and associated outcomes than their white counterparts (Acevedo-Garcia 2000). Many of these racial health disparities were caused by discriminatory practices such as Jim Crow laws in the southern United States. Also, in the first decades of the First Great Migration, over 1.5 million African Americans moved from the agriculture-based southern United States to the densely populated, indus-trialized North. African American arrivals in the North faced segregation and discriminatory policies that limited the housing and employment that was available to them. As a result, they lived in overcrowded conditions and had access only to the lowest-paying jobs (Acevedo-Garcia 2000; Lee et al. 1957).

From 1900 to 1910, average life expectancy for the nation averaged 49.2 years, but for African Americans, it was only 33.5 years (Bureau of the Census 1975, Series B 107–115). In 1914, Dr. Booker T. Washington of Tuskegee In-stitute observed that 450,000 African Americans were consistently seriously ill and that 45% of all African American deaths were preventable (Peterson 1939). These deaths included those resulting from communicable diseases that African Americans experienced at disproportionately high rates (Allen 1915; King and Kiple 1981; Lerner and Anderson 1963). Tuberculosis is a prime example of the widening health disparities of this time. The number of new tuberculosis infections among African Americans steadily increased from 1910 to 1933 while the number of cases among white individuals de-creased (Boyle 1912; Coleman 1903; Zelner, Muller, and Feigenbaum 2017). In some US cities, the rate of tuberculosis mortality among African Ameri-cans in 1930 was three to five times greater than that of whites (Allen 1915; Roberts 2009). Such disparities were exacerbated by some medical profes-sionals' belief at the time that African Americans were not capable of com-prehending information about disease, infection, and treatment (Bean 1906; Terry 1913). This mentality meant that many doctors were disinclined to attempt even basic educational interventions (Allen 1915; Brunner 1915).

The dire need for improvements in African American health was recog-nized, though, and prompted leaders such as Washington to take action. The most significant of these was the establishment of an annual National Negro Health Week. In 1913, the Negro Organization Society of Virginia declared a Clean-Up Day. On that day, African Americans participated in the general cleaning, maintenance, and repair of their homes, neighborhoods, and com-munity buildings (Peterson 1939). The event was so successful that it was extended to Clean-Up Week in 1914. Through the work of the National Negro Business League and Booker T. Washington, a national event called Health Improvement Week was instituted in April 1915 (Beardsley 1987; Moton 1928; Peterson 1939). The aim of this endeavor was to promote the idea of taking personal action to overcome the lack of access to health care that many African Americans experienced (Braff 2020). The event was widely popular, and after Washington died in November 1915, Dr. Robert Moton, Washington's successor as the principal of Tuskegee Institute, continued it (Braff 2020; Pollitt 1996). Under Moton's direction, the week became National Negro Health Week and established partnerships with agencies that included the US Public Health Service to support the initiative, increasing its credibility and expanding its promotion (Braff 2020). Moton described the initiative as "an annual observance in which local, county, state, and national organizations of both races, as well as the Federal Government, now cooperate. The object, of course, is to improve the health of Negroes and the conditions under which they live, in view of the disproportionately high death rate among Negroes in America" (Moton 1928).

The scope of National Negro Health Week increased steadily over the following years. In 1922, almost 130,000 households in 15 states participated, growing to an estimated two million households in thirty-five states by 1939 (Jones 1923). The success of National Negro Health Week was made possible by community-based organizations throughout the United States and contributions from health care professionals, clergy, social workers, and educators, among others (Braff 2020; Moton 1928; Quinn and Thomas 1996). This success included improvements in both short- and long-term health outcomes. A projected reduction in death rates from 24 per 1,000 in 1913 to 12 per 1,000 in 1963 was attributed in part to the event (Quinn and Thomas 1996). National Negro Health Week is also credited with leading to the development of the National Negro Health Movement, which worked to improve the health of African Americans year round (Walker 2016). The US Public Health Service dissolved National Negro Health Week in 1950 as part of its efforts to integrate health and reduce racial barriers (Braff 2020). Historian David McBride argues that ending National Negro Health Week "meant that those black institutions traditionally most effective in stimulating community health projects throughout the nation's black population were merged into larger, predominately white-controlled organizations" (McBride 1991). Even though smaller interventions and outreach programs developed in the following years, the absence of nationally organized, concerted efforts focused on African American health perpetuated racial health disparities in the United States (Braff 2020; National Negro Health News 1950)

Modern Efforts of Interventions to Address the Health of African Americans

In modern times, a stronger emphasis has been placed on reducing racial health disparities through targeted interventions. The Centers for Disease Control and Prevention (CDC) has been actively assessing health disparities since it published its first *CDC Health Disparities and Inequalities Report* in 2011 (Truman 2011). This report corresponds to the Agency for Healthcare Research and Quality's (2019) *National Quality and Disparities Report*, which offers the latest available findings on the quality of and access to health care and focuses on racial and ethnic disparities and other social determinants of health. The CDC's 2011 report assessed disparities across numerous diseases and evaluated behavioral risk factors, environmental exposures, and social determinants of health, including access to health care (Truman 2011). One of the primary goals of this report was to support efforts to reduce—and ultimately eliminate—health disparities on a national scale. It has been followed by assessments that provide detailed information that sheds light on these gaps and identifies areas of need (CDC 2013). These CDC reports provided analyses of health disparities trends and subsequently brought renewed, much-needed attention to racial health inequities that have persisted in the United States for centuries. The high-profile CDC disparity and inequity reports advance these issues by promoting the idea of taking action to reduce disparities, particularly through effective and scalable intervention efforts. Articles within these reports focus on programs and interventions for specific health issues designed to impact factors that contribute to disparate outcomes (CDC 2013; Truman 2011). Among the most prominent strategies that have been identified for accomplishing these goals is using national leaders to engage a broad spectrum of stakeholders, facilitate coordination between partners, champion the implementation of effective policies and programs, and foster multilevel accountability (Meyer et al. 2013).

The CDC has also sponsored numerous interventions that focus on reducing disparities across a variety of health issues (CDC 2014; Penman-Aguilar, Bouye, and Liburd 2016). One initiative that has had success is the Vaccines for Children program, which was created in 1994. It eliminates the cost of vaccines as a barrier to immunization by providing vaccines at no cost to children who may not otherwise be vaccinated because of inability to pay (CDC 2016). Evaluation studies have found that there have been no racial or ethnic disparities in vaccination for measles, mumps, and rubella and poliovirus in the United States since 2005 and a decline in disparities for diphtheria-tetanus-pertussis and diphtheria-tetanus-acellular pertussis vaccination (Walker, Smith, and Kolasa 2014). Other intervention success stories include the development of community-based programs to prevent the spread of HIV and other sexually transmitted infections such as the Healthy Love intervention that focuses on preventing HIV and sexually transmitted infections among heterosexual Black women (Painter et al. 2014) and the highly effective Many Men, Many Voices HIV/STD prevention intervention designed to reduce risky sexual behaviors and increase protective behaviors among Black men who have sex with men (Herbst et al. 2014). These CDC-led interventions emphasize the importance of multidisciplinary collaboration to effectively decrease health disparities. They also demonstrate the importance of approaching these issues on a community level using strategies such as community-based participatory research to achieve the greatest impact. The CDC's endeavors underscore the significance of using evidence-based programs to improve health equity and reduce disparities (CDC 2014; Penman-Aguilar, Bouye, and Liburd 2016)

The Robert Wood Johnson Foundation is another organization that has emphasized eliminating health inequities. From 2005 to 2014, the foundation sponsored the Finding Answers: Disparities Research for Change program (Wilson 2013). Its objective was to pursue the goal of health equity by maintaining a focused commitment to eliminating health and health care disparities (Chin et al. 2012; Wilson 2013). The program published systematic reviews of interventions for reducing disparities in health outcomes and in the delivery of health care services. It also evaluated innovative projects designed to reduce health care disparities across the United States. Perhaps the most significant outcome of this program is that it established best practices and facilitated the development of a disparities reduction framework and a corresponding multistep process (Chin et al. 2012). The program's summary roadmap report illustrated the need for a dynamic process that uses individual-level interventions but also expects organizations and providers to assume ownership for the work of eliminating disparities. The roadmap also stresses the importance of developing infrastructure and social norms that advance equitable care and integrating targeted disparities interventions in quality improvement practices (Chin et al. 2012).

Types of Health Intervention Studies Used to Address the Health of African Americans

Numerous types of health interventions have been used to address the health of African Americans and reduce disparities. These include interventions focused on lifestyle, behaviors, education and awareness, health communications, mobile health initiatives, and community-based participatory research. Cultural appropriateness is a critical aspect that has defined the success of interventions that focus on African American populations (Kreuter et al. 2004; Kreuter et al. 2005; Jackson et al. 2015). Diverse populations have unique needs, motivations, and barriers that contribute to health disparities that are frequently overlooked. Considerable evidence has demonstrated that a one-size-fits-all approach to intervention is not sufficient to make a meaningful impact on behaviors (Archibald 2011). Instead, targeted interventions that are responsive to the needs of a particular population are far more likely to meet needs, improve health, and reduce disparities (Torres-Ruiz et al. 2018). Cultural norms contribute to health behaviors, including risky behaviors that may lead to chronic disease. Attention to these norms is vital for impacting behavior change (Nierkens et al. 2013; Thomas, Fine, and Ibrahim 2004). This can be accomplished, in part, by designing health messages and strategies that uses a group's cultural identity and cultural beliefs, values, and norms as a foundation for providing relevant context about a health problem or behavior (Kreuter et al. 2005; Resnicow, Braithwaite, and Glanz 2002; Resnicow et al. 1999). Cultural tailoring is considered to be highly effective because it focuses on how a population or group's behavior functions in broader cultural and social contexts (Joseph et al. 2017; Krumeich et al. 2001). Research has demonstrated a dire need for culturally tailored interventions for populations at risk of health disparities and that such efforts should incorporate cultural values, traditions, history, beliefs, and practices (Chin et al. 2007; Pasick, D'onofrio, and Otero-Sabogai 1996). Evidence shows that culturally appropriate interventions lead to increased acceptance that increases the likelihood of significantly impacting health outcomes and reducing disparities (Chin et al. 2012; Nierkens et al. 2013). Aligning with the concept of cultural tailoring, many health interventions focused on African Americans have used effective channels such as working with faith-based organizations (Mayo, Scott, and Williams 2009; Stewart 2016; Walsh-Childers et al. 2018). Other successful strategies have incorporated nontraditional locations for intervention implementation such as beauty salons and barbershops (Linnan and Ferguson 2007; Luque et al. 2011; Smith et al. 2020; Wilson et al. 2008).

One of the most noteworthy intervention types used is comparative effectiveness research (CER). This approach identifies treatments and systems-based approaches to reducing and eliminating disparities and is a mainstay of disparities research at the Patient-Centered Outcomes Research Institute (PCORI) (Selby 2017). Cultural tailoring is a core principle of patient-centered outcomes research. One of PCORI's national priorities is attention to a broad range of disparities. This research focuses on identifying possible differences related to prevention, diagnosis, treatment effectiveness, or preferred clinical outcomes across diverse groups of patients and determining what is needed to achieve the best health outcomes in each population (PCORI 2013). PCORI defines CER as "the direct comparison of two or more existing health care interventions to determine which interventions work best for which patients and which interventions pose the greatest benefits and harms" and notes that the core question of CER is "which treatment works best, for whom, and under what circumstances" (PCORI 2014). CER is different from other types of research because it compares multiple interventions. This method enables CER to validate interventions and identify which treatments are most effective for specific populations (PCORI 2014). PCORI has funded studies that tailor or redesign existing care options to be more effective for a particular underserved population and those that develop new approaches with the population of interest by collaborating with researchers and health systems.

PCORI champions the improvement of African Americans' health by promoting interventions related to a diverse range of conditions that disproportionately impact African Americans (e.g., sickle cell anemia, asthma, high blood pressure) (Anise and Hasnain-Wynia 2016; PCORI 2013). These interventions emphasize tailoring health education tools to the target population. They also provide tools to help participants manage their own care and advocate for themselves and their health (Hasnain-Wynia and Beal 2014). These interventions emphasize the importance of valuing the patient's voice. This is particularly crucial for African Americans, who have been underrepresented and/or mistreated in medical research. This is achieved by making patients and participants part of the process and the solution instead of treating them as test subjects. Patients are considered to be valued stakeholders and take part in planning interventions and implementation (Cukor et al. 2016; Sheridan et al. 2017). Evidence shows that this approach is vital to the success of programs because patient buy-in extends to investment in the endeavor, which stimulates creativity and contributes to community engagement and program sustainability (Forsythe et al. 2018; Forsythe et al. 2019; Hasnain-Wynia and Beal 2014; Selby, Forsythe, and Sox 2015). A consistent goal throughout PCORI's disparities work is producing evidence-based results that enable African Americans to make informed decisions that lead to improved health outcomes and reduced disparities (Selby 2017).

Reception of and Accessibility of Health Interventions in African American Populations

African Americans' participation in public health interventions is essential for reducing the health disparities that disproportionately affect them (Freimuth et al. 2001). Currently, minority participation in clinical research is low. Less than 18% of those participating in clinical research are minorities (Vickers and Fouad 2014). To assess the efficacy and effectiveness of health interventions, it is essential that groups that are traditionally underrepresented in research, including women and minorities, are engaged and invited to participate in public health interventions.

Barriers to Participating in Public Health Research and Interventions

African Americans' participation in public health interventions is influenced by a complex and intricate system of individual-, community-, and system-level barriers (Freimuth et al. 2001). Low participation in research interventions cannot simply be attributed to a lack of interest in research. It is driven by structural barriers related to awareness of health interventions, knowledge of research, environmental barriers, and beliefs about the health care system. These barriers are further complicated by the lingering effects of historical examples of mistreatment in clinical and public health research and current examples of discrimination African Americans experience when they seek medical care. In what follows, we highlight a few of the barriers to participating in research that African Americans experience.

Knowledge and Familiarity with Health Interventions

The research process is often vague to individuals who are unfamiliar with the process of conducting public health interventions. While participation rates in public health interventions are traditionally lower among African Americans, studies have shown that African Americans who are informed and knowledgeable about research are more likely to participate in and complete research studies when they are invited to participate (Taani et al. 2020). A study conducted by Freimuth et al. (2001) recruited sixty African American adults to discuss their opinions about participating in research. Participants were asked about their knowledge of research, research terms and procedures, interest in participating in research, motivation for participating, and the researcher's motivation. The study findings revealed that participants valued research, but many were unfamiliar with issues related to the research process, such as informed consent. This study highlighted the importance of providing additional support and education for individuals who are unfamiliar with public health interventions and individuals who have not participated in research interventions in the past (Taani et al. 2020). Education efforts should focus on explaining informed consent, the roles and responsibilities of researchers and study participants, incentives, and how research findings are disseminated (Freimuth et al. 2001).

Lack of Trust in Providers and Health Care

Medical mistrust is a well-established barrier for recruiting African Americans to participate in public health interventions. Medical mistrust among African Americans is associated with refusing to participate in research interventions, concerns about harmful experiences related to research, fears about being exploited, and losing personal privacy (Boulware et al. 2016; LaVeist, Nickerson, and Bowie 2000). Schaff et al. (2010), who conducted focus groups with seventy African American adults to examine their perceptions and concerns about participating in research, found that mistrust was the participants' primary concern. The participants provided insights into the multifaceted nature of mistrust, citing the Tuskegee Syphilis Study, contemporary examples of mistreatment, and fears that researchers often withhold information about the research.

African Americans may also be less likely to participate in research if they perceive that researchers are not interested in establishing a relationship with communities and only engage with communities to recruit for their studies (Otado et al. 2015; Scharff et al. 2010). Researchers may recruit research participants from the community, conduct their study, and leave without sharing research findings with the community residents or empowering them to incorporate research findings into their daily lives so they can make changes (Dancy et al. 2004). These examples of limited investment in communities contribute to the mistrust of researchers and providers that lingers within the African American community.

Provider and Researcher Beliefs about the Interest of African Americans in Participating in Interventions

Health care providers and researchers may have beliefs about African Americans' interest in participating in interventions that are barriers to participating in interventions (Sabin et al. 2009). Providers and researchers may feel that African Americans are less likely to participate and thus are less likely to invite African Americans to participate in interventions. This reduces African Americans' recruitment into health interventions and contributes to unequal access to public health interventions (Boulware et al. 2016).

Social and Environmental Barriers to Participating in Interventions

Social and environmental factors, such as power differences, discrimination, and social capital, are barriers to African Americans participating in research. In medical encounters, there is a power difference between patients and providers. In these settings, patients may be more reluctant to ask questions or question the actions of health researchers and providers (Blair et al. 2013). Socioeconomic factors such as unequal access to jobs and educational opportunities and segregation due to Jim Crow Laws have all contributed to reduced access to quality health care, unequal treatment when seeking care, and differential care (Scharff et al. 2010). This is particularly detrimental in inner-city neighborhoods and low-income communities.

Overcoming Barriers to Public Health Interventions

Several studies have been done to identify approaches to overcoming the many social, structural, and environmental barriers to African American participation in public health interventions. These studies highlight effective and engaging ways to connect with African Americans that may bolster participation in public health interventions. The proposed approaches have focused on recruitment and retention, engaging community members in the research process, and building a meaningful and mutually beneficial relationship with communities. We will highlight a few strategies to build and sustain relationships with the African American community.

Integrating Community Members into Public Health Interventions

Community partnerships may enhance African American's participation and interest in public health interventions by building relationships based on bidirectional exchange, trust, and transparency. Community-based participatory research approaches have been integrated into interventions for African Americans. These interventions invite the participation of African American community members from the tasks that happen during the early stages of the study, such as identifying public health issues in the community, to the tasks that happen at the end of the study, such as disseminating the study findings (Chen et al. 2010). Community members and community health advisors can also facilitate relationships with community leaders, such as spiritual leaders, community activists, social organizations, and community educators (Parrill and Kennedy 2011). Community leaders may help increase awareness about ongoing interventions and provide connections to potential study participants; they can also be called upon to participate on community advisory boards. Studies have shown that practices such as recruiting community members to serve as members of the study staff and hiring a culturally diverse staff increase the participation in and engagement of African Americans with interventions (Taani et al. 2020)

Knowledge of the Community and Community-Based Resources

Effectively engaging with the African American community requires that researchers and providers become familiar with the community and understand the community's needs. Community members have a wealth of anecdotal and historical knowledge of their community that can help elucidate the root causes of health disparities. Partnering with community members and leaders may also provide insights about community resources that can be leveraged to promote and improve community health outcomes.

Conducting Study Activities in the Community

Conducting outreach activities in the community and placing research activities in convenient locations for community members such as community health centers, churches, social and cultural gatherings, and health fairs has been shown to increase recruitment and retention interventions (Sabin et al. 2009). A systematic review found that African Americans preferred having recruitment and retention activities within the community (George, Duran, and Norris 2014). Reducing structural barriers to participating in research such as providing childcare and transportation and reducing the time required to participate may facilitate the recruitment and retention of African Americans (Frosch et al. 2012).

Culturally Appropriate Recruitment and Retention Activities

Several studies have highlighted the importance of investing time and resources in identifying the most effective approaches for recruiting and retaining African American study participants in communities. A 2015 review of 24 studies that explored barriers to African American and Latino participation in research found that the most effective strategies for recruiting African Americans were word of mouth, engaging community agencies, direct marketing, and direct exposure to participants (Lohr et al. 2018). If incentives are used to recruit and retain participants, the researcher should carefully consider whether the incentive is appropriate and whether it reflects the participant's effort and covers any out-of-pocket expenses. However, an incentive should not be so high that it could be perceived as coercive.

Applying community-based participatory research approaches, building and sustaining relationships with communities, and developing interventions that are responsive to the needs of those communities is an effective approach for improving access to, engagement with, and participation in health interventions.

Dissemination and Implementation: Next Steps and Future Directions

A key part of health interventions such as those described above is program evaluation. Evaluation is essential for analyzing a program or intervention to assess whether it has achieved its goals. Evaluations are used to refine and improve program strategies, address concerns and suggest future improvements, assess long-term impacts, show value to stakeholders and funders, seek continued support, and to compile information for dissemination (Rural Health Information Hub 2017). Sharing successful strategies is important for increasing their impact and improving health outcomes on a broader scale. This is the central tenet of dissemination and implementation science, an emerging field of study that explores how scientific evidence and evidence-based strategies are adopted, implemented, and maintained in real-world community and/or clinical settings (Estabrooks, Brownson, and Pronk 2018a). This area of research is critical for advancing public health progress by improving evidence-based interventions and for providing access to interventions to populations that often do not have access to them (Tabak et al. 2017). Previous studies have indicated that approximately 1–5% of the US population has access to health interventions (Clark et al. 2019). This is particularly important for populations such as African Americans that are less likely to have efficacious behavioral and lifestyle interventions delivered to them. Dissemination and implementation studies are guided by over 159 theories, models, and frameworks that are used to inform planning/ design, evaluation, and implementation activities and are used to inform dissemination and sustainability (Strifler et al. 2018). The framework, models and theories include the Consolidated Framework for Implementation Research (CFIR), the PRECEDE-PROCEDE model, the Pragmatic-Explanatory Continuum Indicatory Summary (PRECIS), and the Reach, Effectiveness, Adoption, Implementation, and Maintenance model (RE-AIM).

Interest in dissemination and implementation research has increased over the past 25 years, as has interest in evaluating interventions for African Americans to determine the most effective approaches and to develop plans for disseminating the interventions. Interventions for African Americans have been conducted in barbershops and beauty salons and at health centers and safety-net hospitals. Some interventions have used web-based approaches. However, one of the most effective approaches is faith-based interventions that build on relationships with churches in the African American community. Two examples of faith-based dissemination and implementation interventions are the Project HEAL intervention and the Faith, Activity, and Nutrition (FAN) interventions.

Health through Early Awareness and Learning (Project HEAL)

Project HEAL was a community-based, randomized implementation trial for African American community health advisors in Prince George's County, Maryland (Santos et al. 2017). The project, which was originally developed using three separate trials for breast, prostate, and colorectal cancer, combined all three interventions into one. Project HEAL compared didactic methods to a web-based system for training peer community health advisors. The intervention was guided using the RE-AIM Framework for assessing adoption, reach, and implementation. Adoption was assessed at the church level; 41% of all invited churches participated. The reach of the intervention was examined at the participant level; approximately one-third of eligible people at the churches participated. While the adoption and reach rates were lower than similar faith-based interventions, the researchers believe that the study findings bridge the gap between efficacy and effectiveness. The findings of Project HEAL indicated the intervention is feasible and has strong potential for implementation.

Faith, Activity, and Nutrition (FAN) Dissemination and Implementation Study

The FAN Dissemination and Implementation Study was a group randomized study that targeted churches in rural South Carolina (Wilcox et al. 2018). The FAN study had already proven to be an effective approach for increasing fruit and vegetable intake and physical activity at churches. Some churches received a FAN intervention from the start of the study and a control group of churches received an intervention at a later point. The study, which was guided by the RE-AIM framework, sought to assess participants' intake of fruits and vegetables and their levels of physical activity. The study had high adoption (42%).

Dissemination and implementation research provides opportunities for interventions to become the standard of care and to ensure that the knowledge gained from these interventions is provided to communities and populations in need. Dissemination and implementation studies help reduce barriers to interventions, assess the feasibility and sustainability of interventions, provide insights about the acceptability of the interventions, and provide useful information about their cost effectiveness. Dissemination and implementation studies may help improve health equity and health outcomes and will provide information about the efficacy, effectiveness, and impact of health disparities among African Americans. Future directions for dissemination and implementation might expand on the existing methodologies and develop and apply novel approaches for evaluating intervention effectiveness (Green and Nasser 2017). The findings of dissemination and implementation studies provide insights about the needs of the community, including the value of community partners, the needs of intervention adoptees, the potential burden of interventions, and methods/means of making future interventions more effective, engaging, and sustainable. Study findings must be widely disseminated and available to researchers as they consider adapting interventions for their community of interest. Lastly, future dissemination and implementation studies should focus on which elements are essential for reducing health disparities and promoting health equity, such as conducting community assessments and fostering and building collaborative relationships with communities (Estabrooks, Brownson, and Pronk 2018b).

Case Studies

Community Trial of a Faith-Based Lifestyle Intervention to Prevent Diabetes among African Americans

Approximately 50% of African American adults 20 years or older are obese, putting them at an increased risk for type 2 diabetes mellitus. Lifestyle modifications such as weight loss, increasing physical activity, and modifying diet may help reduce the risk of type 2 diabetes. Lifestyle and behavioral interventions are used to promote healthful behaviors and reduce the risk for type 2 diabetes in the African American community. However, few of these studies have been available in community-based settings.

STUDY OVERVIEW

The goal of this twelve-week, community-based feasibility study was to use a faith-based adaptation of the diabetes prevention program named Fit Body and Soul to lower fasting plasma glucose levels, reduce weight, and increase physical activity among African Americans. Investigators conducted a two-armed cluster randomized trial in churches. Fit Body and Soul, the intervention arm of the study, was a faith-based adaptation of the diabetes prevention intervention. The comparison arm focused on health education and covered topics from the CDC Guide to Community Prevention Services. The research team recruited 20 churches in the Georgia metropolitan area to participate in this study and included churches in urban and rural settings. The churches were stratified by membership size and then randomized into groups. The research team engaged pastors, medical professionals, and other community leaders. The team also assembled an advisory group that provided input for all aspects of the study. It provided suggestions such as scriptures, images of African Americans, and quotes from famous African Americans. The study started in September 2009 with the training of community health advisors at a local church and the recruitment of participants. Baseline data for the study was collected from October 2009 through March 2013.

OVERVIEW OF FINDINGS

Forty participants were enrolled in the study. Eighty-seven percent (n = 35) completed data collection and at least ten sessions. Among the thirty-five participants, 48% experienced a weight loss of at least 5% of baseline weight, 26% of participants lost 7% or more of their baseline weight, and 14% lost more than 10% of baseline weight. The twelve-week program led to a greater reduction in weight in the intervention group than the health education group. Weight loss was modified by the number of sessions attended; those who attended ten or more sessions lost an average of 3.7 kilograms.

STUDY CONCLUSIONS

The study findings indicated that incorporating the diabetes prevention program into a faith-based setting was a feasible and potentially useful approach for addressing type 2 diabetes mellitus among African Americans.

VALUE/CONTRIBUTION OF STUDY AS A TOOL TO ADDRESS HEALTH OF AFRICAN AMERICANS

The study findings highlight the importance of collaborating with African American churches. Church settings may be ideal for reaching and recruiting African Americans and addressing the community's health needs. The effectiveness of church-based intervention may be increased by the support of African American churches that have ministries and committees that are focused on health and wellness.

Mindfulness in Motion and Dietary Approaches to Stop
Hypertension (DASH) in Hypertensive African Americans

African Americans are at greater risk of experiencing late-life cognitive decline than whites. African Americans also report higher rates of essential hypertension. To date, few interventions have addressed both cognitive decline and hypertension. Mindfulness has demonstrated positive
effects in reducing stress, depressive symptoms, and blood pressure among
African Americans. This pilot study examined the feasibility and acceptability of combining a mindfulness intervention (Mindfulness in Motion) with
the Dietary Approaches to Stop Hypertension (DASH) program. The goal
of the study was to improve diet, reduce stress, and lower systolic blood
pressure for African Americans living with mild cognitive impairment and
hypertension.

STUDY OVERVIEW

The study participants were older African Americans living in a midwestern urban setting. The study was designed as a cluster randomized control trial. Participants were divided into six or seven groups and the groups
were randomized into one of three arms: Mindfulness in Motion DASH
(n = 2), attention only (n = 2), and true control (n = 2). The Mindfulness
in Motion DASH group consisted of eight weekly sessions that lasted two
hours. Sessions covered educational information about stress, mindfulness,
the mind-body connection and information about the DASH program to encourage diet modification. Participants in the Mindfulness in Motion DASH
group received a compact disc player with mindfulness recordings and activities for practicing meditation. The attention-only group met for eight weeks
for two-hour sessions that covered fire prevention and personal safety topics.
The true control group received no information between baseline and study
measurements and were given DASH pamphlets at the end of the study.

OVERVIEW OF FINDINGS

The majority of the study participants were women (82%), and the
majority were college educated. Participants in the Mindfulness in Motion
DASH group reported they learned new skills, enjoyed the intervention, and
thought the intervention would help others. There was a clinically significant
reduction in systolic blood pressure in the Mindfulness in Motion DASH

group compared to the attention-only group (17.2 mmHg vs. –0.7mmHg). The change in diastolic blood pressure was not statistically significant.

STUDY CONCLUSIONS

The study findings support that the Mindfulness in Motion DASH intervention was a feasible and acceptable approach for engaging African Americans and contributed to a clinically meaningful decrease in systolic blood pressure. The Mindfulness in Motion DASH intervention did not improve mindfulness, perception of stress, or diet.

VALUE/CONTRIBUTION OF STUDY AS A TOOL FOR
ADDRESSING THE HEALTH OF AFRICAN AMERICANS

The Mindfulness in Motion DASH pilot study was one of the first studies to combine mindfulness and the DASH diet to address health issues among older African Americans with cognitive decline and hypertension. The findings suggest that the Mindfulness in Motion DASH intervention may be an effective approach for reducing systolic blood pressure among African Americans.

Targeting Cancer in Blacks

African Americans face many barriers to receiving cancer screening, including social factors such as skepticism, lack of access, and lack of knowledge about cancer screenings. Many interventions have been developed to provide education about cancer screenings and prevention. It has been hypothesized that culturally sensitive programs that the Black community supports may be the most effective approach for changing knowledge, attitudes, and behaviors related to cancer.

STUDY OVERVIEW

Targeting Cancer in Blacks was a community-based intervention focused on cancer prevention. It promoted the adoption of healthy behaviors that may reduce the risk of cancer among African Americans. The intervention was conducted from 1994 to 1996 in Nashville, Tennessee; Atlanta, Georgia; Chattanooga, Tennessee; and Decatur, Georgia. Participants were African Americans over 18 years old. The multicomponent intervention included educational sessions on cancer risk factors in the community, lectures, presentations on cancer prevention, workshops, and a media campaign. Targeting Cancer in Blacks activities also included a kickoff event to distribute information about the initiative and gain the support of community members who would eventually serve as a steering committee members. Over 100 people attended the kickoff event at each site. At baseline, the sample consisted of 1,461 participants in Atlanta, 1,754 in Decatur, 1,482 in Nashville, and 1,478 in Chattanooga. At follow-up, the survey sample consisted of 1,565 participants in Atlanta, 1,606 in Decatur, 1,561 in Nashville, and 1,537 in Chattanooga.

OVERVIEW OF FINDINGS

The final study sample was 57.6% women in Atlanta with an average age of 41.5, 55.1% women in Decatur with an average age of 39.6, 58.6% women in Nashville with an average age of 42.4, and 59.7% women in Chattanooga with an average age of 44.0. There was a change in knowledge or beliefs about cancer from the preintervention to the postintervention period. The number of participants who consumed more than five servings of fruits and vegetables did not change between preintervention and postintervention. At the Chattanooga site, there was an increase in the percentage of individuals who exercised. There was a statistically significant increase in the number of participants who quit smoking cigarettes at the Decatur site. There was also an increase in the percentage of women in Nashville who had had a Pap test in the previous two years compared to the Chattanooga participants.

VALUE/CONTRIBUTION OF STUDY AS A TOOL FOR
ADDRESSING THE HEALTH OF AFRICAN AMERICANS

The study highlighted the need for longer-term interventions that may be more effective in improving health outcomes and reducing health disparities in the African American community if they are conducted over multiple years.

Testing a Program for Increasing Healthy Behaviors among Black Men

Black men in the United States are more likely to experience chronic health conditions such as diabetes and high blood pressure. The risk of developing a chronic condition can be reduced by increasing access to and promoting a diet of fruits and vegetables and increasing exercise. This study aimed to determine if a lifestyle program, Active and Healthy Brotherhood, would help increase daily exercise among Black men.

STUDY OVERVIEW

The primary objectives of the study were to compare the immediate postintervention effects (six months after randomization) of the Active and Healthy Brotherhood intervention with the control condition on lifestyle behaviors (e.g., physical activity, diet, stress management), health-related outcomes (e.g., blood glucose, hemoglobin A1c [HbA1c] levels, blood pressure), and help-seeking behaviors (e.g., medication adherence) among Black men. The secondary objective was to compare the immediate postintervention effects of the Active and Healthy Brotherhood intervention with the control condition on mediators of behavior change (e.g., social support, motivation, self-efficacy). The final aim was to compare the longer-term effects (twelve months after randomization) of the Active and Healthy Brotherhood intervention with the control condition. Participants were randomly assigned to the Active and Healthy Brotherhood group or the control group (which received education only). Black men were recruited to be a part of the research team and to help design the program. The sessions included a 16-week health education program. The education group received basic health education sessions and information about behaviors that would improve health outcomes. Participants were instructed to wear fitness trackers to measure activity levels and to complete assessments at follow-ups at six and twelve months.

OVERVIEW OF FINDINGS

The study sample included 333 Black men from North Carolina with an average age of 51. Of the 333 participants, 211 completed the six-month follow-up and 218 completed the twelve-month follow-up. At six and twelve months, there were no differences between the Active and Healthy Brotherhood and education groups in terms of physical activity. At six months, participants in the Active and Healthy Brotherhood group showed greater reductions in blood pressure, glucose levels, and HbA1c levels.

VALUE/CONTRIBUTION OF STUDY AS A TOOL FOR ADDRESSING THE HEALTH OF AFRICAN AMERICANS

While the intervention did not improve physical activity levels among Black men, there were important changes among the Active and Healthy

Brotherhood group. Men in this group walked more steps per day and had better nutrition-related outcomes. This study provides valuable insights into managing chronic conditions among Black men and highlights the importance of engaging Black men as study participants and as a part of the research team for interventions.

REFERENCES

Acevedo-Garcia, D. 2000. "Residential Segregation and the Epidemiology of Infectious Diseases." *Soc Sci Med* 51 (8): 1143–1161. https://doi.org/10.1016/s0277-9536(00)00016-2.

Agency for Healthcare Research and Quality. 2019. *2018 National Healthcare Quality and Disparities Report*. Rockville, MD: Agency for Healthcare Research and Quality.

Allen, L. C. 1915. "The Negro Health Problem." *Am J Public Health* 5 (3): 194–203. https://doi.org/10.2105/ajph.5.3.194.

Anise, A., and R. Hasnain-Wynia. 2016. "Patient-Centered Outcomes Research to Improve Asthma Outcomes." *J Allergy Clin Immunol* 138 (6): 1503–1510. https://doi.org/10.1016/j.jaci.2016.10.003.

Archibald, C. 2011. "Cultural Tailoring for an Afro-Caribbean Community: A Naturalistic Approach." *J Cult Divers* 18 (4): 114–119.

Bean, R. B. 1906. "Some Racial Peculiarities of the Negro Brain." *Am J Anat* 5: 353–432.

Beardsley, E. H. 1987. *A History of Neglect: Health Care for Blacks and Mill Workers in the Twentieth-Century South*. Knoxville: University of Tennessee Press.

Blair, Irene V., Edward P. Havranek, David W. Price, Rebecca Hanratty, Diane L. Fairclough, Tillman Farley, Holen K. Hirsh, and John F. Steiner. 2013. "Assessment of Biases against Latinos and African Americans among Primary Care Providers and Community Members." *Am J Public Health* 103 (1): 92–98.

Boulware, L. Ebony, Lisa A. Cooper, Lloyd E. Ratner, Thomas A. LaVeist, and Neil R. Powe. 2016. "Race and Trust in the Health Care System." *Public Health Rep* 118 (4): 358–365.

Boyle, E. M. 1912. "The Negro and Tuberculosis." *J Natl Med Assoc* 4 (4): 344–348.

Braff, P. 2020. "Moving from the National Negro Health Week to the National Public Health Week in the United States." *Am J Public Health* 110 (4): 470–477.

Brunner, W. F. 1915. "The Negro Health Problem in Southern Cities." *Am J Public Health* 5 (3): 183–190. https://doi.org/10.2105/ajph.5.3.183-a.

Bureau of the Census. 1975. *Historical Statistics of the United States: Colonial Times to 1970*. Washington, DC: US Department of Commerce.

CDC. 2013. "CDC Health Disparities and Inequalities Report—United States, 2013." *MMWR Morb Mortal Wkly Rep* 63 (suppl. 3): 1–186.

———. 2014. "Strategies for Reducing Health Disparities—Selected CDC-Sponsored Interventions, United States, 2014." *MMWR Morb Mortal Wkly Rep* 63 (suppl. 1): 1–48.

———. 2016. "Vaccines for Children Program (VFC)." Last modified February 18, 2016. Accessed November 16, 2020. https://www.cdc.gov/vaccines/programs/vfc/index.html.

Chen, Peggy G, Nitza Diaz, Georgina Lucas, and Marjorie S Rosenthal. 2010. "Dissemination of Results in Community-Based Participatory Research." *Am J Prev Med* 39 (4): 372–378.

Chin, M. H., A. R. Clarke, R. S. Nocon, A. A. Casey, A. P. Goddu, N. M. Keesecker, and S. C. Cook. 2012. "A Roadmap and Best Practices for Organizations to Reduce Racial and Ethnic Disparities in Health Care." *J Gen Intern Med* 27 (8): 992–1000. https://doi.org /10.1007/s11606-012-2082-9.

Chin, M. H., A. E. Walters, S. C. Cook, and E. S. Huang. 2007. "Interventions to Reduce Racial and Ethnic Disparities in Health Care." *Med Care Res Rev* 64 (suppl. 5): 7S–28S. https://doi.org/10.1177/1077558707305413.

Clark, Luther T., Laurence Watkins, Ileana L. Piña, Mary Elmer, Ola Akinboboye, Millicent Gorham, Brenda Jamerson, Cassandra McCullough, Christine Pierre, and Adam B. Polis. 2019. "Increasing Diversity in Clinical Trials: Overcoming Critical Barriers." *Curr Prob Cardiology* 44 (5): 148–172.

Coleman, T. D. 1903. "The Susceptibility of the Negro to Tuberculosis." *Trans Am Climatol Assoc* 19: 122–32.

Cukor, D., L. M. Cohen, E. L. Cope, N. Ghahramani, S. S. Hedayati, D. M. Hynes, V. O. Shah, F. Tentori, M. Unruh, et al. 2016. "Patient and Other Stakeholder Engagement in Patient-Centered Outcomes Research Institute Funded Studies of Patients with Kidney Diseases." *Clin J Am Soc Nephrol* 11 (9): 1703–12.

Dancy, Barbara L., JoEllen Wilbur, Marie Talashek, Gloria Bonner, and Cynthia Barnes-Boyd. 2004. "Community-Based Research: Barriers to Recruitment of African Americans." *Nurs Outlook* 52 (5): 234–240.

Estabrooks, P. A., R. C. Brownson, and N. P. Pronk. 2018a. "Dissemination and Implementation Science for Public Health Professionals: An Overview and Call to Action." *Prev Chronic Dis* 15: E162. https://doi.org/10.5888/pcd15.180525.

———. 2018b. "Dissemination and Implementation Science for Public Health Professionals: An Overview and Call to Action." *Prev Chronic Dis* 15: E162.

Forsythe, L., A. Heckert, M. K. Margolis, S. Schrandt, and L. Frank. 2018. "Methods and Impact of Engagement in Research, from Theory to Practice and Back Again: Early Findings from the Patient-Centered Outcomes Research Institute." *Qual Life Res* 27 (1): 17–31. https://doi.org/10.1007/s11136-017-1581-x.

Forsythe, L. P., K. L. Carman, V. Szydlowski, L. Fayish, L. Davidson, D. H. Hickam, C. Hall, G. Bhat, D. Neu, et al. 2019. "Patient Engagement in Research: Early Findings from the Patient-Centered Outcomes Research Institute." *Health Affairs* 38 (3): 359–367. https:// www.healthaffairs.org/doi/10.1377/hlthaff.2018.05067.

Freimuth, Vicki S., Sandra Crouse Quinn, Stephen B. Thomas, Galen Cole, Eric Zook, and Ted Duncan. 2001. "African Americans' Views on Research and the Tuskegee Syphilis Study." *Soc Sci Med* 52 (5): 797–808.

Frosch, Dominick L., Suepattra G. May, Katharine A. S. Rendle, Caroline Tietbohl, and Glyn Elwyn. 2012. "Authoritarian Physicians and Patients' Fear of Being Labeled 'Difficult' among Key Obstacles to Shared Decision Making." *Health Affairs* 31 (5): 1030–1038.

George, Sheba, Nelida Duran, and Keith Norris. 2014. "A Systematic Review of Barriers and Facilitators to Minority Research Participation among African Americans, Latinos, Asian Americans, and Pacific Islanders." *Am J Pub Health* 104 (2): e16–e31.

Green, Lawrence W., and Mona Nasser. 2017. "Furthering Dissemination and Implementation Research." In *Dissemination and Implementation Research in Health: Translating Science to Practice*, ed. Ross C. Brownson, Graham A. Colditz, and Enola K. Proctor, 305–326. Oxford: Oxford University Press.

Hasnain-Wynia, R., and A. C. Beal. 2014. "Role of the Patient-Centered Outcomes Research Institute in Addressing Disparities and Engaging Patients in Clinical Research." *Clin Ther* 36 (5): 619–623. https://doi.org/10.1016/j.clinthera.2014.04.005.

Herbst, J. H., T. M. Painter, H. L. Tomlinson, and M. E. Alvarez. 2014. "Evidence-Based HIV/ STD Prevention Intervention for Black Men Who Have Sex with Men." *MMWR Suppl* 63 (1): 21–27.

Jackson, D. D., O. L. Owens, D. B. Friedman, and R. Dubose-Morris. 2015. "Innovative and Community-Guided Evaluation and Dissemination of a Prostate Cancer Education Program for African-American Men and Women." *J Cancer Educ* 30 (4): 779–85. https://doi .org/10.1007/s13187-014-0774-z.

Jones, E. K. 1923. "The Negroes' Struggle for Health." *Opportunity* (June): 6–7.

Joseph, R. P., C. Keller, O. Affuso, and B. E. Ainsworth. 2017. "Designing Culturally Relevant Physical Activity Programs for African-American Women: A Framework for Intervention Development." *J Racial Ethn Health Disparities* 4 (3): 397–409. https://doi.org/10 .1007/s40615-016-0240-1.

King, V. F., and K. F. Kiple. 1981. *Another Dimension to the Black Diaspora*. Cambridge: Cambridge University Press.

Kreuter, M. W., C. Sugg-Skinner, C. L. Holt, E. M. Clark, D. Haire-Joshu, Q. Fu, A. C. Booker, K. Steger-May, and D. Bucholtz. 2005. "Cultural Tailoring for Mammography and Fruit and Vegetable Intake among Low-Income African-American Women in Urban Public Health Centers." *Prev Med* 41 (1): 53–62. https://doi.org/10.1016/j.ypmed.2004 .10.013.

Kreuter, M. W., C. S. Skinner, K. Steger-May, C. L. Holt, D. C. Bucholtz, E. M. Clark, and D. Haire-Joshu. 2004. "Responses to Behaviorally vs Culturally Tailored Cancer Communication among African American Women." *Am J Health Behav* 28 (3): 195–207. https:// doi.org/10.5993/ajhb.28.3.1.

Krumeich, A., W. Weijts, P. Reddy, and A. Meijer-Weitz. 2001. "The Benefits of Anthropological Approaches for Health Promotion Research and Practice." *Health Educ Res* 16 (2): 121–30. https://doi.org/10.1093/her/16.2.121.

LaVeist, Thomas A., Kim J. Nickerson, and Janice V. Bowie. 2000. "Attitudes about Racism, Medical Mistrust, and Satisfaction with Care among African American and White Cardiac Patients." *Med Care Res Rev* 57 (suppl. 1): 146–161.

Lee, R. E., S. Everett, A. R. Miller, and C. Brainerd. 1957. *Population Redistribution and Economic Growth, United States, 1870–1950*. Vol. 1, *Methodological Considerations and Reference Tables*. Philadelphia: American Philosophical Society.

Lerner, M., and O. Anderson. 1963. *Health Progress in the United States 1890–1960*. Chicago: University of Chicago Press.

Linnan, L. A., and Y. O. Ferguson. 2007. "Beauty Salons: A Promising Health Promotion Setting for Reaching and Promoting Health among African American Women." *Health Educ Behav* 34 (3): 517–530.

Lohr, Abby M., Maia Ingram, Annabelle V. Nuñez, Kerstin M. Reinschmidt, and Scott C. Carvajal. 2018. "Community-Clinical Linkages with Community Health Workers in the United States: A Scoping Review." *Health Promot Pract* 19 (3): 349–360.

Luque, J. S., B. M. Rivers, C. K. Gwede, M. Kambon, B. L. Green, and C. D. Meade. 2011. "Barbershop Communications on Prostate Cancer Screening Using Barber Health Advisers." *Am J Mens Health* 5 (2): 129–139. https://doi.org/10.1177/1557988310365167.

Mayo, R., D. B. Scott, and D. G. Williams. 2009. "The Upstate Witness Project: Addressing Breast and Cervical Cancer Disparities in African American Churches." *J S C Med Assoc* 105 (7): 290–296.

McBride, D. 1991. *From TB to AIDS: Epidemics among Urban Blacks since 1900.* Albany: State University of New York Press.

Meyer, P. A., A. Penman-Aguilar, V. A. Campbell, C. Graffunder, A. E. O'Connor, and P. W. Yoon. 2013. "Conclusion and Future Directions: CDC Health Disparities and Inequalities Report—United States, 2013." *MMWR Suppl* 62 (3): 184–186.

Moton, R. R. 1928. "Organized Negro Effort for Racial Progress." *Ann Am Acad Polit SS* 140: 257–263.

National Negro Health News. 1950. "Special Notice." *National Negro Health News* 18 (2): 1.

Nierkens, V., M. A. Hartman, M. Nicolaou, C. Vissenberg, E. J. Beune, K. Hosper, I. G. van Valkengoed, and K. Stronks. 2013. "Effectiveness of Cultural Adaptations of Interventions Aimed at Smoking Cessation, Diet, and/or Physical Activity in Ethnic Minorities: A Systematic Review." *PLOS ONE* 8 (10): e73373. https://doi.org/10.1371/journal.pone.0073373.

Otado, Jane, John Kwagyan, Diana Edwards, Alice Ukaegbu, Faun Rockcliffe, and Nana Osafo. 2015. "Culturally Competent Strategies for Recruitment and Retention of African American Populations into Clinical Trials." *Clin Transl Sci* 8 (5): 460–466.

Painter, T. M., J. H. Herbst, D. D. Diallo, and L. D. White. 2014. "Community-Based Program to Prevent HIV/STD Infection among Heterosexual Black Women." *MMWR Suppl* 63 (1): 15–20.

Parrill, Rachel, and Bernice Roberts Kennedy. 2011. "Partnerships for Health in the African American Community: Moving toward Community-Based Participatory Research." *J Cult Divers* 18 (4): 150–154.

Pasick, R. J., C. N. D'onofrio, and R. Otero-Sabogai. 1996. "Similarities and Differences across Cultures: Questions to Inform a Third Generation for Health Promotion Research." *Health Educ Quart* 23: 142–161.

PCORI. 2013. "National Priorities and Research Agenda." Patient-Centered Outcomes Research Institute. Last modified August 21, 2014. Accessed November 21, 2020. https://www.pcori.org/research-results/about-our-research/research-we-support/national-priorities-and-research-agenda.

———. 2014. "Research We Support." Patient-Centered Outcomes Research Institute. Last modified July 25, 2018. Accessed August 13, 2020. https://www.pcori.org/research-results/about-our-research/research-we-support#content-3697.

Penman-Aguilar, A., K. Bouye, and L. Liburd. 2016. "Strategies for Reducing Health Disparities—Selected CDC-Sponsored Interventions, United States, 2016." *MMWR Morb Mortal Wkly Rep* 65 (suppl. 1): 1–69.

Peterson, F. D. 1939. "Statement Concerning National Negro Health Week." *National Negro Health News* 7 (2): 13.

Pollitt, P. A. 1996. "From National Negro Health Week to National Public Health Week." *J Commun Health* 21 (6): 401–407. https://doi.org/10.1007/bf01702601.

Quinn, S. C., and S. B. Thomas. 1996. "The National Negro Health Week, 1915 to 1951: A Descriptive Account." *J Wellness Perspect* 12 (4): 172–179.

Resnicow, K., T. Baranowski, J. S. Ahluwalia, and R. L. Braithwaite. 1999. "Cultural Sensitivity in Public Health: Defined and Demystified." *Ethn Dis* 9 (1): 10–21.

Resnicow, K., R. L. Braithwaite, and K. Glanz, eds. 2002. *Health Behavior and Health Education: Theory, Research, and Practice*. San Francisco: Jossey-Bass.

Roberts, S. K. 2009. *Infectious Fear: Politics, Disease, and the Health Effects of Segregation*. Chapel Hill: University of North Carolina Press.

Rural Health Information Hub. 2017. "Importance of Evaluation." Rural Health Information Hub. Last modified September 14, 2017. Accessed December 12, 2020. https://www.ruralhealthinfo.org/toolkits/rural-toolkit/4/evaluation-importance.

Sabin, J., B. A. Nosek, A. Greenwald, and F. P. Rivara. 2009. "Physicians' Implicit and Explicit Attitudes about Race by MD Race, Ethnicity, and Gender." *J Health Care Poor U* 20 (3): 896–913. https://www.ncbi.nlm.nih.gov/pmc/articles/PMC3320738/.

Santos, Sherie Lou Zara, Erin K. Tagai, Mary Ann Scheirer, Janice Bowie, Muhiuddin Haider, Jimmie Slade, Min Qi Wang, and Cheryl L. Holt. 2017. "Adoption, Reach, and Implementation of a Cancer Education Intervention in African American Churches." *Implement Sci* 12 (1): 36.

Scharff, Darcell P., Katherine J. Mathews, Pamela Jackson, Jonathan Hoffsuemmer, Emeobong Martin, and Dorothy Edwards. 2010. "More than Tuskegee: Understanding Mistrust about Research Participation." *J Health Care Poor U* 21 (3): 879–897.

Selby, J. V. 2017. "Improving the Health of African Americans." Patient-Centered Outcomes Research Institute. Last modified February 17, 2017. Accessed August 13, 2020. https://www.pcori.org/blog/improving-health-african-americans.

Selby, J. V., L. Forsythe, and H. C. Sox. 2015. "Stakeholder-Driven Comparative Effectiveness Research: An Update From PCORI." *JAMA* 314 (21): 2235–2236. https://doi.org/10.1001/jama.2015.15139.

Sheridan, S., S. Schrandt, L. Forsythe, T. S. Hilliard, and K. A. Paez. 2017. "The PCORI Engagement Rubric: Promising Practices for Partnering in Research." *Ann Fam Med* 15 (2): 165–170. https://doi.org/10.1370/afm.2042.

Smith, C., A. Porter III, J. Biddle, A. Balamurugan, and M. R. Smith. 2020. "The Arkansas Minority Barber and Beauty Shop Health Initiative: Meeting People Where They Are." *Prev Chronic Dis* 17: E153. https://doi.org/10.5888/pcd17.200277.

Stewart, J. M. 2016. "Faith-Based Interventions: Pathways to Health Promotion." *West J Nurs Res* 38 (7): 787–789. https://doi.org/10.1177/0193945916643957.

Strifler, Lisa, Roberta Cardoso, Jessie McGowan, Elise Cogo, Vera Nincic, Paul A. Khan, Alistair Scott, Marco Ghassemi, Heather MacDonald, et al. 2018. "Scoping Review Identifies Significant Number of Knowledge Translation Theories, Models, and Frameworks with Limited Use." *J Clin Epidemiol* 100 (August): 92–102.

Taani, Murad H., Bev Zabler, Michael Fendrich, and Rachel Schiffman. 2020. "Lessons

Learned for Recruitment and Retention of Low-Income African Americans." *Contemp Clin Trials Comm* 17: 100533.

Tabak, Rachel G., Margaret M. Padek, Jon F. Kerner, Kurt C. Stange, Enola K. Proctor, Maureen J. Dobbins, Graham A. Colditz, David A. Chambers, and Ross C. Brownson. 2017. "Dissemination and Implementation Science Training Needs: Insights from Practitioners and Researchers." *Am J Prev Med* 52 (3): S322–S329.

Terry, C. E. 1913. "The Negro: His Relation to Public Health in the South." *Am J Public Health* 3 (4): 300–306.

Thomas, S. B., M. J. Fine, and S. A. Ibrahim. 2004. "Health Disparities: The Importance of Culture and Health Communication." *Am J Public Health* 94 (12): 2050.

Torres-Ruiz, M., K. Robinson-Ector, D. Attinson, J. Trotter, A. Anise, and S. Clauser. 2018. "A Portfolio Analysis of Culturally Tailored Trials to Address Health and Healthcare Disparities." *Int J Environ Res Public Health* 15 (9): 1859.

Truman, B. 2011. "CDC Health Disparities and Inequalities Report—United States, 2011." *MMWR Morb Mortal Wkly Rep* 60 (suppl. 1): 1–113.

Vickers, Selwyn M., and Mona N. Fouad. 2014. "An Overview of EMPaCT and Fundamental Issues Affecting Minority Participation in Cancer Clinical Trials: Enhancing Minority Participation in Clinical Trials (EMPaCT): Laying the Groundwork for Improving Minority Clinical Trial Accrual." *Cancer* 120: 1087–1090.

Walker, A. T., P. J. Smith, and M. Kolasa. 2014. "Reduction of Racial/Ethnic Disparities in Vaccination Coverage, 1995–2011." *MMWR Suppl* 63 (1): 7–12.

Walker, T. 2016. "'National Negro Health Week': 1915 to 1951." National Archives: Rediscovering Black History, March 29, 2016. https://rediscovering-black-history.blogs.archives.gov/2016/03/29/national-negro-health-week-1915-to-1951/.

Walsh-Childers, K., F. Odedina, A. Poitier, E. Kaninjing, and G. Taylor 3rd. 2018. "Choosing Channels, Sources, and Content for Communicating Prostate Cancer Information to Black Men: A Systematic Review of the Literature." *Am J Mens Health* 12 (5): 1728–1745.

Wilcox, Sara, Ruth P. Saunders, Andrew T. Kaczynski, Melinda Forthofer, Patricia A. Sharpe, Cheryl Goodwin, Margaret Condrasky, Vernon L. Kennedy Sr., Danielle E. Jake-Schoffman, et al. 2018. "Faith, Activity, and Nutrition Randomized Dissemination and Implementation Study: Countywide Adoption, Reach, and Effectiveness." *Am J Prev Med* 54 (6): 776–785.

Wilson, L. 2013. "Finding Answers: Disparities Research for Change." Robert Wood Johnson Foundation. Accessed September 2, 2020. https://www.rwjf.org/en/library/research/2013/10/finding-answers—disparities-research-for-change.html.

Wilson, T. E., M. Fraser-White, J. Feldman, P. Homel, S. Wright, G. King, B. Coll, S. Banks, D. Davis-King, et al. 2008. "Hair Salon Stylists as Breast Cancer Prevention Lay Health Advisors for African American and Afro-Caribbean women." *J Health Care Poor U* 19 (1): 216–226. https://doi.org/10.1353/hpu.2008.0017.

Zelner, J. L., C. Muller, and J. J. Feigenbaum. 2017. "Racial Inequality in the Annual Risk of Tuberculosis Infection in the United States, 1910–1933." *Epidemiol Infect* 145 (9): 1797–1804. https://doi.org/10.1017/s0950268817000802.

5

Faith-Based Interventions

CHARLTON COLES, PhD,

and VERONICA PARKER, PhD

The Black church is the oldest and most respected institution in the Black community.[1] The origins of the Black church can be traced to slaves seeking temporary refuge from the brutality of slavery in the swamps or woods surrounding plantations. Then, as now, the Black church served multiple functions for the Black community. During the institution of slavery, the church enabled enslaved people to construct a common social reality, establish a common language from disparate African dialects (at a time when reading and writing were generally outlawed for slaves), explore spirituality, and continue the process of establishing a collectivist culture.[2] The church eventually enabled Black Americans to share liberation strategies and communicate with outside groups such as abolitionist organizations. These liberation strategies continued through the abolition of slavery, the Reconstruction period, and the Civil Rights Movement of the 20th century and they continue today. The Black church has long represented a place of refuge and healing for an oppressed and marginalized population hungry for social, political and economic change.[3] From its inception, the church has embodied kinship, social connectivity and shared resources. These resources have enabled congregations to engage in capacity-building efforts and allowed for resilience under extremely adverse social, political, and economic conditions. The Black church's long-term engagement with healing and resilience has led to partnerships with community and government agencies and has provided a basis for community-based interventions.

The success of a society is linked to the well-being of its citizens. Because Black Americans continue to suffer disproportionally from chronic health conditions, social development initiatives and community engagement for the purpose of achieving long-term and sustainable outcomes are particularly important for improving the health and well-being of this group. Community-based interventions are typically preferred over individual-level interventions for Black Americans because community-level interventions are better able to address the social and environmental determinants of poor health and disease.[4,5] A community approach to health with a broad focus can better recognize that individuals are embedded within social-cultural, economic, and political systems that influence health-related behaviors and provide access to resources that are necessary for maintaining good health. The health ministries of the Black church are the most likely community resources for bridging the gaps between these systems.

Health Ministries

Because of the vast scope of health disparities and health inequalities in the United States, more churches are offering structured activities that promote health. Examples include health fairs, health screenings, and other health-related efforts.[6] Structured and informal attempts to address health-related matters within church settings are often referred to as health ministries. These ministries are critically important for addressing the concerns of vulnerable populations, but they have a limited recorded history in Black churches.[4] Most of the history of Black health ministries relates to parish nursing programs. These programs have been largely successful but can also be limited. Health ministries exist only if pastors and other church leaders perceive them as essential, as effective in reducing disease risk, and as consistent with the mission of the church.[7] Lay health leaders and staff are key to the successful implementation of health ministries in Black churches, but they have to serve under the church leadership structure. It is important to understand health ministries in the overall context of faith-based organizations.[6]

Faith-Based Organizations

Faith-based organizations (FBOs) maintain a religious identity in their activities, decision-making, and staffing.[8] FBO types include congregations, national networks (e.g., Lutheran Social Services), or religious organizations that have incorporated outside the structures of congregations and national networks. FBOs have a rich tradition in the United States. Historically, the earliest hospitals in the United States were associated with Catholic and Protestant churches, Jewish synagogues, and other religious bodies. The health-related activities FBOs sponsor may originate internally through health ministries within churches or through external partners (e.g., health departments or university-led research projects). Health-related church activities can range from the distribution of health education pamphlets to church-based health clinics. Churches and other FBOs have played a major role in health promotion since the 1970s and have become important vehicles for health promotion in underserved and vulnerable communities.[9,10] Black churches, in particular, can be an important type of FBO that can incorporate health promotion in their overall mission.[11] However, even to this day, faith-based organizations in the Black community remain an underutilized resource for providing leadership and guidance for public health programming, policymaking, and research to identify public health needs and build strong, healthy, and productive communities.[12]

Although Black FBOs have tremendous potential, barriers still exist that can limit their true effectiveness. One is the lack of knowledge about how health ministries and activities are established and maintained within the Black church.[6] This lack of awareness has limited the scope of health-related efforts. For example, most of the activities performed have had the simple goal of distributing health-related print materials and bringing in speakers to address health conditions. Few health ministries are aware of evidence-based interventions or how to access these interventions. Moreover, health ministries in Black churches can experience digital divide issues.[13] Such issues must be addressed in order to diminish racial disparities regarding access to health information.

The challenges to conducting health promotion activities within the Black church occur at both the organizational (e.g., church) and individual levels (e.g., parishioners). Organizational challenges can include maintaining a volunteer base that is sufficient for carrying out the activities of the health ministry over time.[6] Another organizational challenge is a lack of financial resources in Black churches. Only a few Black churches have earmarked sufficient funds for health ministry activities. Technology-related issues can exist at both the organizational and individual levels. Black churches in rural areas may lack broadband internet access, and even urban churches can lack access and the financial resources necessary to livestream or maintain an online presence. Black church members can also lack internet access and financial resources. Church members can also face individual-level barriers to engagement in long-term health efforts, such as issues related to childcare, lack of time, and lack of transportation. Few research studies have focused on understanding these issues in the proper context. It is important to know about the history of FBOs overall and the Black FBOs in particular.

Recent History of FBOs

Although faith-based organizations have played a role in health promotion since the 1970s, these health-based institutions did not move into the public sphere until President George W. Bush's executive orders that established the White House Office of Faith-based and Community Initiatives.[14] These executive orders mandated that the Department of Health and Human Services explore the means to fund such initiatives. Because the links between spiritual, physical and psychological health are important to people of faith, faith-based partnerships are opportunities to expand on holistic notions of health.[15] Faith-based organizations within Black congregations tend to be similar to parish nursing programs, in which nurses of a particular denomination provide care to members of a congregation. However, faith-based organizations and faith-based initiatives tend to be more expansive than the program offered by parish nurses; they tend to include all health professionals within a congregation as well as health advocates, church leaders, and health coaches who run different programs. Faith-based organizations can play a role in improving the overall health of vulnerable Black communities by educating and encouraging people and by engaging church and community members.[3] Black churches are uniquely positioned to play a role in improving the health of Black communities because they serve many social, organizational and religious functions and can provide multiple opportunities for promoting health behaviors.[16]

Health ministries seek to address the spiritual, physical, and psychological health of congregations. To address these areas, Black pastors often have to serve multiple roles. For example, Black pastors can be educators, politicians and health agents.[17,18] Black congregations often rely on culturally based and evidence-based interventions to address health issues such as heart disease,[19] HIV/AIDS prevention,[20] diabetes prevention,[21] vaccinations,[22] and fruit and vegetable consumption,[23] among others. Respecting a church's spiritual culture in all activities[24] and involving community stakeholders and member participation using the community-based participatory research

(CBPR) model is central to establishing successful health promotion programs in Black Churches.[25] CBPR acknowledges that community participants are equal partners in knowledge and skill development and seeks the help of community members when assessing the effectiveness of programs.[26,27] In addition to measuring change, the CBPR approach can be used to inform sustainable empirically based action.[28] Table 5.1 presents examples of culturally based and evidence-based interventions that used elements of the CBPR model to address obesity (a major risk factor for many chronic diseases) in adults in predominantly Black churches. In all of the studies listed, weight loss was a primary outcome.

Dodani and Fields conducted a feasibility study, Fit Body and Soul, to determine the effects of a spiritually based lifestyle modification program for diabetes prevention that included diet, nutrition, physical activity, and weight control.[29] The participants included 40 adult members of a church in Evans County, Georgia, who were overweight (19.5%), obese (48.8%), or morbidly obese (31.7%). The mean age of the participants was 46 years and most were female (85.3%). CBPR principles were followed to deliver the spiritually based lifestyle modification program for diabetes prevention. Of the 35 participants who attended at least ten sessions and provided information required for the study, 48% lost at least 5% of their baseline weight, 26% lost 7% or more, and 14% lost over 10% of their baseline weight. Generalizability was limited by the small sample size and lack of a comparison group. Findings of this pilot study suggested that implementing a larger Fit Body and Soul study in a faith-based setting using behavioral lifestyle interventions for African American communities is feasible and could lead to a clinically significant degree of weight loss.

In conjunction with a coalition of community and academic leaders, Goldfinger et al. conducted a pilot study, Project HEAL (Healthy Eating, Active Lifestyles), to assess the effects of a peer-led, community-based course on healthy eating and active living using a pre-post design to assess weight change as the primary outcome.[30] The sample (mean age of 68 years) consisted of 26 overweight and obese African American adult members of a church in Harlem, New York. Participants lost a mean of 4.4 pounds at 10 weeks, 8.4 pounds at 22 weeks, and 9.8 pounds at 1 year. Because of the small sample size and lack of a randomized controlled design, generalizability was limited. However, the findings indicated that a peer-led, community-based

Table 5.1. Examples of weight-loss interventions conducted in Black churches using the community-based participatory research model

Study	Sample description	Setting & location	Design	Weight-loss results & limitations	Limitations
Fit Body and Soul[29]	N = 40 Mean age: 46 yrs.	Semi-urban church in Evans County, Georgia	Pre-post test of a behavioral faith-based lifestyle modification program for diabetes prevention	Of 35 participants who provided information required for the study, 48% lost at least 5% of their baseline weight, 26% lost 7% or more, and 14% lost over 10% of their baseline weight	Small sample size, lack of a comparison group
Project HEAL[30]	N = 26 Mean age: 68 yrs.	Local church in Harlem, New York	Pre-post test of a peer-led, community-based course on healthy eating and active living	Participants lost a mean of 4.4 pounds at 10 weeks, 8.4 pounds at 22 weeks, and 9.8 pounds at 1 year	Small sample size, lack of a randomized controlled design
The LIFE Project[31]	N = 35 Mean age: 51.14 yrs.	3 rural churches in South Carolina	Pre-post evaluation of a spiritually based vs. non-spiritually based intervention	For the 28 participants with complete data, both nonspiritual ($p < 0.05$) and spiritual interventions ($p < 0.01$) led to significant reductions in weight. The spiritually based intervention led to a significant reduction in BMI ($p < 0.05$).	Small sample size, nonrandomized design
The WORD[32]	N = 73 Mean age: 54.1 yrs.	4 rural churches in North Carolina	Quasi-experimental design with an intervention group and a delayed intervention control group	The mean weight loss in the intervention group was 3.60 lbs. compared to 0.59 lbs. in the control group ($p < 0.001$)	Small sample size, non-randomized design
Living Well by Faith[33]	N = 106 adults Age 45+ yrs.	5 churches in Denver, Colorado	Small-scale randomized trial of diet, nutrition, and physical activity intervention (small group educational sessions, demonstrations of healthy food preparation, and physical activities)	At two months follow-up, the intervention group showed greater decreases in weight ($p < 0.02$), BMI ($p < 0.05$), and % body fat ($p < 0.03$) than the control groups	Small sample size, limited number of male participants

course can foster behavioral change and weight loss. Moreover, predominantly minority communities plagued by overweight and obesity can benefit from culturally appropriate and low-cost weight loss interventions.

In three rural counties of South Carolina, Parker et al. conducted the LIFE Project, a church-based weight loss intervention using CBPR principles. (L = Love, for self, family and God; I = Inspiration, from friends, God and family; F = Feedback; E = Education, about dietary practices, daily physical activities, and discussions with health care providers). The participants were 35 African American women.[31] Two different ten-week interventions (on spiritually based and the other not spiritually based) were pilot tested using a pre-post design. The final sample size was 28 due to incomplete data. The mean age of participants (n = 9) was 52.4 years for the nonspiritually based intervention group and 49.8 for the spiritually based group (n = 19). Both interventions led to significant reductions in weight ($p < 0.05$ for the nonspiritually based intervention group and $p < 0.01$ for the spiritually based intervention group). In addition, body mass index was significantly reduced in the spiritually based intervention ($p < 0.05$). Although this study provided important information about a lifestyle intervention for achieving weight reduction among overweight and obese rural African American women, the generalizability of the findings is limited by the small sample size and the nonrandomized design. A measure of stage of readiness to change should be incorporated to provide greater understanding of how women progress from disinterest in weight loss to participation in a weight-loss program to sustaining their weight loss. Further studies with larger samples should incorporate rural African American women with no religious affiliation both to address their health care needs and to better test the difference in effectiveness, if any, between the spiritual and nonspiritual LIFE Project curricula.

Kim et al. conducted a quasi-experimental study of a faith-based weight-loss intervention that used a delayed-intervention control group protocol.[32] The Wholeness, Oneness, Righteousness, Deliverance (WORD) program was an eight-week intervention designed to address obesity in rural Black Americans using a community-based participatory research (CBPR) approach. The initial sample consisted of 73 participants from rural churches in North Carolina. The majority (71%) of the participants in the study were women; the mean age was 54.1 years. Because of attrition, the final sample size for analyses was 61 (n = 27 in the intervention group and n = 34 in the control group).

The mean weight loss in the intervention group was 3.60 lbs. compared to 0.59 lbs. in the control group ($p < 0.001$). The program may have limited generalizability beyond the rural Black community because of purposive sampling and the small sample size. Although the study design included a control group and controlled for baseline differences between treatment and control in the analyses, the lack of randomization and subsequent differences in baseline characteristics between groups indicated that treatment effects could have occurred because of demographic characteristics. However, the authors felt that the WORD program showed promise that a faith-based weight-loss program using a CBPR approach can be effective in a rural African American faith community. Future CBPR-based weight-loss studies that test the WORD program should use a larger and more representative sample and a longer time frame.

Using CBPR as a guiding framework, Woods et al. conducted a small-scale randomized trial of diet, nutrition, and physical activity called the Living Well by Faith Health and Wellness Program.[33] The 106 adults (73% female) were from five churches (3 intervention, 2 control) in Denver, Colorado. The control group (n = 32) received a minimal intervention consisting of one educational workshop and the intervention group (n = 74) received a more intensive eight-week program. At two months follow-up, the intervention group showed greater decreases in weight ($p < 0.02$), body mass index ($p < 0.05$), and % body fat ($p < 0.03$) than the control groups. While the sample mainly consisted of African Americans, care should be taken in generalizing the findings since participants were highly educated, were mostly female, were not underserved based on family income, and had access to a primary care physician who signed a medical release form. Despite these limitations, this study can serve as a model for the use of CBPR for developing a successful community-based health and wellness intervention. Moreover, the findings provide a strong foundation for conducting a larger and longer-duration study that would incorporate more diversity among participants (e.g., socioeconomic status, gender).

Critiques of Faith-Based Interventions
Relative Strengths of Culturally Tailored
Evidence-Based Interventions

The main strength of the spiritually based faith-based interventions reviewed above is that they were successful in addressing weight loss as a primary outcome for a vulnerable population. The programs demonstrated varying degrees of efficacy, but all had a demonstrated level of effectiveness. For example, each program revealed reductions in weight regardless of design. The programs were also well received within church congregations, although the participation rates differed. The success of these programs also translated across different settings (e.g., rural and urban). Each program used elements of the CBPR model, indicating that CBPR principles should be considered when designing church-based interventions for predominantly Black congregants. All of these areas are important to a population that is susceptible to health disparities. A final strength is the overall ability of these programs to successfully translate health information to a vulnerable population. Proper translation is key if successful preventive health programs are to be developed and maintained over time.

Relative Weaknesses of Culturally Tailored Evidenced-Based Interventions

The interventions reviewed above had some weaknesses. For example, the participants in these programs tended to be Black women in midlife. Although this population is vulnerable to health disparities, it is still relatively unknown if these programs would be attractive to other subpopulations, such as Black men. One area of particular concern in this subpopulation is Black men's low rates of participation in health-related interventions. Black men are a difficult population to engage in research, particularly in terms of recruitment and retention.[34] They are unlikely to participate in interventions due to a number of factors, including distrust, especially in light of the Tuskegee Syphilis Study.[35,36] In that study, African American men with cases of syphilis were left untreated so researchers could study the long-term effects of the disease. This case of unethical research is well known in the Black community. Other reasons why Black men decline to participate in research studies include a perceived lack of concern about the community on the part of researchers and a lack of personal time to participate in research studies.[37,38] Another research gap in this subpopulation concerns the paucity of successful wellness promotion programs that target African American men. More exploratory research that incorporates CBPR principles is needed in this area. One unpublished focus group conducted with church-going Black men revealed that an evidence-based intervention could be effective but would have to be modified to include fewer sessions, incorporate more technology, and explore more male-centric health issues. However, more qualitative work is needed to support these conclusions. Exploratory research would also have to be quantitative, particularly in terms of testing pilot programs and comparing health-related results of providing evidence-based interventions with merely delivering health-related information to Black churchgoers.

The direct dissemination of health-related information to churches is another limitation of faith-based interventions.[39] These programs tend to remain within the congregations in which they were originally tested. In fact, many congregations are not allowed to keep the original intervention content.[39] Plans for larger dissemination to similar FBOs or health ministries is often not an option or is not presented as an option.[6] This lack of a dissemination strategy is particularly problematic given that churches and community researchers have characteristics that make them ideal health partners. For instance, churches have a history of effectively addressing the community concerns of Black residents. These organizations are also effective at translating health-related content into health prevention and promotion efforts and they have valuable resources that are needed to carry out effective prevention efforts. FBOs are also effective at addressing related issues, such as social and spiritual support and mental health concerns. Academic researchers would be natural partners, but concerns about dissemination and content ownership would have to be resolved before these partnerships could be truly successful. The principles of CBPR provide some strategies about how to resolve these issues, but all partners have to be willing to negotiate.

Barriers to Culturally Tailored Evidenced-Based Interventions

The research literature has consistently identified many barriers to the successful delivery and translation of health prevention information to the Black community. These barriers have mainly been divided into the two main categories of provider barriers and patient barriers.[6] Provider barriers can include a lack of provider knowledge about educational standards, cultural differences with patients, time constraints, a lack of sufficient support staff, and low provider reimbursement rates.[40,41] Patient barriers can include economic limitations, general distrust of the health care system, and a lack of access to or sustained engagement with health care providers. To varying degrees, these barriers appear to at least be mitigated by using culturally appropriate evidence-based interventions through health ministries. More research is needed to determine if intervention results can be sustained over time and if these interventions can effectively reduce health disparities at the community level.

Overcoming Barriers to Culturally Tailored Evidenced-Based Interventions

One strategy for addressing the issue of disseminating health content would be enhanced networking between Black FBOs and campus partners. These networks could be formally established and maintained through the use of the internet and social media outlets. Networks of this nature could be maintained primarily through FBOs because that would allow for expanding networks and partnering with other community and government networks. Evidence-based interventions could then more freely share successes and challenges with the whole network. The network could more effectively address sustainability and/or translation issues by spotlighting them and discussing effective ways to address them through supportive community discussions. Having a firmly established network could also aid in the allocation of material, spiritual, supportive, or professional resources, particularly to congregations in vulnerable communities in dire need of such resources.

Ownership is an issue that might negatively impact successful dissemination of health-related content. For example, if a campus-community partnership successfully develops an evidence-based intervention, who "owns" the intervention? Questions like this should be addressed before a formal dissemination strategy can be drafted. Portability is another issue, particularly for community residents who do not attend church or who belong to a different faith. This outreach issue can be brought up to the entire network so it can brainstorm and find effective solutions.

One strategy for addressing the issue of capacity in Black FBOs is the Faith-Based Organization Capacity Inventory (FBO-CI).[42] This instrument assesses main components of a conceptual model designed for FBOs: System Antecedents for Innovation (staffing and space), System Readiness for Innovation (health promotion experience), and Outer Context (external collaboration).[43] Staffing and space are the stable components of FBOs that usually do not change with the introduction of an intervention. Health promotion experience relates to activities specifically related to a health ministry. External collaboration includes collaborations or partnerships and involvement in research and technical assistance from outside organizations or individuals.

The FBO-CI is a paper-and-pencil inventory that is completed by a pastor or returned by a community partner by interview. The administration time of the FBO-CI is usually 30 to 60 minutes. Initial results suggest that the interview format tends to yield higher-quality information and more timely data collection.[38] This instrument typically classifies FBOs as low, medium, or high in terms of capacity. It can be useful for researchers, FBO leaders, and practitioners. It can help researchers identify the FBOs that are most open to partnerships on health-related initiatives and the type and amount of technical assistance that a FBO might need. It can help FBO leaders identify their strengths and areas of future development. It can help practitioners and researchers working with FBOs assess capacity-building initiatives over time.

Summary

Health disparities among Black Americans are an ongoing problem in the United States. Disparities in health are a major impediment to reaching the health goals outlined in Healthy People 2030.[44] Health disparities within the Black community are pervasive enough that there has been a general call for more community-based health projects instead of projects based on individual effort.[5,25] A research emphasis on individual-level risk factors can overlook the contributions of social and environmental determinants of health and disease.[25] A community approach to health with a broader focus recognizes that individuals are embedded in sociocultural, economic, and political systems that influence both health-related behaviors and access to the resources necessary to maintain health. The Black church is a natural community partner for addressing health and health-related concerns.

The Black church is generally the most respected entity in the Black community. In addition, it has many resources that can be allocated to using FBOs to create successful health ministries that can then collaborate with other partners, such as universities or government agencies, that test and evaluate effective health programs. However, capacity is an issue that would have to be addressed.

Future Directions

The evidence-based interventions reviewed in this chapter have all demonstrated effectiveness and have the potential to expand the capabilities of health ministries, such as training lay health educators. These interventions have also been effective at addressing other health issues for a population that is vulnerable to health disparities and health inequities. More FBOs and health ministries in Black churches should have access to existing evidence-based interventions. Awareness of such interventions can be increased through the expansion of FBO networks. Questions and concerns will naturally arise about who is primarily responsible for maintaining networks and disseminating the information gained from evidence-based interventions. Questions of content ownership would also have to be addressed. However, more access to established evidence-based interventions has tremendous potential to address long-standing health disparities and health inequities in the Black community.

If an effective network of FBOs could be expanded and maintained, the issue of translation beyond the church will have to be addressed, particularly to community residents who are not churchgoers. Gender is another important issue, particularly in terms of translating successful health-related content to adult Black males. Outreach to other community partners and government agencies would help meet these goals. If these barriers can be addressed, more access to and successful translation of health-related content to the Black community could have tremendous positive impact in reducing health disparities and inequities.

Assessment instruments (such as the FBO-CI) can be useful to networks of FBOs by assessing the initial capacity of FBOs within a network. One drawback to this instrument is that it has not been extensively used outside a limited geographical area.[38] More work is also needed with larger samples to examine the true factor structure of the FBO-CI. Having more established networks of available Black FBOs would better address this limitation. Developing more community-level assessment instruments can also aid in evaluating the success of Black FBOs. A well-established capacity-assessing instrument and community-level assessment tools would increase our understanding of the links between capacity and FBO success and how capacity could be increased. These instruments would allow for better assessment of how Black FBOs can reduce racial health disparities in Black communities over time.

REFERENCES

1. Avent, Janeé R., and Craig S. Cashwell. "The Black Church: Theology and Implications for Counseling African Americans." *Professional Counselor* 5, no. 1 (2015): 81–90. https://doi.org/10.15241/jra.5.1.81.

2. Holmes, Barbara A. *Joy Unspeakable*. 2nd ed. Minneapolis: Fortress Press, 2017.

3. Brewer, LaPrincess C. and David R. Williams. "We've Come this Far by Faith: The Role of the Black Church in Public Health." *American Journal of Public Health* 109, no. 3 (2019): 385–386. https://doi.org/10.2105/AJPH.2018.304939.

4. Carter-Edwards, Lori, Yhenneko B. Jallah, Moses V. Goldmon Jr., J. T. Roberson, and Cathrine Hoyo. "Key Attributes of Health Ministries in African American Churches: An Exploratory Survey." *North Carolina Medical Journal* 67, no. 5 (2006): 345–350. https://www.ncbi.nlm.nih.gov/pubmed/17203634.

5. Wing, Rena R., Melissa M. Crane, J. Graham Thomas, Rajiv Kumar, and Brad Weinberg. "Improving Weight Loss Outcomes of Community Interventions by Incorporating Behavioral Strategies." *American Journal of Public Health* 100, no. 12 (2010): 2513–2519. https://doi.org/10.2105/AJPH.2009.183616.

6. Holt, Cheryl L., Anita L. Graham-Phillips, C. Daniel Mullins, Jimmie L. Slade, Alma Savoy, and Roxanne Carter. "Health Ministry and Activities in African American Faith-Based Organizations: A Qualitative Examination of Facilitators, Barriers, and Use of Technology." *Journal of Health Care for the Poor and Underserved* 28, no. 1 (2017): 378–388. https://doi.org/10.1353/hpu.2017.0029.

7. Williams, Quantara, Penny A. Ralston, Iris Young-Clark, and Catherine Coccia. "Establishing Health Ministries: Leaders' Perceptions of Process and Effectiveness." *International Quarterly of Community Health Education* 34, no. 2 (2014): 139–157. https://doi.org/10.2190/IQ.34.2.c.

8. Bielefeld, Wolfgang and William Suhs Cleveland. "Defining Faith-Based Organizations and Understanding Them through Research." *Nonprofit and Voluntary Sector Quarterly* 42, no. 3 (2013): 442–467. https://doi.org/10.1177/0899764013484090.

9. Anderson, Carolyn M. "The Delivery of Health Care in Faith-Based Organizations: Parish Nurses as Promoters of Health." *Health Communication* 16, no. 1 (2004): 117–128. https://doi.org/10.1207/S15327027HC1601_8.

10. Campbell, Marci Kramish, Marlyn Allicock Hudson, Ken Resnicow, Natasha Blakeney, Amy Paxton, and Monica Baskin. "Church-Based Health Promotion Interventions: Evidence and Lessons Learned." *Annual Review of Public Health* 28, no. 1 (2007): 213–234. https://doi.org/10.1146/annurev.publhealth.28.021406.144016.

11. Parrill, Rachel, and Bernice Roberts Kennedy. "Partnerships for Health in the African American Community: Moving toward Community-Based Participatory Research." *Journal of Cultural Diversity* 18, no. 4 (2011): 150–154. https://www.ncbi.nlm.nih.gov/pubmed/22288213.

12. Levin, Jeff and Jay Hein. "A Faith-Based Prescription for the Surgeon General: Challenges and Recommendations." *Journal of Religion and Health* 51, no. 1 (2012): 57–71.

13. Lorence, Daniel, Heeyoung Park, and Susannah Fox. "Racial Disparities in Health Information Access: Resilience of the Digital Divide." *Journal of Medical Systems* 30, no. 4 (2006): 241–249. https://doi,org/10.1007/s10916-005-9003-y.

14. Bush, George W. "Executive Order 13199—Establishment of White House Office of Faith-Based and Community Initiatives." The American Presidency Project, January 29, 2001. https://www.presidency.ucsb.edu/documents/executive-order-13199-establishment -white-house-office-faith-based-and-community.

15. Levin, Jeff. "Partnerships between the Faith-Based and Medical Sectors: Implications for Preventive Medicine and Public Health." *Preventive Medicine Reports* 4 (2016): 344–350. https://doi.org/10.1016/j.pmedr.2016.07.009.

16. Baruth, Meghan, Sara Wilcox, Marilyn Laken, Melissa Bopp, and Ruth Saunders. "Implementation of a Faith-Based Physical Activity Intervention: Insights from Church Health Directors." *Journal of Community Health* 33, no. 5 (2008): 304–312. https://doi.org /10.1007/s10900-008-9098-4.

17. Levin, J. S. "The Role of the Black Church in Community Medicine." *Journal of the National Medical Association* 76, no. 5 (1984): 477–483. https://www.ncbi.nlm.nih.gov/pub med/6737505.

18. Levin, Jeffrey S. "Roles for the Black Pastor in Preventive Medicine." *Pastoral Psychology* 35, no. 2 (1986): 94–103. https://doi.org/10.1007/BF01768709.

19. Parry, Monica and Judy Watt-Watson. "Peer Support Intervention Trials for Individuals with Heart Disease: A Systematic Review." *European Journal of Cardiovascular Nursing* 9, no. 1 (2010): 57–67. https://doi.org/10.1016/j.ejcnurse.2009.10.002.

20. Wingood, Gina and Ralph DiClemente. "The ADAPT-ITT Model: A Novel Method of Adapting Evidence-Based HIV Interventions." *Journal of Acquired Immune Deficiency Syndromes* 47, suppl. 1 (2008): S40–S46. https://doi.org/10.1097/QAI.0b013e3181605df1.

21. Parikh, Punam, Ellen P. Simon, Kezhen Fei, Helen Looker, Crispin Goytia, and Carol R. Horowitz. "Results of a Pilot Diabetes Prevention Intervention in East Harlem, New York City: Project HEED." *American Journal of Public Health* 100, suppl. 1 (2010): S232–S239. https://doi.org/10.2105/AJPH.2009.170910.

22. Gilkey, Melissa B., Michael J. Parks, Marjorie A. Margolis, Annie-Laurie McRee, and Jason V. Terk. "Implementing Evidence-Based Strategies to Improve HPV Vaccine Delivery." *Pediatrics* 144, no. 1 (2019): e20182500. https://doi.org/10.1542/peds.2018-2500.

23. Kothe, E. J., B. A. Mullan, and P. Butow. "Promoting Fruit and Vegetable Consumption: Testing an Intervention Based on the Theory of Planned Behaviour." *Appetite* 58, no. 3 (2012): 997–1004. https://doi.org/10.1016/j.appet.2012.02.012.

24. Austin, Sandra A. and Nancy Claiborne. "Faith Wellness Collaboration: A Community-Based Approach to Address Type II Diabetes Disparities in an African-American Community." *Social Work in Health Care* 50, no. 5 (2011): 360–375. https://doi.org/10.1080/0098 1389.2011.567128.

25. Israel, B. A., A. J. Schulz, E. A. Parker, and A. B. Becker. "Review of Community-Based Research: Assessing Partnership Approaches to Improve Public Health." *Annual Review of Public Health* 19, no. 1 (1998): 173–202. https://doi.org/10.1146/annurev.publhealth .19.1.173.

26. Alvarez, Ann Rosegrant and Lorraine M. Gutiérrez. "Choosing to do Participatory

Research." *Journal of Community Practice* 9, no. 1 (2001): 1–20. https://doi.org/10.1300/J125v09n01_01.

27. Israel, B. A., A. J. Schulz, E. A. Parker, A. B. Becker, A. Allen, and J. R. Guzman. "Critical Issues in Developing and Following Community-Based Participatory Research Principles." In *Community-Based Participatory Research for Health*, ed. Meredith Minkler and Nina Wallerstein, 53–76. San Francisco: Jossey-Bass, 2003.

28. Avent Harris, Janeé R. "Community-Based Participatory Research with Black Churches." *Counseling and Values* 66, no. 1 (2021): 2–20. https://doi.org/10.1002/cvj.12141.

29. Dodani, S., and J. Z. Fields. "Implementation of the Fit Body and Soul, a Church-Based Life Style Program for Diabetes Prevention in High-Risk African Americans: A Feasibility Study." *Diabetes Educator* 36, no. 3 (2010): 465–472. https://doi.org/10.1177/0145721710366756.

30. Goldfinger, Judith Z., Guedy Arniella, Judith Wylie-Rosett, and Carol R. Horowitz. "Project HEAL: Peer Education Leads to Weight Loss in Harlem." *Journal of Health Care for the Poor and Underserved* 19, no. 1 (2008): 180–192. https://doi.org/10.1353/hpu.2008.0016.

31. Parker, Veronica, Charlton Coles, Barbara Logan, and Leroy Davis. "The LIFE Project: A Community-Based Weight Loss Intervention Program for Rural African American Women." *Family & Community Health* 33, no. 2 (2010): 133–143. https://doi.org/10.1097/FCH.0b013e3181d594d5.

32. Kim, Karen Hye-cheon, Laura Linnan, Marci Kramish Campbell, Christine Brooks, Harold G. Koenig, and Christopher Wiesen. "The WORD (Wholeness, Oneness, Righteousness, Deliverance): A Faith-Based Weight-Loss Program Utilizing a Community-Based Participatory Research Approach." *Health Education and Behavior* 35, no. 5 (2008): 634–650. https://doi.org/10.1177/1090198106291985.

33. Woods, Gaye, Arnold H. Levinson, Grant Jones, Ralph L. Kennedy, Lucille C. Johnson, Zung Vu Tran, Tondeleyo Gonzalez, and Alfred C. Marcus. "The Living Well by Faith Health and Wellness Program for African Americans: An Exemplar of Community-Based Participatory Research." *Ethnicity & Disease* 23, no. 2 (2013): 223–229. https://www.ncbi.nlm.nih.gov/pubmed/23530305.

34. Yancey, Antronette K., Alexander N. Ortega, and Shiriki K. Kumanyika. "Effective Recruitment and Retention of Minority Research Participants." *Annual Review of Public Health* 27, no. 1 (2006): 1–28. https://doi.org/10.1146/annurev.publhealth.27.021405.102113.

35. Bates, Benjamin R. and Tina M. Harris. "The Tuskegee Study of Untreated Syphilis and Public Perceptions of Biomedical Research: A Focus Group Study." *Journal of the National Medical Association* 96, no. 8 (2004): 1051–1064. https://www.ncbi.nlm.nih.gov/pubmed/15303410.

36. LaVeist, T. A., K. J. Nickerson, and J. V. Bowie. 2000. "Attitudes about Racism, Medical Mistrust, and Satisfaction with Care among African American and White Cardiac Patients." *Medical Care Research and Review* 57 suppl. 1: 146–161. https://doi.org/10.1177/107755800773743637.

37. Corbie-Smith, G., S. Thomas, and D. St. George. "Distrust, Race and Research." *Archives of Internal Medicine* 162, no. 21 (2002): 2458–2473. https://jamanetwork.com/journals/jamainternalmedicine/fullarticle/214437.

38. Moser, Debra, Kathleen Dracup, and Lynn Doering. "Factors Differentiating Drop-

outs from Completers in a Longitudinal, Multicenter Clinical Trial." *Nursing Research* 49, no. 2 (2000): 109–116. https://doi.org/10.1097/00006199-200003000-00008.

39. Newlin, Kelley, Susan MacLeod Dyess, Emily Allard, Susan Chase, and Gail D'Eramo Melkus. "A Methodological Review of Faith-Based Health Promotion Literature: Advancing the Science to Expand Delivery of Diabetes Education to Black Americans." *Journal of Religion and Health* 51, no. 4 (2012): 1075–1097. https://doi.org/10.1007/s10943-011-9481-9.

40. Chin, Marshall H., Sandy Cook Lei Jou, Melinda L. Drum, James F. Harrison, Julie Kopport, Fay Thiel, Anita G. Harrand, Cynthia T. Schaefer, Herbert T. Takashima, and Sin-Ching Chiu. "Barriers to Providing Diabetes Care in Community Health Centers." *Diabetes Care* 24, no. 2 (2001): 268–274. https://doi.org/10.2337/diacare.24.2.268.

41. Larme, Anne C., and Jacqueline A. Pugh. "Evidence-Based Guidelines Meet the Real World: The Case of Diabetes Care." *Diabetes Care* 24, no. 10 (2001): 1728–1733. https://doi.org/10.2337/diacare.24.10.1728.

42. Tagai, Erin Kelly, Mary Ann Scheirer, Sherie Lou Z. Santos, Muhiuddin Haider, Janice Bowie, Jimmie Slade, Tony L. Whitehead, Min Qi Wang, and Cheryl L. Holt. "Assessing Capacity of Faith-Based Organizations for Health Promotion Activities." *Health Promotion Practice* 19, no. 5 (2018): 714–723. https://doi.org/10.1177/1524839917737510.

43. Greenhalgh, Trisha, Glenn Robert, Fraser MacFarlane, Paul Bate, and Olivia Kyriakidou. "Diffusion of Innovations in Service Organizations: Systematic Review and Recommendations." *Milbank Quarterly* 82, no. 4 (2004): 581–629. https://doi.org/10.1111/j.0887-378X.2004.00325.x.

44. Office of Disease Prevention and Health Promotion. "Healthy People 2030 Framework." HealthyPeople.gov. Last modified February 6, 2022. https://www.healthypeople.gov/2020/About-Healthy-People/Development-Healthy-People-2030/Framework.

6

Clinical and Community-Based Research Networks for Addressing Health Disparities

LUFEI YOUNG, PhD, APRN

The determinants of health disparities that affect populations such as African Americans in the Southern United States are complex. They include biological and behavioral factors related to individual behavior, provider behavior, and health care system actions.[1] Studying the determinants of racial disparities requires interdisciplinary research collaborations and experienced and knowledgeable investigators, who are often available in academic health systems. However, the majority of racial disparities in health care occur in community-based primary and specialty clinics. Clinical or community-based research networks (CBRNs) are the most effective way to connect clinicians and researchers so they can identify the factors that influence racial disparities in health care.[2] Such networks are an integral part of translating discovery to practice. CBRNs can gather and link data from communities and community-based practices, public health surveillance data from local or national health care organizations, and patient medical record data from tertiary medical centers in order to address health disparities across the full spectrum of public health to clinical care. This chapter will describe two major types of CBRNs: practice-based research networks (PBRNs) and community-based participatory research (CBPR). It will briefly outline the history and characteristics of these two types of CBRNs and their implications for health disparity research. It will also describe current challenges and barriers to success in each type of CBRN and new CBRN strategies and opportunities for advancing implementation research. At the end of the chapter, readers will be challenged and motivated to consider ways to engage CBRN in their health equity efforts through several case studies.

Historical Background

The History of Practice-Based Research Networks

PBRNs developed because of the inconsistency in scientific evidence between research conducted in controlled specialty settings and real-world practices.[2-5] In the United States, PBRNs were developed in the 1970s.[2-5] The number of networks in the United States has grown substantially in the past few decades.[2-5] Factors that have contributed to the advancement of PBRNs are national initiatives, federal funding, shared electronic health records, and the use of a broad range of research methodologies.[2-5] Early networks tended to be regional in scope and to focus on the epidemiology, natural history, and diagnosis of common problems encountered in ambulatory care. The first groups of regional PBRNs in the United States were created in 1978.[6] These networks involved partnerships with community clinics.[2-5] The research and leadership of the Ambulatory Sentinel Practice Network, which was established in 1981, played a critical role in the early development of PBRNs.[2-5]

The Agency for Healthcare Research and Quality (AHRQ) recognizes the vital role of PBRNs in health care research. In 2002, it supported the establishment of a PBRN Resource Center.[7] Today, over 180 active networks are registered with the PBRN Resource Center. Health care professionals from a variety of disciplines who conduct clinically relevant research projects and quality-improvement initiatives engage with the PBRN Resource Center.[7] PBRN centers, which operate in all 50 US states and internationally, serve over 24 million patients and interact with tens of thousands of physicians and advanced practice providers throughout the United States and around the world. Many PBRNs received AHRQ funding for infrastructure support and pilot projects. In addition, AHRQ supports PBRN centers through educational, technical, and consultative services. In the past 40 years, PBRNs have provided an important infrastructure for encouraging interdisciplinary research and partnership between academicians and practices or communities that seek to reduce racial disparities in health care, conduct comparative effectiveness and patient-centered outcomes research, and study health policy reform. PBRNs are a crucial component of translating research evidence to clinical practice.[7]

History of Community-Based Participatory Research

CBPR began with the participatory action research developed by Kurt Lewin and the popular education movement in Latin America associated with Paulo Freire in Brazil.[8] In the 1940s, Kurt Lewin, a social scientist, developed a research method that combined action research with the experimental approach to addressing social injustice and disparity.[8] In 1970, in *Pedagogy of the Oppressed*, Paulo Freire suggested that study subjects were not empty vessels and objects of research inquiry.[8] He argued that subjects should be able to determine their own needs as full participants in research projects. Researchers and international organizations used Freire's ideas to work with disenfranchised communities in order to generate evidence to force policy changes and to acquire funding.[8] In the 1990s, the Centers for Disease Control and Prevention (CDC) funded prevention research centers and community-based advisory boards that consisted of community members, volunteers, health and educational professionals, and policy makers.[8] In the 1990s, many health care researchers adopted CBPR. In 1998, the North American Primary Care Research Group was the first high-level research organization to adopt a policy that promoted CBPR.

In the 2000s, the US Institute of Medicine (now the National Academy of Medicine) supported CBPR that was both methodologically rigorous and most beneficial to communities.[8-10] In accord with the national goal of eliminating health disparities, the National Institute of Nursing Research and the National Center for Minority Health and Health Disparities adopted the use of community-partnered interventions in research that targeted minority populations. In 2002, the National Institute of Nursing Research began funding applications for community-partnered interventions that seek to reduce health disparities in racial and ethnically diverse minority populations.[10] Many CBPR projects were multisite and were linked by overarching academic-community boards and successful large randomized controlled trials. As a result of these positive research outcomes, many national and international granting agencies (i.e., the Patient Centered Outcomes Research Institute) began funding CBPR researchers with the goal of strengthening research quality, credibility, and impact on policy and practice.[10]

Characteristics of CBRN
Characteristics of PBRN

AHRQ defines PBRNs as a group of community-based clinician researchers who conduct studies in real-world practices of clinically meaningful questions with the goal of improving the quality of care.[7] The Institute of Medicine called PBRN the most promising infrastructure for supporting research in primary care.[3] PBRNs help link relevant clinical questions with rigorous research methods in community settings to produce scientific evidence that is generalizable and can easily be translated into daily practice.[2-5]

In response to shifting funding opportunities and changes in the health care landscape, some PBRNs have incorporated CBPR research methodologies and others have focused on conducting comparative-effectiveness research or developing the capacity to extract or modify data from various clinical databases.[6,13,14] The essential functions of PBRNs include supporting project development, building sustainable relationships with principal investigators and funders, recruiting and retaining clinicians and practices, managing staff and governance groups, performing research activities, maintaining a membership roster, supporting multiple methods of communication with key stakeholders, hosting regular meetings, meeting member needs, creating networking opportunities for investigators with similar topical interests, and responding to funding announcements in a timely fashion.[12]

To accomplish these functions, PBRNs create organizational structures and core infrastructure. The typical core elements of a PBRN include a minimum of 15 member practices, a formal mission and purpose statement, established leadership, administrative staff, a mechanism for feedback from PBRN clinicians and communities, organizational structure, two-way communication, and research and/or quality improvement infrastructure.[12-13] At a minimum, a PBRN includes a network director (often an MD or PhD) and a coordinator who are operationally responsible for the day-to-day operations of the network and research initiatives. Network leadership may also sustain an advisory board that consists of representative members of the PBRN to guide network activities and inform research. In order to accomplish network goals and support research studies, many PBRNs hire core and study-specific university staff for portions of their time. This can be economically beneficial for both developed and developing networks.[6,12,13]

Characteristics of CBPR

CBPR is a partnership approach to research that equitably involves community members, organizational representatives, researchers, and others in all aspects of the research process. All partners in the process contribute expertise and sharing in decision-making and ownership.[9] The Kellogg Foundation's definition of CBPR is a "collaborative approach to research that equitably involves all partners in the research process and recognizes the unique strengths that each brings. CBPR begins with a research topic of importance to the community, works in partnership with members of marginalized communities, combines scientific evidence with action, and achieves social justice to improve health outcomes and eliminate health disparities."[14] In addition to quantitative research, CBPR uses a wide variety of qualitative research methods, including photo elicitation, focus groups, semi-structured interviews, participatory mapping, photovoice, and digital storytelling.[13]

The core character of CBPR is a commitment to decentered research expertise. knowledge of community members is viewed as research expertise and community members are involved at every stage of the research process. The aim of CBPR is to empower research participants to design and develop research studies and become the users of research products.[14] In 1998, Israel et al. outlined the eight key components of CBPR: (1) it recognizes community as a unit of identity; (2) it builds on strengths and resources within the community; (3) it facilitates collaborative partnerships in all phases of the research; (4) it integrates knowledge and action for the mutual benefit of all partners; (5) it promotes a co-learning and empowering process that attends to social inequalities; (6) it involves a cyclical and iterative process; (7) it addresses health from both positive and ecological perspectives; and (8) it disseminates findings and knowledge gained to all partners.[8,10] Taking a CBPR approach results in the increased capacity of community members and researchers, increases the quality of research outputs and outcomes over time, increases sustainability, and integrates the generation of evidence with implementation.[10,14]

The strengths of CBPR are listed below.

- It is feasible because it adapts existing resources in innovative ways and empowers community members to investigate their own situations.
- It is sustainable and credible because of community input.
- It is useful because it aligns with what the community perceives as social and health goals.
- It is rigorous because it joins research partners with varied skills, knowledge, and expertise to address complex problems in complex situations.
- It adds more resources for the communities involved.
- It can bridge cultural differences and increase cultural knowledge through collaborations among the participants.

- It helps dismantle the lack of trust between communities and the research team.[10]

Challenges and Barriers
Challenges of PBRN

PBRNs play a critical role in the study of care delivery and the application of these approaches to daily practice.[6,12-13] However, PBRNs face the following critical challenges:

- Adapting to a changing health care landscape: PBRN leadership may be challenged to identify and sustain a shared vision that can motivate participation and secure the infrastructure capacity needed to respond to more diverse stakeholders in an ever-changing health care landscape. Because many PBRNs cover large geographic regions with diverse populations, they can be impractical, they can be costly in terms of both time and money, and they may not be representative of PBRN as a whole.
- Recruiting and retaining membership: Changing practice structures and growing competing demands may make it more difficult to recruit and sustain practice membership. It is becoming increasingly difficult to negotiate, reframe, and renew the benefits of PBRNs offered to individual clinicians and to engage administrative and executive staff.
- Securing infrastructure support: Many PBRNs struggle to finance core infrastructure. Building a robust research capacity is difficult when networks are dependent only on grant funds for core staff support. In an increasingly competitive grant environment, PBRNs may seek nontraditional funding from state governments, insurance companies, and health care systems. Working with new partners to secure financing needs to be carefully balanced with the mission and credibility of the PBRN.
- Managing the expectations of both academics and the community: The resource demands, priorities, and core measures of quality achievement are different in community and academic environments. Community-based practices work at a fast pace and are often focused on providing services at the individual level, while academic research teams follow funding timelines from idea to funding to project completion and can last for years. Networks may struggle to balance a clinic's

or a community's need for action with a researcher's timeline. In addition, the expectations from community members may be higher than what university partners can commit to, leading to broken trust.[13]

- Preparing for work force transitions: The PBRN leadership is aging. Developing transition plans so that networks can be sustained as current network directors retire will be crucial. Because many networks have a lean infrastructure, there are often no people in the ranks who have been mentored over time to take on leadership roles. Such transitions may challenge network stability.

- Developing trusting relationships. Establishing trust between the community members and academic research team is difficult because PBRNs are geographically distributed and involve multiple communities with diverse cultural, racial, and economic backgrounds. Especially in minority and underserved communities, there is a long-standing lack of trust in and negative beliefs about health care systems and research.[13,14]

Challenges of CBPR

CBPR also poses the following special challenges, which relate to functioning within a cross-cultural setting, the quality and equality of collaborative partnerships, ethics, and methodological issues:[10]

- The recruitment of participants to CBPR research is labor intensive.
- Retaining participants in community-based research is a great challenge especially among low-income and less-educated participants. Continued participation is often a low priority for participants, especially since the benefits to them may not be apparent. Low income, less education, and African American race have been associated with increased attrition rates in research projects.[11] Common reasons for a high attrition rate include a lack of awareness of research benefits, lack of transportation, interference with work or family responsibilities, financial costs, negative side effects, and burdensome procedures.
- CBPR teams need to balance research rigor and feasibility. To improve research rigor, academic research teams select the strongest study design, the most comprehensive measures, the strongest data collection plan, and the analytic procedures that will provide some benefit to all participants from the community. Because of difficulties in recruit-

ment and high attrition rates, CBPR research can encounter challenges in balancing research rigor and feasibility.

- The fact that most minority communities lack resources and funding is a barrier to building research capacity.
- Both funding organizations and communities lack knowledge of and experience with conducting CBPR.

Implications of CBRN for Health Disparity Research
Implications of PBRN

Most people go to community-based primary care or specialty care clinics for their health care needs, which makes PBRN an ideal infrastructure for addressing health disparities.[12] They are positioned in the local community and their infrastructure represents and can adapt to the diverse nature and specific health issues of communities and their members.[12] Because PBRN enables clinician researchers to conduct research projects in the real world instead of in the rigid academic environment, it provides an opportunity to investigate the impacts of race, ethnicity, and social determinants on health.[12] PBRNs are also an ideal laboratory for studying interventions to address health equity issues, particularly those that are well suited to delivery in primary care settings. Finally, PBRN practices can alert investigators to the presence of important health disparity issues while also providing a laboratory for investigating and confirming suspected health equity issues.[12]

The Southeast Regional Clinicians Network (SERCN) is a PBRN in eight southeastern states (Georgia, Florida, Mississippi, Alabama, North Carolina, South Carolina, Kentucky, and Tennessee).[12] SERCN is administered at the National Center for Primary Care at Morehouse School of Medicine, a historically Black school of medicine that was ranked number one in social mission in the country and whose mission is to "lead the creation and advancement of health equity." SERCN, which is funded by the Patient-Centered Outcomes Research Institute, explicitly prioritizes health equity in their mission statement.[12] Its current priority is to promote equity for medically and socially complex patients who are served by federally qualified health centers. Currently, SERCN includes 203 federally qualified health centers at over 1,700 primary care sites that serve over 4 million patients. These clinics provide comprehensive primary care, dental, and mental health services to a high-risk population that is disproportionately poor, minority, and medically underserved. SERCN clinics help clinician investigators identify important health disparity issues and generate support data and findings that help develop effective system interventions to address these health equity issues. One of their research priorities is developing practical measures to ensure primary care continuity for Medicaid enrollees from underserved racial/ethnic groups.

Because PBRNS are based in communities, they can often address community needs as well as clinic-based research. Some studies have focused on understanding cancer mortality inequalities from the perspectives of patients and primary care providers in order to inform interventions designed to reduce mortality disparities.[12] Other PBRN projects have focused on identifying a community's health care priorities, the sources of health disparities, and opportunities to leverage community-based resources with the goal of improving health equity in their communities. By moving research into the community, PBRNs offer the opportunity to identify and study health issues relevant to the community and patient. PBRNs are a vital component of the pathway from discovery to implementation and dissemination.[12] PBRNs play a vital role in promoting health equity for underserved populations and communities that participate in research studies, in selecting patient-centered health outcomes, and in ensuring access to health care providers.[12]

Implications of CBPR

Unlike traditional research aimed at adding new evidence to advance a specific field, CBPR is an iterative process, incorporating research, reflection, and action in a cyclical process. The fact that people of ethnically and racially diverse minority groups experience poorer health than the majority population is well documented. Research projects that have been developed by investigators outside the minority group and community have often failed to address the issues related to racial and ethnic health disparities. It is clear that new methods and models for conducting research among people of minority groups and marginalized communities are needed. CBPR recognizes that if the research process is to be a means of facilitating change, it is important to involve members of a study population as active and equal participants in all phases of the research project. CBPR shows promise as an approach to reducing health disparities.[10]

Future Directions

There are striking similarities between PBRN research and CBPR. Both strive to use ground-up rather than top-down approaches (the traditional research approach) to address common life experiences among minority groups such as African Americans in the South. Both recognize and emphasize the strengths of minority people and communities (including the community of clinicians) and their capacity for solving problems. In addition, both strive to be driven by local priorities rather than solely by the priorities of academic researchers. Interest in combining PBRN and CBPR to address health disparities is increasing. However, to date, there is a lack of understanding about how to integrate these two types of CBRN. Substantial barriers to involving community members in PBRN research have been reported.[2] There are no commonly accepted guidelines for combining CBPR and PBRN. Guidelines are needed to help increase community participation at all stages of the research process, from development of the research question to analysis of the data and presentation of the results. A community guidebook can provide assistance to PBRNs as they plan, implement, and evaluate participatory CBPR projects.[2] There are little or no data on the benefits of combining CBPR and PBRN in health disparity research. Based on the CBPR literature and findings, however, it seems clear that community involvement will enhance PBRN research.

Involving members of marginalized communities served by PBRN physicians may be the logical next step to asking important clinical questions that matter to patients and are relevant to physicians. Community members can help prioritize research projects conducted in PBRNs. Community members can also help generate research ideas, ground the research in real patient experiences, help refine research methods, interpret findings, and assist in local dissemination of results.[2]

The terminology of CBPR continues to grow with the added focus of community and patient engagement.[8] There is a significant need for conversations that lead to clarity and agreement on taxonomy and terminology. Other major needs include more rigorous CBPR reviews in order to document the benefits and pitfalls of this research approach; to increase the understanding of how to achieve designs that accomplish the goals and translate findings into action and innovation; to increase capacity for all team members, including academics and policy makers; to incorporate partners in the process of developing guiding principles and ethical guidelines for research teams and authors and for journal submissions.[8] Training is also needed for journal editors and ethics boards, as is guidance for authors about how to include the key partnership elements in their articles in order to facilitate systematic reviews. Changes in university promotion and tenure guidelines would accommodate the additional time required for all the partnership meetings and the varied—and often very significant—outcomes beyond scientific publications.

Finally, funding is needed for projects based outside universities.[8] Funding agencies need to change their funding mechanisms to support the development of infrastructure for CBPR. Recently, federal funding agencies have begun to recognize that CBPR plays a vital role in health disparity research. Two of the national funding priorities of the Patient-Centered Outcomes Research Institute are to improve health equity and eliminate disparities in areas of health care outcomes related to racism, discrimination, and bias and to integrate the implementation of scientific findings and empower the public to access, understand, and act on research findings. These two goals cannot be achieved without CBPR. In addition, the strategic plans of National Institutes of Health include improving minority health, reducing health disparities, and leveraging community partnerships in order to increase the public's engagement with research activities. Given these goals, this is an ideal time to move forward with CBPR.

Case Studies
Counseling African Americans to Control Hypertension (CAATCH)
BACKGROUND

Data is limited on implementation of evidence-based multilevel interventions targeted at blood pressure control in hypertensive low-income African Americans who have multiple comorbidities and receive care in low-resource community-based primary care practices. The CAATCH trial was designed to compare the effectiveness of a multilevel, multicomponent, evidence-based intervention to usual care targeted at improving blood pressure control in hypertensive African Americans who receive care in community health centers.[15,16]

STUDY METHODS

CAATCH was a two-arm cluster-randomized controlled trial that was implemented in community health centers that are members of Clinical Directors Network, a PBRN in New York City. The eligible study participants were patients who self-identified as black or African American, had received care at the community health center for ≥ 6 months, and had uncontrolled hypertension. Thirty paired community health centers were randomly assigned to provide the intervention condition or usual care. Participants at the intervention condition sites received: (1) four modules of interactive computerized patient education; (2) six behavioral lifestyle telephone or group counseling sessions; (3) free automated home blood pressure monitors; and (4) encouragement to record their weekly blood pressure readings in a diary and bring it to each study visit. Physicians at the intervention condition sites attended monthly hypertension case rounds and received feedback on their patients' home blood pressure readings and chart audits. Patients and physicians at the usual care sites received a single hypertension patient education session and printed patient education material. The primary outcome was blood pressure control and secondary outcomes were mean changes in systolic and diastolic blood pressure at twelve months that was assessed with an automated blood pressure device.

STUDY FINDINGS

A total of 1,059 patients (mean age 56 years; 28% men, 59% obese, and 36% diabetic) were enrolled. In an unadjusted intent-to-treat analysis, blood pressure control at twelve months was 50.2% at the intervention condition sites and 45.3% at the usual care sites (odds ratio [OR] 1.22; 95% confidence interval [CI] 0.92–1.63; $p = 0.18$). These results showed no significant intervention effect. After adjusting for baseline blood pressure, comorbidity, diabetes, and resistant hypertension status, the blood pressure control rate at the intervention condition sites was 49.3% and 44.5% at the usual care sites (OR 1.21; 95% CI 0.90–1.63, $p = 0.21$). The between-group difference in blood pressure control favored the intervention for 73% of the community health center pairs (11 of the 15 randomized pairs; $p = 0.06$, one-tailed). The pre-specified subgroup analyses indicated that the intervention was associated with significantly greater blood pressure control at twelve months in patients without diabetes (54.0% in the intervention condition group and 44.7% in the usual care group; OR 1.45, 95% CI 1.02–2.06); and in those who received care in small-sized community health centers (51.1% in the intervention condition and 39.6% in the usual care group; OR 1.60, 95% CI 1.04–2.45). The multicomponent intervention was associated with marginally significantly greater blood pressure control in patients with moderate to good health literacy (50.6% in the intervention condition group and 40.8% in the usual care group; OR 1.48, 95% CI 0.99–2.22). Depressive symptoms, comorbidity, and medication adherence at baseline did not moderate the intervention effects.

STUDY CONCLUSIONS

A practice-based multicomponent intervention was no better than usual care in improving blood pressure control among hypertensive African Americans. Future research on implementation of behavioral modification strategies for hypertension control in low-resource settings should focus on the development of interventions that are more efficient and more tailored for this high-risk population.

CONTRIBUTIONS

CAATCH is the largest practice-based implementation trial of a multilevel evidence-based intervention targeted at blood pressure control in hypertensive African Americans in community health centers. It targeted both patients and physicians in practice-based settings. Compared to other trials, the participants had higher levels of poverty, obesity, and resistant hypertension and significantly more comorbidity. These factors enhance the potential to generalize these findings to a broader population who receive care in low-resource settings. In addition, this trial expands our understanding of barriers and facilitators of intervention implementation in real-world clinical settings. It also increases our understand of the strategies for implementing behavioral modification interventions in previously understudied and underserved populations.

Race and Preventive Services Delivery among Black Patients and White Patients Seen in Primary Care

Studies have demonstrated that Black patients are less likely than whites to receive a wide range of treatment. Date relating the extent of racial disparities in preventive services are more limited. The purpose of this study was to compare rates of preventive service delivery to Black and white patients in a primary care setting.

STUDY METHODS

This study was a cross-sectional, multimethod study. The study participants were physicians from the 531 members of the Ohio Academy of

Family Physicians, a PBRN in northeast Ohio.[17] Data were collected on 4,454 consecutive office visits to 138 family physicians in 84 practices between October 1994 and August 1995 using direct observation of the patient visit, patient exit questionnaires, and medical record review. Physicians and patients were blinded to research questions regarding race or preventive service delivery. Preventive service deliveries included 15 screenings, 24 health habit counseling sessions, and 11 immunization services recommended by the United States Preventive Services Task Force.

STUDY FINDINGS

A total of 138 physicians and 4,454 patient visits were observed. Multilevel linear regression analysis found no significant racial differences in rates of delivery of screening services or immunizations. However, Black patients were more likely to receive preventive health habit counseling (mean percent of patients who were up to date on all recommended counseling services, adjusted for covariates: 11.6% for Black patients, 9.5% for white patients, $p = 0.003$).

CONCLUSIONS

Black patients were able to access primary care receive preventive services at rates equal to or greater than those of white patients. This suggests that efforts to increase delivery of preventive care in Black patients need to focus on access to primary care.

CONTRIBUTIONS

Using the PBRN approach, the study design overcame the underreporting bias often seen in other studies conducted in the controlled research setting rather than in the real-world setting of primary. The findings contrast with those of other studies that report racial differences in a wide range of treatment services.

A Trial of Three Interventions to Promote Colorectal Cancer Screening in African Americans

Colorectal cancer is the second leading cause of cancer death in the United States. The rates of incidence and mortality from colorectal cancer are higher for Blacks than for whites. Colorectal cancer screening reduces morbidity and mortality. However, the rates of screening are lower for Blacks than they are for whites. The purpose of this study was to test three interventions to increase colorectal cancer screening rates among African Americans.[18,19]

STUDY METHODS

The study was a randomized community intervention trial to assess the efficacy of two behavioral and educational counseling interventions and a financial support intervention to promote screening for colorectal cancer. The project used CBPR methods that involved a community coalition board; the Morehouse School of Medicine Prevention Research Center; the CDC; the Metropolitan Atlanta Coalition on Cancer Awareness, part of the Atlanta-based National Black Leadership Initiative on Cancer; and other community organizations (e.g., churches and clinics).[18,19]

The eligible patients were African American over age 49 who had no history of colorectal cancer and no previous colorectal cancer screening test within the recommended time interval. Three interventions were chosen to address evidence gaps in the Guide to Community Preventive Services: one-on-one education, group education, and reducing out-of-pocket costs. Data sources included medical records and a questionnaire survey (which was administered both before and after screening) to assess knowledge, attitudes, beliefs, and practices regarding general health issues and screening for colorectal cancer risk. Screening status for colorectal cancer was assessed by phone and/or mail at the follow-up assessment periods at three and, if necessary, six months after the intervention. A total of 369 African American men and women aged ≥ 50 years were enrolled in this randomized controlled community intervention trial. The main outcome measures were a post-intervention increase in colorectal cancer knowledge and obtaining a screening test within six months after completing the interventions.

STUDY FINDINGS

During two years of the study period, 645 eligible participants were recruited from 34 churches, 13 senior residences, 11 community senior centers, 3 medical clinics, and 4 men's groups in counties in the Atlanta metropolitan area. A total of 369 entered the study. They were randomized into four cohorts. The participants assigned to the one-on-one education cohort received three 45-minute education sessions over three weeks about CRC risk and screening recommendations. The participants in the group education cohort received four education sessions over four weeks. The participants in the financial support cohort were offered financial reimbursement up to $500 for out-of-pocket expenses for CRC screening. The fourth cohort was the control group. The participants in this group attended the introductory session but received no intervention other than accepting the contents of the gift bag and educational pamphlets. There was substantial attrition: 257 participants completed the intervention and were available for follow-up three to six months later. Among completers, there were significant increases in knowledge in the two cohorts that received education but in neither of the other two. By the six-month follow-up, 17.7% (11/62) of control group members reported having undergone screening, compared to 33.9% (22/65) of the group education cohort ($p = 0.039$). Screening rate increases in the other two cohorts were not statistically significant.

CONCLUSIONS

The most successful intervention was group education, which suggested that the information and emotional support received in a support network may reduce participants' barriers related to colorectal cancer screening. The involvement of family members, friends, volunteers, and others can promote cancer early detection and augment treatment. However, only about a third of the individuals that participated in the group education intervention obtained screening after the study, indicating that more effective interventions are needed.[18,19]

CONTRIBUTIONS

The success of this study demonstrates that CBPR partnership played a major role in health disparity research in community settings.

REFERENCES

1. Braveman, P., and L. Gottlieb. 2014. "The Social Determinants Of Health: It's Time to Consider the Causes of the Causes." *Public Health Reports* 129 (suppl. 2): 19–31.

2. Westfall, J. M., R. F. VanVorst, D. S. Main, and C. Herbert, 2006. "Community-Based Participatory Research in Practice-Based Research Networks." *Annals of Family Medicine* 4 (1): 8–14.

3. Green, L. A., and J. Hickner. 2006. "A Short History of Primary Care Practice-Based Research Networks: From Concept to Essential Research Laboratories." *Journal of the American Board of Family Medicine* 19 (1): 1–10.

4. Lanier, D. 2005. "Primary Care Practice-Based Research Comes of Age in the United States." *Annals of Family Medicine* 3 (suppl. 1): S2–S4.

5. Niebauer, L., and P. A. Nutting. 1994. "Primary Care Practice-Based Research Networks Active in North America." *Journal of Family Practice* 38 (4): 425–427.

6. Davis, M. M., S. Keller, J. E. DeVoe, and D. J. Cohen. 2012. "Characteristics and Lessons Learned from Practice-Based Research Networks (PBRNs) in the United States." *Journal of Healthcare Leadership* 4: 107.

7. U.S. Department of Health and Human Services. "Projects Funded Under RFA: Primary Care Practice-Based Research Networks (PBRNs) III." Part of "Fiscal Year 2002: Research on Children's Health: New Starts." Agency for Healthcare Research and Quality. https://archive.ahrq.gov/research/findings/factsheets/children/new-starts/2002.html #capacity.

8. Macaulay, A. C. 2017. "Participatory Research: What Is the History? Has the Purpose Changed?" *Family Practice* 34 (3): 256–258.

9. Israel, B. A., A. J. Schulz, E. A. Parker, and A. B. Becker. 1998. "Review of Community-Based Research: Assessing Partnership Approaches to Improve Public Health." *Annual Review of Public Health* 19 (1): 173–202.

10. Holkup, P. A., T. Tripp-Reimer, E. M. Salois, and C. Weinert. 2004. "Community-Based Participatory Research: An Approach to Intervention Research with a Native American Community." *ANS: Advances in Nursing Science* 27 (3): 162.

11. Flores, G., A. Portillo, H. Lin, C. Walker, M. Fierro, M. Henry, and K. Massey. 2017. "A Successful Approach to Minimizing Attrition in Racial/Ethnic Minority, Low-Income Populations." *Contemporary Clinical Trials Communications* 5 (March 1): 168–174.

12. Westfall, J. M., R. Roper, A. Gaglioti, and D. E. Nease Jr. 2019. "Practice-Based Research Networks: Strategic Opportunities to Advance Implementation Research for Health Equity." *Ethnicity & Disease* 29 (suppl. 1): 113.

13. Gaglioti, A. H., J. J. Werner, G. Rust, L. J. Fagnan, and A. V. Neale. 2016. "Practice-Based Research Networks (PBRNs) Bridging the Gaps between Communities, Funders, and Policymakers." *Journal of the American Board of Family Medicine* 29 (5): 630–635.

14. Jull, J., A. Giles, and I. D. Graham. 2017. "Community-Based Participatory Research and Integrated Knowledge Translation: Advancing the Co-Creation of Knowledge." *Implementation Science* 12 (1): 1–9.

15. Sankaré, I. C., R. Bross, A. F. Brown, H. E. Del Pino, L. F. Jones, D. A. M. Morris, C. Porter, A. Lucas-Wright, R. Vargas, N. Forge, and K. C. Norris. 2015. "Strategies to Build Trust and Recruit African American and Latino Community Residents for Health Research: A Cohort Study." *Clinical and Translational Science* 8 (5): 412–420.

16. Ogedegbe, G., J. N. Tobin, S. Fernandez, A. Cassells, M. Diaz-Gloster, C. Khalida, T. Pickering, and J. E. Schwartz. 2014. "Counseling African Americans to Control Hypertension: Cluster-Randomized Clinical Trial Main Effects." *Circulation* 129 (20): 2044–2051.

17. Williams, R. L., S. A. Flocke, and K. C. Stange. 2001. "Race and Preventive Services Delivery among Black Patients and White Patients Seen in Primary Care." *Medical Care* 39 (11): 1260–1267.

18. Blumenthal, D. S., S. A. Smith, C. D. Majett, and E. Alema-Mensah. 2010. "A Trial

of 3 Interventions to Promote Colorectal Cancer Screening in African Americans." *Cancer: Interdisciplinary International Journal of the American Cancer Society* 116 (4): 922–929.

19. Smith, S. A., M. S. Whitehead, J. Q. Sheats, B. E. Ansa, S. S. Coughlin, and D. S. Blumenthal. 2015. "Community-Based Participatory Research Principles for the African American Community." *Journal of the Georgia Public Health Association* 5 (1): 52.

III HEALTH DISPARITIES

7

Hypertension

GEORGIANA LOGAN, PhD, MS

Historically, African Americans have borne a disproportionate burden of risk factors for and incidence, morbidity, and mortality rates associated with chronic diseases. This chapter provides an overview of hypertension among African Americans including behavioral, biological, and psychosocial risk factors for the disease. It considers the epidemiological data, social determinants, and lived experiences of African Americans. It seeks to provide a better understanding of hypertension among this group by offering a lifespan approach to the topic of African Americans and hypertension.

Hypertension Guidelines

Hypertension, or high blood pressure, is defined as the amount of force or pressure it takes to pump blood from the heart to the rest of the body. Blood pressure is measured by two numbers: systolic, the upper number of the blood pressure measurement, which represents the amount of force that blood exerts on the arteries as the heart contracts while delivering blood to the rest of the body and diastolic, the lower number of the blood pressure measurement, which represents the amount of force that blood exerts on the arteries as the heart rests between beats and the coronary artery resupplies blood to the heart.[3] A diagnosis of high blood pressure must be confirmed by a medical professional and is based on a set of guidelines.

Periodically, the Joint National Committee on Prevention, Detection, Evaluation, and Treatment of High Blood Pressure revises it hypertension guidelines, and in 2017, the American College of Cardiology and the American Heart Association revised its blood pressure guidelines and defined several distinct categories of hypertension (see table 7.1).

Table 7.1. Revised blood pressure guidelines from the American College of Cardiology and American Heart Association, 2017

Category	Systolic (mm Hg)		Diastolic (mm Hg)
Normal	Less than 120	and	Less than 80
Elevated	120–129	and	Less than 80
High (hypertension stage 1)	130–139	or	80–89

Source: "New ACC/AHA High Blood Pressure Guidelines Lower Definition of Hypertension," American College of Cardiology, November 3, 2017, https://www.acc.org/latest-in-cardiology /articles/2017/11/08/11/47/mon-5pm-bp-guideline-aha-2017.

Hypertension usually presents little to no warning signs or symptoms and is often dubbed the silent killer. Thus, hypertension is often undiagnosed, untreated, and unmanaged.

Prevalence and Incidence of Hypertension

Hypertension is a leading cause of preventable disease and death in the United States. Every year, thousands of Americans are diagnosed with hypertension. Recent reports suggests that 45% of adults in the United States have hypertension. Close to 500,000 deaths are primarily attributable to hypertension in the United States[3,22] African Americans disproportionally experience higher incidence, prevalence, and mortality rates of hypertension across every US state, especially in the southern regions of the United States.[18,20,55] The southern region is most commonly known as the Bible Belt, the Black Belt and the Stroke Belt. Within this region, hypertension prevalence is higher among African Americans than it is among their white, Asian, and Hispanic counterparts.[22] Literature suggests that African American men experience hypertension at much higher rates than both white men and African American women. Moreover, African American men are less likely (40%) to have their blood pressure under control than white men (48%).[39] When we examine hypertension across the lifespan, the prevalence of hypertension and high blood pressure levels among African American children and adolescents mirror what we see in African American adults in relation to their white counterparts.[47] Close to 46% of African Americans ≥ 19 years of age suffer from cardiovascular disease.[3] African Americans are more likely to experience complications from hypertension such as heart attack, stroke, and chronic kidney disease and die at an earlier age than their white counterparts.[16,61,62]

Historical and Theoretical Perspectives of Hypertension

Why do racial disparities in hypertension across the lifespan exist? Since the early 1800s theorists have described several etiologies to explain the origin and development of hypertension among individuals. Theories have proposed that various biological perspectives, health behaviors, and social determinants of health influence or increase a person's risk of developing and controlling hypertension.[34,41,68]

Promising population-based epidemiological studies such as the Jackson Heart Study, the Coronary Artery Risk Development in Young Adults Study (CARDIA study), the Framingham Heart Study, the Bogalusa Heart Study, the Atherosclerosis Risk in Communities Study (ARIC study), and REasons for Geographic and Racial Differences in Stroke (REGARDS) offer insights into the risk of developing hypertension and theories about the factors associated with hypertension risk and cardiovascular health.[5,14,46,51,56,67,70] These studies offered key insights about the health disparities observed among racial/ethnic groups and offer a platform for future interventions.

Several theorists suggest biopsychosocial, positive health models as a means of promoting targeted interventions for addressing health and disease. These have been used to address chronic disease such as cancer and adolescent health and are starting to garner attention among health education and health promotion professionals as culturally appropriate models for hypertension interventions and strategies. Biopsychosocial interventions that focus on positive health offer promise as interventions that may be able to reduce hypertension disparities. Two models can be used to address various diseases and chronic conditions: the resiliency theory and the culture and social class model.[38,64] Resilience describes an individual's ability to bounce back and overcome adverse circumstances and situations.[74] The role of resiliency as a protective factor in relation to chronic health conditions and health behaviors and their associated health outcomes in relation to length of life and quality of life has not been well studied. The culture and social class model suggests that social class and culture are co-constructed and that "socioeconomic factors and social class are fundamental determinants of human functioning across the life span, including development, well-being, and physical and mental health."[4,53] Both theories offer a strengths-based approach to understanding risk exposure and disease as they relate to hypertension.

Nutrition (Behavioral Risk Factor)

Numerous studies have shown that diet plays a mediating role in the risk of developing hypertension.[11] Currently, 78.5% of African Americans consume less than the recommended five servings of fruits and vegetables a day and 69% of African Americans report that they consume more than 30% of their calories from fat.[21] The amount and types of food people consume are often influenced by culture, family traditions, geographic region, food accessibility, and religious practices. Those influences relate to taste (e.g., spices and seasonings), meat preferences (e.g., red meat, fish, chicken, and pork), fillers (e.g., starches and root vegetables), and other factors. These dietary habits have been linked to a higher prevalence of obesity and hypertension within the African American population. However, African American dietary practices and the incidence of hypertension has not been extensively studied.[24]

The Western diet and the southern diet are key contributors to hypertension among African Americans. The Western diet is associated with low consumption of fruits and vegetables and a high consumption of meats, high-fat processed meats, high cholesterol, high sugar, and high sodium foods. Poor dietary patterns in the US South (e.g., processed foods, high sodium, high-fat food, fried foods, excess sugar, red meat, and pork) have been cited as a key risk factor for hypertension.[32,45] These dietary patterns symbolize comfort food or soul food in the South. Today, African Americans are more likely to consume large amounts of salt and have poorer dietary practices (e.g., eating processed food, fatty foods, and high caloric and high cholesterol foods) due to neighborhood environment (e.g., ease of access to fast food and convenience stores) and because they may lack access to places that sell healthier foods (e.g., farmer's markets and grocery stores).[57]

A reduction in sodium intake is highly recommended as a lifestyle behavioral change for the prevention and treatment of hypertension. The American Heart Association recommends that adults limit the amount of sodium they consume daily to less than 1,500 mg.[32] An increase in potassium has also been shown to be effective in reducing blood pressure and lowering mortality among hypertensive adults. Potassium has been shown to have a number of key benefits such as inhibiting sodium reabsorption and increasing urine excretion and offers protection against vascular injury in salt-sensitive hypertensive adults. Daily dietary consumption of fish that is high in omega-3 polyunsaturated fatty acids has also been to help reduce blood pressure. Two diets that curtail the prevalence and incidence of hypertension are the Dietary Approaches to Stop Hypertension (DASH) diet and the Mediterranean diet.

The DASH diet was first introduced in the 1990s by the National Heart, Lung and Blood Institute to help control incidence and prevalence of hypertension by recommending that adults consume at least four or five servings per day of fruits and vegetables, increase their consumption of lean meats or fish and whole grains, and limit their consumption of red meats and refined sugar.[15] This diet is also rich in essential nutrients (e.g., potassium, magnesium, calcium, fiber) that help lower blood pressure. DASH has been cited as an effective dietary intervention to lower blood pressure in African Americans.[15]

Much like the DASH diet, the Mediterranean diet has been identified as one of the healthiest dietary patterns to adopt when trying to improve health and lower risk for disease. It suggests that adults consume higher amounts of vegetables, fruits, whole grains, beans, nuts, and olive oil or grapeseed oil while limiting consumption of foods high in sugar, fat, and sodium and processed meats/foods. Both diets introduced healthy alternatives for cooking and eating. Interventions that incorporate nutrition education using these two diets have been shown to be effective in changing behaviors while reducing the risk for hypertension, lowering blood pressure, and reducing obesity.[8] African Americans, however, are less likely to adhere to both diets due to economic barriers, cultural influences, and food preferences that are often associated with how foods taste and their perceptions about healthy eating practices.[33,36,49,63] Interventions that are culturally appropriate and aim to modify traditional recipes and food preferences may offer some success in meeting current nutritional guidelines and modifying health behaviors among this group. Additional focus should be placed on addressing nutrition environment, food insecurity, food assistance programs, and policies that address the root causes of poor diet quality and cardiovascular health.

Physical Activity (Behavioral Risk Factor)

The United States Department of Health and Human Services and the American Heart Association recommend that adults participate in 75 minutes of vigorous physical activity, such as running or participation in active sports at least three days per week or 30 minutes of moderate physical activity, defined as activities such as brisk walking for at least 10 minutes at a time on at least five days per week and performing muscle-strengthening exercises on two or more days per week.[26,60] Physical activity provides many benefits; it helps improve weight management, lower blood pressure, and reduce cardiovascular disease risk.

Many African Americans do not participate in the recommended minutes of physical activity per week. Physical inactivity is an important modifiable risk factor associated with hypertension. Physical inactivity is often defined as a sedentary lifestyle in which individuals sit for long periods of time while participating in leisure activities (e.g., watching TV, playing video games, sitting at a computer, or using a mobile phone for extended periods of time).[31,71] Modifying sedentary behaviors and participating in moderate-intensity physical activities can help reduce incidence of hypertension.

POTENTIAL BARRIERS TO PHYSICAL ACTIVITY AND POTENTIAL STRATEGIES FOR OVERCOMING BARRIERS

The rate of physical activity compliance is documented to be lowest for African American populations (40%).[52] African Americans are more likely to engage in physical activity as a planned activity instead of as a primary mechanism for preventing chronic disease.

Barriers to physical activity including the lack of a suitable environment (e.g., safe, and green spaces), lack of access to facilities (e.g., location and cost), not knowing what to do (e.g., education and awareness), discomfort with sweating, lack of time, negative body image (e.g., weight perceptions), physical limitations (e.g., disabilities), and lack of social support (e.g., family, friends, and other supportive networks).

African Americans underestimate their body size and are more likely to report body satisfaction regardless of size. Both men and women prefer larger body sizes, especially in the South.[6,19,47,48,59] Most body image studies have focused on African American women and adolescents. Few studies have addressed African American men's attitudes and perceptions related to physical activity in relation to their understanding of its protective factors in relation to obesity and hypertension. Studies that focus on interventions to address physical activity compliance in efforts to reduce hypertension and cardiovascular events (i.e., stroke and heart attack) report that many participants understand that physical activity is important but do not mention specific strategies for overcoming barriers associated with physical activity compliance. Such studies are likely to suggest group workouts (e.g., gender-based, age-specific, and church-based) walking or running groups.[32,43]

Obesity (Health Outcome as a Result of Behavioral Risk Factors)

Obesity is a major contributing risk factor for hypertension and is associated with poor health outcomes. Obesity is a modifiable risk factor that can be managed through diet and exercise. The National Health and Nutrition Examination Survey suggests that over 30% of adults in the United States are considered overweight or obese measured by a body mass index ≥ 30. Obesity is the number-one risk factor for hypertension and diabetes. Almost 40% of African Americans in the United States are considered obese (the highest prevalence among all racial/ethnic groups): 37.5% of African American men are considered obese while 56.1% African American women are considered obese.[22]

Numerous risks factors such as genetics, culture, poor nutrition, sedentary lifestyle, and environment lead to increased risk of obesity, a comorbidity of hypertension among African Americans.[20,71] Health inequities and disparities are closely linked with the social determinants of health—that is, the social, economic, and/or environmental disadvantages associated with where a person lives, works, learns, prays, and plays. These disadvantages may help explain disparities in obesity prevalence among African Americans.

Built, Physical, and Social Environments

The environment plays a major role in health and well-being. This concept of environment must include the physical (i.e., nature), built (i.e., infrastructures and greenspaces), and social environments (i.e., cultural, and social institutions, norms, beliefs, and policies) and the interactions and connections between each environment.

The physical and built environments are of primary concern in relationship to obesity. Minority communities in both urban and rural locations tend to be less invested in and offer little to no resources to help lower risks of obesity across the lifespan. Many of these communities in every state have poor built or unsafe spaces (e.g., inadequate parks or green spaces, inadequate sidewalks, poor lighting, and crime), limited access to full-service grocery stores, and limited access to fresh and nutritious foods. Many low-income, minority, and rural neighborhoods lack full-service grocery stores and famer's markets where healthy food can be purchased. These areas are commonly known as food deserts. Instead, such neighborhoods often feature an abundance of convenience stores and fast-food options in place of grocery stores. Convenience stores often charge twice as much for the groceries they supply and often offer only poor-quality food.

Biological and Psychosocial Risk Factors
INTERGENERATIONAL HYPERTENSION

African Americans tend to present with an earlier onset and severity of hypertension that begins in childhood and a higher incidence and prevalence of hypertension across the lifespan.[50,58,69,73] Two potential explanations for intergenerational hypertension are epigenetics and intergenerational health practices.

Biology may be influenced by lifestyle behaviors that affect health for multiple generations via epigenetic modifications (i.e., DNA methylation and histone modification).[49,68] These gene variations are bidirectionally related to various epigenetic factors that occur across the lifespan because of life circumstances and personal health behaviors and because the environment in which one is born, lives, and grows leave epigenetic footprints in the DNA. Epigenetic changes may present in subsequent generations (transgenerational).[49,68]

Epigenetic gene variations can be influenced by changes in lifestyle behaviors. Adopted behaviors are often learned across generations. In the late 1970s, Albert Bandura proposed the social cognitive theory, which posits that people learn through observing the behavior and attitudes of others and then imitating and modeling what they observe based on perceived outcomes of those behaviors.[10] According to Bandura, the influential models in our lives that we observe consciously or unconsciously influence our adoption of the observed behaviors, attitudes, and practices of those models. One key risk factor for hypertension involves behavioral choices that place an individual at risk for the disease. This is important because culturally and intergenerational health-related practices, beliefs, and messages are often transferred between family members of different generations and influence health and well-being.

Intergenerational learning is a transformative and informal process that takes place through multigenerational interactions. It is a cultural exchange of knowledge, customs, beliefs, and practices between generations.[65,66] Intergenerational practices involve participating in activities that bridge across multiple generations and builds on the positive resources that each generation has to offer other generations and the broader community.[10,65]

Family history plays a crucial role in the development of hypertension. If you have a mother, father, sister, or brother with hypertension, you are more likely to get hypertension yourself and more likely to be pre-hypertensive. African American beliefs, practices, and customs are often passed across generations. Many of these practices and beliefs are rooted in history. Moreover, historical psychosocial factors such as racism and discrimination play a mediating role in the development of hypertension for African Americans.[13,17,25]

RACISM AND STRESS

The cumulative burden of biological and environmental epigenetics across the lifespan has direct implications for health disparities and health inequities for African Americans. Psychosocial factors such as perceived racial discrimination as a result of these burdens is often associated with physical and psychological trauma that leads to poorer health outcomes among this group.[17] Racism is "the beliefs, attitudes, institutional arrangements, and acts that tend to denigrate individuals or groups because of phenotypic characteristics or ethnic group affiliation."[25] Racism, which has many dimensions and can be perpetuated across many levels of influence simultaneously, results in acute exposure to stress over the lifespan that impacts health. Studies have suggested a possible association between racial discrimination and hypertension.[34] Racial discrimination leads to inequitable access to social resources (i.e., education, health care, and monetary resources) that impact health and well-being across the lifespan.

SOCIOECONOMIC STATUS

The wealth gap between the self-reported median household income of African Americans and whites and income-related socioeconomic stressors are associated with disparities in health and chronic health conditions such as hypertension.[28,44] When education level is factored in, the wealth gap widens. Currently, the median African American household income is about $43,000, in contrast to the median white household income of about

$71,000, a $28,000 difference.[30] African Americans are twice as likely as whites to live in poverty. They are less likely to own a home and more likely to be unemployed or lack stable employment than whites.

SOCIAL SUPPORT

Social support may buffer the negative effects of psychosocial factors that impact health.[28] Stress-buffering theory posits that interpersonal social supports (e.g., family, friends, co-workers, peers, community members, and religious associations) may attenuate societal and systemic stressors that lead to "weathering" or wear and tear on marginalized populations over the lifespan through lived experiences.[40] Studies show an inverse relationship between social support and blood pressure.[7,27,40] This inverse relationship suggests that various forms of social support promotes increased participation in physical activity and consumption of good nutrition.[27] Physical activity and nutrition are important behavioral risk factors of hypertension and decrease rates of obesity.

Access to and Use of Health Care to Manage Hypertension

Racial and ethnic differences in access to and use of health care have been extensively documented as key contributors to how well hypertension is managed. Literature suggests that adherence to hypertension treatment recommendations are lower among African Americans than other racial/ethnic groups. Health inequities in access to, use of, and quality of health care by race/ethnicity are apparent from assessments of patient experiences and perceptions about health care. Studies have examined various correlates of poor hypertension management among racial/ethnic groups, including non-adherence (e.g., failure to keep appointments or take medication), uncomfortable patient-provider communication, the absence of shared decision making, discrimination within health care practices, poor access to health care, inability to afford or continue pharmacotherapy regimens, and poor quality health care.[1,2,12,13]

Patients' knowledge of and beliefs about their susceptibility to and the severity of hypertension are significant predictors of effective hypertension management.[2,37] Achieving successful hypertension management remains a challenge, especially among African Americans. This is problematic because African Americans have a greater burden of cardiovascular disease (e.g., heart attacks, stroke, etc.). Because African Americans encounter barriers to effective hypertension management at multiple levels, interventions that address access to and use of health care should target multiple levels of the socioecological model (i.e., intrapersonal, interpersonal, institutional, and community factors and policies) in order to address barriers to blood pressure control for African Americans across the lifespan.

In order to fully understand health disparities and inequities among marginalized populations, it is necessary to understand the intersections of health, race/ethnicity, access to health care services, use of health care, and bias among health care providers.[23] These intersections are primary concerns for African Americans in the South because of the historical treatment of African Americans within health care and among health care providers. Distrust, poor patient-provider communication, lack of shared decision making, and discrimination are key barriers to successful control of hypertension.

Implications for Public Health

African Americans bear the burden of disease for many health indicators in the United States. Disparities among the leading causes of death between African Americans and whites are significant across the lifespan, especially deaths as a result of cardiovascular disease, which is the leading cause of death in the United States and often begins in youth. Roughly 50% of African Americans ≥ 19 years of age in the United States suffer from cardiovascular disease.[23] African Americans have a higher incidence of all health issues related to cardiovascular disease than their white counterparts. This disparity leads to disproportionate disparities in life expectancy.[20,42] Premature death and excess death from cardiovascular disease is attributable to preventable and controllable diseases such as hypertension. Recent findings suggest that in the United States, "attributable risk for hypertension and 30-year mortality among white men was 23.8% compared with 45.2% among African American men and 18.3% for white women compared with 39.5% for African American women."[39] Moreover, African American men suffer from increased rates of age- and cause-specific morbidity and mortality than African American women and white Americans.[16]

Despite reductions in the disparity gap in death rates between African Americans and whites, African Americans continue to die at higher rates than their white counterparts.[29] African Americans are more likely to die at an earlier age and experience diminished quality of life than whites across the life span and across generations. Programs, services, and interventions to reduce cardiovascular disease burden among African Americans offer promise for eradicating health disparities among African Americans.

Lifespan Perspective

This chapter concludes by offering final thoughts regarding hypertension across the lifespan for African Americans. Martinson suggests that "health over the lifespan is a dynamic process that is shaped by when health conditions first appear, how soon conditions are diagnosed, how conditions are managed and treated, and the extent to which symptoms are experienced."[54] African Americans bear the disproportionate burden of chronic diseases across the lifespan Poor dietary practices, lack of physical activity, high rates of obesity, and disproportionate rates of hypertension begin in youth and impact overall life expectancy and quality of life for this group.

Health inequities associated with hypertension that are characterized by behavioral, biologica;, and psychosocial risk factors accumulate, persist, or diminish across the lifespan. A lifespan perspective sheds light on premature death and excess death associated with hypertension for African American. Recent advances that have declared that racism is a public health issue offer hope that efforts will increase to improve the social determinants of health and dismantle the systemic racism that have led to health inequities for many African Americans. In addition, it presents a call to clinicians, public health professionals, and policy makers to target interventions that educate, advocate, motivate, and provide an opportunity for successful lifestyle changes; social, systemic, and environmental policy initiatives, and modifications in health care.

REFERENCES

1. Abegaz, Tadesse Melaku, Abdulla Shehab, Eyob Alemayehu Gebreyohannes, Akshaya Srikanth Bhagavathula, and Asim Ahmed Elnour. "Nonadherence to Antihypertensive Drugs: A Systematic Review and Meta-Analysis." *Medicine* 96, no. 4 (2017): e5641. https://doi.org/10.1097/md.0000000000005641.

2. Al-Noumani, H., J. R. Wu, D. Barksdale, G. Sherwood, E. AlKhasawneh, and G. Knafl. "Health Beliefs and Medication Adherence in Patients with Hypertension: A Systematic Review of Quantitative Studies." *Patient Educ Couns* 102, no. 6 (2019): 1045–1056. https://doi.org/10.1016/j.pec.2019.02.022.

3. American Heart Association. "High Blood Pressure." American Heart Association, 2022. https://www.heart.org/en/health-topics/high-blood-pressure.

4. American Psychological Association. *2007 Annual Report*, July-August 2008. Washington, DC: American Psychological Association. https://www.apa.org/pubs/info/reports/2007-annual.pdf.

5. Arnett, D. K., H. A. Tyroler, G. Burke, R. Hutchinson, G. Howard, and G. Heiss. "Hypertension and Subclinical Carotid Artery Atherosclerosis in Blacks and Whites: The Atherosclerosis Risk in Communities Study." *Arch Intern Med* 156, no. 17 (1996): 1983–1989.

6. Awad, G. H., C. Norwood, D. S. Taylor, M. Martinez, S. McClain, B. Jones, A. Holman, and C. Chapman-Hilliard. "Beauty and Body Image Concerns among African American College Women." *J Black Psychol* 41, no. 6 (2015): 540–564.

7. Baghi, V., and E. Baghban Karimi. "Predicting the Quality of Life of Patients with Hypertension Based on Resilience and Social Support." *J Nurs Educ* 5, no. 6 (2018): 24–30. https://doi.org/10.21859/ijpn-05064.

8. Baker, E. A., E. K. Barnidge, M. Schootman, M. Sawicki, and F. L. Motton-Kershaw. "Adaptation of a Modified Dash Diet to a Rural African American Community Setting." *Am J Prev Med* 51, no. 6 (2016): 967–974. https://doi.org/10.1016/j.amepre.2016.07.014.

9. Baltes, Paul B., Ulman Lindenberger, and Ursula M. Staudinger. "Life Span Theory in Developmental Psychology." In *Handbook of Child Psychology: Theoretical Models of Human Development*, vol. 1, 6th ed., ed Richard M. Lerner, 569–664. Hoboken, NJ: John Wiley & Sons, 2006. https://onlinelibrary.wiley.com/doi/full/10.1002/9780470147658.chpsy0111.

10. Bandura, Albert. *Social Learning Theory*. Oxford: Prentice-Hall, 1977.

11. Bazzano, L. A., T. Green, T. N. Harrison, and K. Reynolds. "Dietary Approaches to Prevent Hypertension." *Curr Hypertens Rep* 15, no. 6 (2013): 694–702. https://doi.org/10.1007/s11906-013-0390-z.

12. Beckie, T. M. "Ethnic and Racial Disparities in Hypertension Management among Women." *Semin Perinatol* 41, no. 5 (2017): 278–286. https://doi.org/10.1053/j.semperi.2017.04.004.

13. Ben, Jehonathan, Donna Cormack, Ricci Harris, and Yin Paradies. "Racism and Health Service Utilisation: A Systematic Review and Meta-Analysis." *PLOS ONE* 12, no. 12 (2017): e0189900. https://doi.org/10.1371/journal.pone.0189900.

14. Berenson, G. S. "Bogalusa Heart Study: A Long-Term Community Study of a Rural Biracial (Black/White) Population." *Am J Med Sci* 322, no. 5 (2001): 293–300. https://doi.org/10.1097/00000441-200111000-00007.

15. Bertoni, A. G., C. G. Foy, J. C. Hunter, S. A. Quandt, M. Z. Vitolins, and M. C. Whitt-Glover. "A Multilevel Assessment of Barriers to Adoption of Dietary Approaches to Stop Hypertension (DASH) among African Americans of Low Socioeconomic Status." *J Health Care Poor U* 22, no. 4 (2011): 1205–1220. https://doi.org/10.1353/hpu.2011.0142.

16. Bond, M. Jermane, and Allen A. Herman. "Lagging Life Expectancy for Black Men: A Public Health Imperative." *Am J Public Health* 106, no. 7 (2016): 1167–1169. https://doi.org/10.2105/AJPH.2016.303251.

17. Brondolo, Elizabeth, Erica E. Love, Melissa Pencille, Antoinette Schoenthaler, and Gbenga Ogedegbe. "Racism and Hypertension: A Review of the Empirical Evidence and Implications for Clinical Practice." *Am J Hypertens* 24, no. 5 (2011): 518–529. https://doi.org/10.1038/ajh.2011.9.

18. Brown, Alison G. M., Robert F. Houser, Josiemer Mattei, Dariush Mozaffarian,

Alice H. Lichtenstein, and Sara C. Folta. "Hypertension among US-Born and Foreign-Born Non-Hispanic Blacks: National Health and Nutrition Examination Survey 2003–2014 Data." *J Hypertens* 35, no. 12 (2017): 2380–2387. https://doi.org/10.1097/hjh.0000000000001489.

19. Bruce, M. A., B. M. Beech, D. M. Griffith, and R. J. Thorpe Jr. "Weight Status and Blood Pressure among Adolescent African American Males: The Jackson Heart Kids Pilot Study." *Ethn Dis* 25, no. 3 (2015): 305–312. https://doi.org/10.18865/ed.25.3.305.

20. Carnethon, M. R., J. Pu, G. Howard, M. A. Albert, C. A. M. Anderson, A. G. Bertoni, M. S. Mujahid, L. Palaniappan, H. A. Taylor Jr., et al. "Cardiovascular Health in African Americans: A Scientific Statement from the American Heart Association." *Circulation* 136, no. 21 (2017): e393–e423. https://doi.org/10.1161/CIR.0000000000000534.

21. CDC (Centers for Disease Control and Prevention). "A Closer Look at African American Men and High Blood Pressure Control: A Review of Psychosocial Factors and Systems-Level Interventions." CDC: High Blood Pressure. Last reviewed November 2, 2020. https://www.cdc.gov/bloodpressure/aa_sourcebook.htm.

22. CDC. "National Center for Health Statistics: Health Data Interactive." Accessed in 2019. www.cdc.gov/nchs/hdi.htm.

23. CDC. "Youth Risk Behavior Surveillance System." CDC: Adolescent and School Health, 2019. https://www.cdc.gov/healthyyouth/data/yrbs/index.htm.

24. Chan, Q., J. Stamler, and P. Elliott. "Dietary Factors and Higher Blood Pressure in African-Americans." *Curr Hypertens Rep* 17, no. 2 (2015): 10. https://doi.org/10.1007/s11906-014-0517-x.

25. Clark, R., N. B. Anderson, V. R. Clark, and D. R. Williams. "Racism as a Stressor for African Americans. A Biopsychosocial Model." *Am Psychol* 54, no. 10 (1999): 805–816. https://doi.org/10.1037//0003-066x.54.10.805.

26. Cogbill, S. A., V. L. Thompson, and A. D. Deshpande. "Selected Sociocultural Correlates of Physical Activity among African-American Adults." *Ethn Health* 16, no. 6 (2011): 625–641. https://doi.org/10.1080/13557858.2011.603040.

27. Coulon, S. M., D. K. Wilson, and B. M. Egan. "Associations among Environmental Supports, Physical Activity, and Blood Pressure in African-American Adults in the Path Trial." *Soc Sci Med* 87 (2013): 108–115. https://doi.org/10.1016/j.socscimed.2013.03.018.

28. Coulon, S. M., and D. K. Wilson. "Social Support Buffering of the Relation between Low Income and Elevated Blood Pressure in At-Risk African-American Adults." *J Behav Med* 38, no. 5 (2015): 830–834. https://doi.org/10.1007/s10865-015-9656-z.

29. Cunningham, T. J., J. B. Croft, Y. Liu, H. Lu, P. I. Eke, and W. H. Giles. "Vital Signs: Racial Disparities in Age-Specific Mortality among Blacks or African Americans—United States, 1999–2015." *MMWR Morb Mortal Wkly Rep* 66, no. 17 (2017): 444–456.

30. "Demographic Trends and Economic Well-Being." Pew Research Center, August 20, 2020. https://www.pewsocialtrends.org/2016/06/27/1-demographic-trends-and-economic-well-being/.

31. Dempsey, P. C., R. N. Larsen, D. W. Dunstan, N. Owen, and B. A. Kingwell. "Sitting Less and Moving More: Implications for Hypertension." *Hypertension* 72, no. 5 (2018): 1037–1046. https://doi.org/10.1161/hypertensionaha.118.11190.

32. Der Ananian, Cheryl, Donna M. Winham, Sharon V. Thompson, and Megan E.

Tisue. "Perceptions of Heart-Healthy Behaviors among African American Adults: A Mixed Methods Study." *Int J Env Res Pub He* 15, no. 11 (2018): 2433. https://doi.org/10.3390/ijer ph15112433.

33. Divens, L. L., and D. V. Carter-Holmes. "Optimizing Blood Pressure in African American Women with Dietary Approaches to Stop Hypertension (DASH)." *J Natl Black Nurses Assoc* 30, no. 1 (2019): 1–6.

34. Dolezsar, C. M., J. J. McGrath, A. J. M. Herzig, and S. B. Miller. "Perceived Racial Discrimination and Hypertension: A Comprehensive Systematic Review." *Health Psychol* 33, no. 1 (2014): 20–34. https://doi.org/10.1037/a0033718.

35. Epstein, D. E., A. Sherwood, P. J. Smith, L. Craighead, C. Caccia, P. H. Lin, M. A. Babyak, J. J. Johnson, A. Hinderliter, and J. A. Blumenthal. "Determinants and Consequences of Adherence to the Dietary Approaches to Stop Hypertension Diet in African-American and White Adults with High Blood Pressure: Results from the ENCORE Trial." *J Acad Nutr Diet* 112, no. 11 (2012): 1763–1773. https://doi.org/10.1016/j.jand.2012.07.007.

36. FitzGerald, Chloë, and Samia Hurst. "Implicit Bias in Healthcare Professionals: A Systematic Review." *BMC Med Ethics* 18 (2017): article 19. https://doi.org/10.1186/s12910 -017-0179-8.

37. Fitzpatrick, T., ed. *Treating Vulnerable Populations of Cancer Survivors: A Biopsychosocial Approach*. Cham: Springer International Publishing, 2016.

38. Fryar, C. D., Y. Ostchega, C. M. Hales, G. Zhang, and D. Kruszon-Moran. "Hypertension Prevalence and Control among Adults: United States, 2015–2016." *NCHS Data Brief* 289 (October 2017): 1–8. https://pubmed.ncbi.nlm.nih.gov/29155682/.

39. Geronimus, A. T., M. Hicken, D. Keene, and J. Bound. "'Weathering' and Age Patterns of Allostatic Load Scores among Blacks and Whites in the United States." *Am J Public Health* 96, no. 5 (2006): 826–833. https://doi.org/10.2105/ajph.2004.060749.

40. Glanz, K., B. K. Rimer, and K. Viswanath, eds. *Health Behavior: Theory, Research, and Practice*. 5th ed. San Francisco: Jossey-Bass, 2015.

41. Graham, G. "Disparities in Cardiovascular Disease Risk in the United States." *Curr Cardiol Rev* 11, no. 3 (2015): 238–245. https://doi.org/10.2174/1573403x11666141122220003.

42. Griffith, D. M., E. M. Bergner, E. K. Cornish, and C. M. McQueen. "Physical Activity Interventions with African American or Latino Men: A Systematic Review." *Am J Mens Health* 12, no. 4 (Jul 2018): 1102–1117. https://doi.org/10.1177/1557988318763647.

43. Herring, C., and L. Henderson. "Wealth Inequality in Black and White: Cultural and Structural Sources of the Racial Wealth Gap." *Race Soc Probl* 8 (2016): 4–17. https://doi.org /10.1007/s12552-016-9159-8.

44. Howard, G., M. Cushman, C. S. Moy, S. Oparil, P. Muntner, D. T. Lackland, J. J. Manly, M. L. Flaherty, S. E. Judd, et al. "Association of Clinical and Social Factors with Excess Hypertension Risk in Black Compared with White Us Adults." *JAMA* 320, no. 13 (2018): 1338–1348. https://doi.org/10.1001/jama.2018.13467.

45. Howard, V. J., M. Cushman, L. Pulley, C. R. Gomez, R. C. Go, R. J. Prineas, A. Graham, C. S. Moy, and G. Howard. "The Reasons for Geographic and Racial Differences in Stroke Study: Objectives and Design." *Neuroepidemiology* 25, no. 3 (2005):135–143. https://doi:10 .1159/000086678.

46. Jackson, S. L., Z. Zhang, J. L. Wiltz, F. Loustalot, M. D. Ritchey, A. B. Goodman, and Q. Yang. "Hypertension among Youths—United States, 2001–2016." *MMWR Morb Mortal Wkly Rep* 67, no. 27 (2018): 758–762. https://doi.org/10.15585/mmwr.mm6727a2.

47. Jones, LaShanda R., Elizabeth Fries, and Steven J. Danish. "Gender and Ethnic Differences in Body Image and Opposite Sex Figure Preferences of Rural Adolescents." *Body Image* 4, no. 1 (2007): 103–108. https://doi.org/10.1016/j.bodyim.2006.11.005.

48. Kris-Etherton, P. M., K. S. Petersen, G. Velarde, N. D. Barnard, M. Miller, E. Ros, and A. M. Freeman. "Barriers, Opportunities, and Challenges in Addressing Disparities in Diet & Related Cardiovascular Disease in the United States." *J Am Heart Assoc* 9, no. 7 (2020): E014433. https://doi.org/10.1161/JAHA.119.014433.

49. Liang, M. "Epigenetic Mechanisms and Hypertension." *Hypertension* 72, no. 6 (2018): 1244–1254. https://doi.org/10.1161/HYPERTENSIONAHA.118.11171.

50. Mahmood, S. S., D. Levy, R. S. Vasan, and T. J. Wang. "The Framingham Heart Study and the Epidemiology of Cardiovascular Disease: A Historical Perspective." *Lancet* 383, no. 9921 (2014): 999–1008. https://doi.org/10.1016/S0140-6736(13)61752-3.

51. Mansyur, C. L., V. N. Pavlik, D. J. Hyman, W. C. Taylor, and G. K. Goodrick. "Self-Efficacy and Barriers to Multiple Behavior Change in Low-Income African Americans with Hypertension." *J Behav Med* 36, no. 1 (2013): 75–85. https://doi.org/10.1007/s10865-012-9403-7.

52. Marshall, C. A., L. K. Larkey, M. A. Curran, K. L. Weihs, T. A. Badger, J. Armin, and F. García. "Considerations of Culture and Social Class for Families Facing Cancer: The Need for a New Model for Health Promotion and Psychosocial Intervention." *Fam Sys Health* 29, no. 2 (2011): 81–94. https://doi.org/10.1037/a0023975.

53. Martinson, Melissa L., Julien O. Teitler, Rayven Plaza, and Nancy E. Reichman. "Income Disparities in Cardiovascular Health across the Lifespan." *SSM Popul Health* 2 (2016): 904–913. https://doi.org/10.1016/j.ssmph.2016.10.009.

54. Mensah, George A. "Hypertension in African Americans." In *Hypertension: A Companion to Braunwald's Heart Disease*, 3rd ed., ed. George L. Bakris and Matthew Sorrentino, 383–392. Philadelphia: Elsevier. https://doi.org/10.1016/b978-0-323-42973-3.00041-x.

55. Muntner, P., M. Abdalla, A. Correa, M. Griswold, J. E. Hall, D. W. Jones, G. A. Mensah, M. Sims, D. Shimbo, et al. "Hypertension in Blacks: Unanswered Questions and Future Directions for the JHS (Jackson Heart Study)." *Hypertension* 69, no. 5 (2017): 761–769. https://doi.org/10.1161/HYPERTENSIONAHA.117.09061.

56. Nguyen, H., O. A. Odelola, J. Rangaswami, and A. Amanullah. "A Review of Nutritional Factors in Hypertension Management." *Int J Hypertens* 2013 (2013): 698940. https://doi.org/10.1155/2013/698940.

57. Niiranen, T. J., E. L. McCabe, M. G. Larson, M. Henglin, N. K. Lakdawala, R. S. Vasan, and S. Cheng. "Risk for Hypertension Crosses Generations in the Community: A Multi-Generational Cohort Study." *Eur Heart J* 38, no. 29 (2017): 2300–2308. https://doi.org/10.1093/eurheartj/ehx134.

58. Parham-Payne, Wanda. "Weight Perceptions and Desired Body Size in a National Sample of African-American Men and Women with Diabetes." *J Afr Am Stud* 17, no. 4 (2013): 433–443. https://doi.org/10.1007/s12111-012-9239-9.

59. Piercy, Katrina L., Richard P. Troiano, Rachel M. Ballard, Susan A. Carlson, Janet E.

Fulton, Deborah A. Galuska, Stephanie M. George, and Richard D. Olson. "The Physical Activity Guidelines for Americans." *JAMA* 320, no. 19 (2018): 2020–2028. https://doi.org/10.1001/jama.2018.14854.

60. Rader, F., R. M. Elashoff, S. Niknezhad, and R. G. Victor. "Differential Treatment of Hypertension by Primary Care Providers and Hypertension Specialists in a Barber-Based Intervention Trial to Control Hypertension in Black Men." *Am J Cardiol* 112, no. 9 (2013): 1421–1426. https://doi.org/10.1016/j.amjcard.2013.07.004.

61. Ravenell, J., H. Thompson, H. Cole, J. Plumhoff, G. Cobb, L. Afolabi, C. Boutin-Foster, M. T. Wells, M. Scott, et al. "A Novel Community-Based Study to Address Disparities in Hypertension and Colorectal Cancer: A Study Protocol for a Randomized Control Trial." *Trials* 14 (2013): 287. https://doi.org/10.1186/1745-6215-14-287.

62. Sotos-Prieto, M., and J. Mattei. "Mediterranean Diet and Cardiometabolic Diseases in Racial / Ethnic Minority Populations in the United States." *Nutrients* 10, no. 3 (2018): 352. https://doi.org/10.3390/nu10030352.

63. Spikes, T., M. Higgins, T. Lewis, and S. B. Dunbar. "The Associations among Illness Perceptions, Resilient Coping, and Medication Adherence in Young Adult Hypertensive Black Women." *J Clin Hypertens* 21, no. 11 (2019): 1695–1704. https://doi.org/10.1111/jch.13712.

64. Springate, I., M. Atkinson, and K. Martin. *Intergenerational Practice: A Review of the Literature*. LGA Research Report F/SR262. Slough, Berkshire: National Foundation for Educational Research, 2008. https://files.eric.ed.gov/fulltext/ED502358.pdf.

65. Taylor, J., K. Price, A. Braunack-Mayer, M. T. Haren, and R. McDermott. "Intergenerational Learning about Keeping Health: A Qualitative Regional Australian Study." *Health Promot Int* 29, no. 2 (2012): 361–368. https://doi:10.1093/heapro/das068.

66. Thomas, S. Justin, John N. Booth, Chen Dai, Xuelin Li, Norrina Allen, David Calhoun, April P. Carson, Samuel Gidding, Cora E. Lewis, et al. "Cumulative Incidence of Hypertension by 55 Years of Age in Blacks and Whites: The Cardia Study." *J Am Heart Assoc* 7, no. 14 (2018): e007988. https://doi.org/10.1161/JAHA.117.007988.

67. Tudge, Jonathan, Irina Mokrova, Bridget Hatfield, and Rachana Karnik. "Uses and Misuses of Bronfenbrenner's Bioecological Theory of Human Development." *J Fam Theor Rev* 1, no. 4 (2009): 198–210. https://doi.org/10.1111/j.1756-2589.2009.00026.x.

68. Wise, I. A., and F. J. Charchar. "Epigenetic Modifications in Essential Hypertension." *Int J Mol Sci* 17, no. 4 (2016): 451. https://doi.org/10.3390/ijms17040451.

69. Wyatt, S. B., E. L. Akylbekova, M. R. Wofford, S. A. Coady, E. R. Walker, M. E. Andrew, W. J. Keahy, H. A. Taylor, and D. W. Jones. "Prevalence, Awareness, Treatment, and Control of Hypertension in the Jackson Heart Study." *Hypertension* 51, no. 3 (2008): 650–656. https://doi:10.1161/HYPERTENSIONAHA.107.100081.

70. Young, D. R., M. F. Hivert, S. Alhassan, S. M. Camhi, J. F. Ferguson, P. T. Katzmarzyk, C. E. Lewis, N. Owen, C. K. Perry, et al. "Sedentary Behavior and Cardiovascular Morbidity and Mortality: A Science Advisory from the American Heart Association." *Circulation* 134, no. 13 (2016): e262–e79. https://doi.org/10.1161/cir.0000000000000440.

71. Young, Deborah Rohm, Heidi Fischer, David Arterburn, Daniel Bessesen, Lee Cromwell, Matthew F. Daley, Jay Desai, Assiamira Ferrara, Stephanie L. Fitzpatrick, et al. "Associations of Overweight/Obesity and Socioeconomic Status with Hypertension Prevalence

across Racial and Ethnic Groups." *J Clin Hypertens* 20, no. 3 (2018): 532–540. https://doi.org /10.1111/jch.13217.

72. Zilbermint, M., F. Hannah-Shmouni, and C. A. Stratakis. "Genetics of Hypertension in African Americans and Others of African Descent." *Int J Mol Sci* 20, no. 5 (2019): 1081. https://doi.org/10.3390/ijms20051081.

73. Zimmerman, M. A. "Resiliency Theory: A Strengths-Based Approach to Research and Practice for Adolescent Health." *Health Educ Behav* 40, no. 4 (2013): 381–383. https:// doi.org/10.1177/1090198113493782.

8

Myocardial Infarction

ANNA KUCHARSKA-NEWTON, PhD, MPH

Historical Perspective

Data from the past several decades point clearly to sustained race disparities in mortality from coronary heart disease (CHD) in the United States. Rates of angina and fatal and non-fatal myocardial infarction remain consistently higher among Black (African American) than among white and Hispanic residents of the United States.[1,2] Yet in the 1960s and 1970s, the picture was considerably different. Early clinical studies from the 1950s consistently reported a lower burden of CHD among Blacks than among whites. This was the impetus for a seminal study conducted in Evans County, Georgia, the Evans County Cardiovascular and Cerebrovascular Health Study.[3,4] Taking the lead from a primary care physician, Dr. Curtis Hames, who observed in his practice that African Americans had lower rates of CHD even though they had higher rates of hypertension and a diet high in fat, Evans County study investigators systematically examined the incidence of CHD and rates of death attributable to CHD among residents of Evans County during the years 1960–1962 and 1967–1969.[5] The study recruited participants from all county residents age 40 or older and targeted 50% of those aged 15–39 years. At the time the study began, 33.4% of Evans County residents were Black.

Study results confirmed Dr. Hames's observations and suggested that the Black residents of the county experienced rates of CHD, defined as angina or myocardial infarction, that were half the rates observed among white residents. Race differences in CHD mortality were most evident among men: white men died from CHD at a rate of 70 per 1,000, but Black men died from the same cause at a rate of 20 per 1,000. In an attempt to overcome the effect of potential survival bias on the observed rates of death attributable to CHD, an incidence study was conducted in Evans County during the years 1967–1969.[6] Results of that study were consistent with mortality data, again suggesting a greater rate of CHD incidence among white than among Black study participants.[7]

At the time, the reasons for the observed race differences in the burden of CHD were attributed primarily to a greater level of physical activity among Black residents of Evans County. This was evidenced, among other factors, by the strong effect of social class on CHD-related mortality and comparable rates of CHD observed among Black and white sharecroppers.[7] The critique of the Evans County study was its focused location in the South, which limited the generalizability of the study to other parts of the country. Nevertheless, the study was a landmark in drawing attention to differences in CHD risk among whites and Blacks and the need to ascertain antecedent factors.

Trends in CHD Burden

The patterns of mortality from the 1950s to the present suggest that the rates of CHD incidence and mortality reported in Evans County masked an appreciable increase in CHD mortality observable from the late 1940s to the mid-1960s.[8] Vital statistics data for the 35–74 year age groups suggest that this increase was most pronounced among non-white men and women, who experienced a 78.7% and 50.7% increase in CHD mortality, respectively, during that time. Compared to white men, who experienced a 28.6% increase in CHD mortality rates during the same period and white women, who experienced a 9.1% decrease in CHD mortality, these trends were dramatic, although they were not yet reflected in overall disease prevalence. Looking further in time from the late 1960s we will see a profound shift in rates of CHD incidence, prevalence, and associated mortality.

In the absence of a national CHD surveillance system, data on the incidence of CHD are more difficult to obtain than mortality data. The trends in CHD incidence presented here constitute a compilation of information gathered from longitudinal cohort studies, community surveillance studies, disease registries, and proprietary health system data. Most of the information concerning CHD incidence is available from the late 1980s; there is little data on disease incidence before that time.

Data from the surveillance of acute myocardial infarction incidence in four geographically distinct communities conducted through the Atherosclerosis Risk in Communities Study (ARIC study) suggest that from 1987 through 2008, there has been a decline in acute myocardial infarction rates among adults 35–74 years of age.[1] The overall relative age-standardized decline was 4.3% among white men, 3.8% among white women, 1.5% among Black men, and 2.9% among Black women. The greatest decline was observed during the years 1997–2008. In contrast to observations made only 20 years before the initiation of the ARIC study, rates of CHD remained higher among Black men and women than among white men and women during the years 1987–2008.

Persistent discrepancies in CHD incidence were also observed in trends in subtypes of acute myocardial infarction, ST-elevation myocardial infarction (STEMI) and non-STE-elevation myocardial infarction (NSTEMI), within a population of beneficiaries of the Kaiser Permanente health care system.[9] From 2000 to 2014, the overall percent annual change in myocardial infarction incidence was –4.75% among white Medicare beneficiaries. Among Black beneficiaries, the annual percent change in CHD incidence was –5.31% in the period 2000–2009, but only –1.05% during 2010–2014.

Using the Centers for Medicaid & Medicare Services Medicare claims for adults 65 years and older, Choudry and colleagues examined race differences in the rate of hospital readmissions within one year after hospitalization for acute myocardial infarction.[10] Recurrent hospitalization rates were overall higher among Black than among white Medicare beneficiaries. A 27.7% decline was observed among white beneficiaries, but a decrease of only 13.6% was observed among Black beneficiaries during that same time period.

Most recent statistics from the Centers for Disease Control and Prevention for the years 2016–2018 estimate a comparable rate of acute myocardial infarction hospitalizations among Medicare beneficiaries by race, with 7.9 events per 1,000 observed among Black beneficiaries and 7.5 events per 1,000 among white beneficiaries.[11] These data belie significant disparity among women, of whom 7.5 per 1,000 Black beneficiaries experienced an acute myocardial infarction hospitalization, while during that same period, 5.3 per 1,000 white beneficiaries had an acute myocardial infarction. Among men, the rates of acute myocardial infarction during 2016–2018 were 8.6 per 1,000 Black beneficiaries and 9.6 per 1,000 white beneficiaries.

Deaths attributable to CHD among adults 35 years and older, identified from the underlying cause of deaths registered in the National Vital Statistics Surveillance System from 1979 through 2017 show a persistent decline

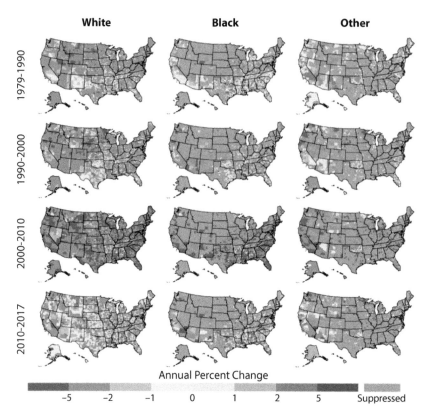

Figure 8.1. County-level annual percent change in coronary heart disease death rate by year and race, United States, 1979–2017. Reproduced with permission from A. S. Vaughan, L. Schieb, and M. Casper, "Historic and Recent Trends in County-Level Coronary Heart Disease Death Rates by Race, Gender, and Age Group, United States, 1979–2017," *PLos One* 15, no. 7 (2020): e0235839, https://doi.org/10.1371/journal. pone.0235839.

in all age and sex-race groups.[12] The relative advantage in CHD mortality observed among Black, as compared to white, men and women during the years 1979–1990 and again in 1990–2000, was reversed during the 2000–2010 period, continuing into the next decade. However, the observed overall trends in CHD mortality mask important differences by state and county. During the almost four decades from 1979 to 2017 there was a sustained shift in the burden of CHD mortality from northern states to the south, with an increase in CHD-related deaths observed among nonwhite populations in the South during the years 2010–2017 (fig. 8.1).

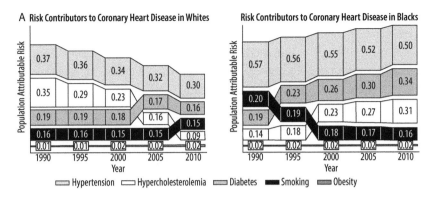

Figure 8.2. Temporal trends in the contributions of major risk factors to coronary heart disease in whites and Blacks. Reproduced with permission from W. Nadruz Jr., B. Claggett, M. Henglin, A. M. Shah, H. Skali, W. D. Rosamond, A. R. Folsom, S. D. Solomon, and S. Cheng, "Widening Racial Differences in Risks for Coronary Heart Disease," *Circulation* 137, no. 11 (2018): 1195–1197, https://doi.org/10.1161/CIRCULATIONAHA.117.030564.

Risk Factor Burden

Disparities in CHD incidence, prevalence, and mortality are reflected in persistent and widening racial disparities in the burden of cardiovascular disease risk factors. Longitudinal data from the ARIC study, which spans 21 years of follow-up (1990 through 2010), suggest that while the contribution of hypertension and hypercholesterolemia to CHD risk decreased among white men and women, those two factors gained in significance for Black men and women (fig. 8.2).[13]

The contribution of type 2 diabetes to CHD risk increased for both race groups, although the proportion of variance attributable to diabetes was greater among Black men and women than it was for white men and women. Interestingly, the contribution of smoking to CHD risk decreased among Black men and women but not white men and women. It is important to note that because the Black population of the ARIC study derives from Jackson, Mississippi, and Forsyth County, North Carolina, the findings pertain to Black men and women residing in the South. Although the burden of hypertension and diabetes is concentrated in similar geographic regions of the United States—primarily in the southern states—the prevalence of smoking is greatest in the North and the northern Midwest among Black men and women, but it is greatest in the southern Midwest among white men and women.[14]

A detailed comparison of cardiovascular disease risk factor distribution across states and regions in the United States is available from a study by Parcha and colleagues, who used Behavioral Risk Factor Surveillance System data to examine the distribution of lipid levels, hypertension, obesity, diabetes, smoking, and physical activity by state.[15] Not unexpectedly, the group's findings confirmed extant findings of high risk factor levels in the southern-most states, often described as the Stroke Belt. (The Stroke Buckle, a sub-category of the Stroke Belt, refers to the coastal plains of Georgia, North Carolina, and South Carolina.)[16] Parcha et al. also examined the prevalence of cardiovascular health, defined as guideline-established optimal levels of blood pressure, blood glucose levels, body mass index, smoking patterns, physical activity, and diet, by state and geographic region.[17] They concluded that the highest prevalence of poor cardiovascular health, which was observed in southern states, was further associated with an overall highest risk of mortality observed in Louisiana, Mississippi, Alabama, West Virginia, Tennessee, Kentucky, Oklahoma, and Arizona. This pattern was consistent within sex groups and among white men and women. Among Black men and women, the positive relationship between poor cardiovascular health and mortality that was prevalent in the southern states extended into the Midwest.

Socioeconomic Determinants of Myocardial Infarction

The literature on the contribution of socioeconomic factors to the risk of myocardial infarction is extensive, although the contribution of socioeconomic disparities to the risk of coronary heart disease is not unique to the United States population.[18,19] Nevertheless, in the United States, the combination of the polarization of the risk of myocardial infarction by race persistent disparities in socioeconomic position by race, and prevalent structural racism, presents challenges that are especially significant and warrant special attention.[20]

Both individual socioeconomic factors (e.g., education, income, and occupation) and contextual community characteristics (e.g., access to resources such as healthy food, health care, green spaces; levels of air pollution; prevalence of violence) play important roles in the risk of myocardial infarction. These factors influence lifestyle and individual behaviors that collectively determine health behaviors and outcomes.[21]

Of the individual socioeconomic factors, low education is consistently associated with an increased risk of acute myocardial infarction.[22] In the

ARIC study cohort, low education was associated with a modestly increased risk of fatal and nonfatal myocardial infarction among Black men and women residing primarily in Jackson, Mississippi, and among white women, but not among white men.[23]

Despite long-standing nationwide initiatives to improve cardiovascular health and to reduce health disparities[17,24,25] and the resulting noticeable overall decrease in myocardial infarction incidence,[26] US counties with the lowest median household income consistently lag by approximately four years in the risk of fatal and nonfatal myocardial infarction.[27] Despite regional differences in mean household income, the lack of geographic variation in this relationship makes these findings particularly relevant to the South, where the concentration of counties with the lowest median household income level and the high proportion of Black men and women is the highest.

Racial segregation compounds the detrimental effects of individual and neighborhood socioeconomic position on the risk of myocardial infarction and post-acute outcomes. According to findings from the Multi-Ethnic Study of Atherosclerosis, each standard deviation in racial segregation increases the risk of incident cardiovascular disease by 12%, even after adjusting for neighborhood characteristics, individual socioeconomic position, and risk factor burden.[28] An examination of the income inequality index based on race differences in the proportion of aggregate income derived from net earnings, unemployment benefits and income maintenance, and the diversity index, which measures racial diversity at the level of local jurisdictions, reveals persistent racial segregation in the southernmost regions of Virginia, North Carolina, South Carolina, Georgia, Alabama, and Mississippi, which have the highest rates of myocardial infarction hospitalizations.[29]

Data from the ARIC study and the Reasons for Geographic and Racial Differences in Stroke study (REGARDS) suggest that social determinants of health and of cardiovascular disease risk factor burden account for the majority of race differences in the risk of fatal CHD. Those factors, however, do not fully explain the paradoxically persistently lower risk of nonfatal CHD among Black men and women than among white men and women.[30]

Person-Level Factors Contributing to Race Disparities in the Risk of Myocardial Infarction and Post-Acute Outcomes

Socioeconomic measures, such as level of education and indicators of neighborhood socioeconomic position, are beginning to be incorporated into health care guidelines. The most recent American College of Cardiology and American Heart Association guideline recommendations for primary prevention of cardiovascular disease emphasize the importance of social determinants of health in risk of cardiovascular disease and suggest that researchers include a patient's socioeconomic and educational status in the assessment of risk.[31] Specifically, the guideline recommends the use of the Centers for Medicare & Medicaid Services tool for screening for patients' nonmedical health-related social risk factors, including housing instability, food insecurity, transportation difficulties, utility assistance needs, and interpersonal safety.[32] However, primary and secondary prevention strategies rarely address depression, loneliness, and social isolation.

Time and again, studies have presented evidence that a high risk of incident and recurrent CHD is associated with low income. However, information regarding the effect of acute and chronic financial hardships on heart health, especially among African Americans, is sparse. Data from the Jackson Heart Study suggest that although financial stress may be associated with an increased risk of acute myocardial infarction among Black men and women, psychosocial (e.g., depression) and lifestyle factors (e.g., smoking) as well as cardiovascular risk factor burden may contribute to the observed associations.[33]

The examination of dietary patterns among REGARDS study participants who did not have CHD revealed that compared to a plant-based diet, the highly calorific Southern diet, which includes high consumption of eggs, fried and processed food, and sugar-sweetened beverages, was associated with an increased risk of incident CHD.[34] The study confirmed the findings of a meta-analysis of multiple studies that sugar-sweetened beverages are the dietary element most detrimental to the risk of CHD.[35] The focus of the REGARDS study on the southern states makes these results especially relevant to Black men and women residing in the South.

Considerable differences in adherence to guideline-based recommendations for the treatment of myocardial infarction have been observed. Early extensive examination of Medicare claims conducted by the Dartmouth Institute suggests that in the South, a lower proportion of myocardial infarction patients are prescribed guideline-based medications, including aspirin and beta blockers, during hospitalization and at discharge.[36] Regional differences in in-hospital and post-acute care accentuate race differences in post-myocardial infarction outcomes. For example, a comparison of care delivered to acute coronary syndrome patients in Massachusetts and Georgia that was conducted as part of the Transitions, Risks, and Actions in Coronary Events Center for Outcomes Research and Education study[37] suggests that Black patients in Georgia receive on average less evidence-based care than whites in Georgia and whites in Massachusetts.[38]

An analysis of a national sample of fee-for-service Medicare claims provides a summary of data regarding regional variation in racial differences in the treatment for patients with myocardial infarction.[39] Whereas rates of guideline-based medication use were found to be similar between Black and white acute myocardial infarction patients in the Northeast, Black patients in the South were less likely to receive guideline-recommended medication than white patients in the South. Racial differences in the use of coronary revascularization were greatest in the South.

Reasons for the observed variation in racial differences are unclear. Attribution of those differences to region-specific symptom perceptions that may differ by race is one of the explanations suggested,[40,41] but relevant studies were small and subject to low generalizability.

Post-Acute Outcomes

Data from the REGARDS study, one of the few studies to focus on the health of populations in the South, suggest that following hospitalization for acute-incident myocardial infarction, the risk of recurrent cardiovascular events is 42% greater among Black men and women than it is for white men and women.[42] This risk difference, which is modestly attenuated following adjustment for socioeconomic status, appears to be a result of the severity of a myocardial infarction and overall health status prior to the event.

In an attempt to understand factors contributing to race disparities in post-myocardial infarction outcomes, investigators from the REGARDS study also examined race differences in the proportion of study participants with prevalent coronary artery disease who met American Heart Association/American College of Cardiology guideline-recommended secondary prevention goals, including aspirin use, maintenance of systolic/diastolic blood pressure at 130/85 mm Hg, optimal lipid levels, fasting glucose at less than 126 mg/dL, body mass index of less than 25 kg/m^2, and an exercise regimen of at least four days a week of moderate to vigorous physical activity.[43] These goals are also relevant for primary prevention. Only 1% of the study participants satisfied all seven guideline recommendations. On average, participants met four of the seven prevention goals. Black study participants were 36% less likely to achieve goals for decreasing risk factors and 33% less likely to maintain blood pressure and lipid control and use aspirin than white participants. Living in the Stroke Belt or the Stroke Buckle region was not associated with control of risk factors, but low educational attainment and low income were independently associated with low adherence to guideline recommendations. Data from the Jackson Heart Study confirm the REGARDS study's finding of an inverse association of ideal cardiovascular health with the risk of myocardial infarction.[44]

Adherence to discharge medication recommendations at one year after discharge is lower among Black patients, especially Black women, that it is for patients of other races and ethnicities; this can contribute to observed differences in outcomes.[45] However, regional data on race differences in medication adherences are not available.

Cardiac rehabilitation, an American Heart Association Class 1 recommendation, has proven lifestyle and health benefits for myocardial infarction survivors, yet its uptake remains remarkably low.[46] During 2017, 24.4% of eligible fee-for-service Medicare beneficiaries participated in at least one cardiac rehabilitation session.[47] Uptake of cardiac rehabilitation was found to be the lowest among non-Hispanic Black beneficiaries (13.6%) and those residing in the southern and southwestern states.[48] A linkage of the Get With the Guidelines data with Medicare claims for the years 2003–2009 points to the low (40% overall) rate of referral for cardiac rehabilitation as a factor that contributes to low enrollment in the program.[49] During the study period, cardiac rehabilitation referral rates were the lowest among Black myocardial infarction patients (20%).

In conclusion, despite significant advances in the prevention and treatment of acute myocardial infarction, Black men and women carry a disproportionately high burden of the disease. Differences by race in the management of the acute event and post-acute care are most evident in the South and point to the need for interventions that specifically target southern US communities at greatest risk.

REFERENCES

1. Rosamond, W. D., L. E. Chambless, G. Heiss, T. H. Mosley, J. Coresh, E. Whitsel, L. Wagenknecht, H. Ni, and A. R. Folsom. "Twenty-Two-Year Trends in Incidence of Myocardial Infarction, Coronary Heart Disease Mortality, and Case Fatality in 4 US Communi-

ties, 1987–2008." *Circulation* 125, no. 15 (2012): 1848–1857. https://www.ahajournals.org/doi/10.1161/circulationaha.111.047480.10.1161/CIRCULATIONAHA.111.047480.

2. CDC. "Heart Disease Facts." Last reviewed February 7, 2022. Accessed July 2021. https://www.cdc.gov/heartdisease/facts.htm.

3. Cassel, J. C. "Summary of Major Findings of the Evans County Cardiovascular Studies." *Arch Intern Med* 128, no. 6 (1971): 887–889.

4. Crook, E. D., B. L. Clark, S. T. Bradford, R. Calvin, H. S. Taylor Jr., B. L. Clark, and E. D. Crook. "From 1960s Evans County Georgia to Present-Day Jackson, Mississippi: An Exploration of the Evolution of Cardiovascular Disease in African Americans." *Am J Med Sci* 325, no. 6 (2003): 307–314. https://www.amjmedsci.com/article/S0002-9629(15)34262-2/fulltext.

5. Hames, C. G. "Evans County Cardiovascular and Cerebrovascular Epidemiologic Study. Introduction." *Arch Intern Med* 128, no. 6 (1971): 883–886. https://pubmed.ncbi.nlm.nih.gov/5132443/.

6. Cornoni, J. C., L. E. Waller, J. C. Cassel, H. A. Tyroler, and C. G. Hames. "The Incidence Study—Study Design and Methods." *Arch Intern Med* 128, no. 6 (1971): 896–900.

7. Cassel, J., S. Heyen, A. G. Bartel, B. H. Kaplan, H. A. Tyroler, J. C. Cornoni, and C. G. Hames. "Incidence of Coronary Heart Disease by Ethnic Group, Social Class, and Sex." *Arch Intern Med* 128, no. 6 (1971): 901–906.

8. Stamler, J. "The Marked Decline in Coronary Heart Disease Mortality Rates in the United States, 1968–1981: Summary of Findings and Possible Explanations." *Cardiology* 72, nos. 1–2 (1985): 11–22.

9. Chi, G. C., M. H. Kanter, B. H. Li, L. Qian, S. R. Reading, T. N. Harrison, S. J. Jacobsen, R. D. Scott, J. J. Cavendish, et al. "Trends in Acute Myocardial Infarction by Race and Ethnicity." *J Am Heart Assoc* 9, no. 5 (2020): e013542. https://www.ahajournals.org/doi/10.1161/JAHA.119.013542.

10. Chaudhry, S. I., R. F. Khan, J. Chen, K. Dharmarajan, J. A. Dodson, Y. Wang, and H. M. Krumholz. "National Trends in Recurrent AMI Hospitalizations 1 Year after Acute Myocardial Infarction in Medicare Beneficiaries: 1999–2010." *J Am Heart Assoc* 3, no. 5 (2014): e001197. https://www.ahajournals.org/doi/10.1161/JAHA.114.001197.

11. CDC. Interactive Database of Heart Disease and Stroke: Atlanta, Georgia. 2021 Accessed July 9, 2021. https://nccd.cdc.gov/DHDSPAtlas/Reports.aspx.

12. Vaughan, A. S., L. Schieb, and M. Casper. "Historic and Recent Trends in County-Level Coronary Heart Disease Death Rates by Race, Gender, and Age Group, United States, 1979–2017." *PLOS ONE* 15, no. 7 (2020): e0235839. https://journals.plos.org/plosone/article?id=10.1371/journal.pone.0235839.

13. Nadruz, W., Jr., B. Claggett, M. Henglin, A. M. Shah, H. Skali, W. D. Rosamond, A. R. Folsom, S. D. Solomon, and S. Cheng. "Widening Racial Differences in Risks for Coronary Heart Disease." *Circulation* 137, no. 11 (2018): 1195–1197. https://www.ahajournals.org/doi/10.1161/CIRCULATIONAHA.117.030564.

14. Loop, M. S., G. Howard, G. de Los Campos, M. Al-Hamdan, M. M. Safford, E. B. Levitan, and L. A. McClure. "Heat Maps of Hypertension, Diabetes Mellitus, and Smoking in the Continental United States." *Circ Cardiovasc Qual Outcomes* 10, no. 1 (2017). https://www.ahajournals.org/doi/10.1161/circoutcomes.116.003350.

15. Parcha, V., R. Kalra, S. S. Suri, G. Mala, T. J. Wang, G. Arora, and P. Arora. "Geographic Variation in Cardiovascular Health among American Adults." *Mayo Clin Proc* 96, no. 7 (2021): 1770–1781. https://www.mayoclinicproceedings.org/article/S0025-6196(21)00053-7/fulltext.

16. Howard, V. J., M. Cushman, L. Pulley, C. R. Gomez, R. C. Go, R. J. Prineas, A. Graham, C. S. Moy, and G. Howard. "The Reasons for Geographic and Racial Differences in Stroke Study: Objectives and Design." *Neuroepidemiology* 25, no. 3 (2005): 135–143. https://doi.org/10.1159/000086678.

17. Lloyd-Jones, D. M., Y. Hong, D. Labarthe, D. Mozaffarian, L. J. Appel, L. Van Horn, K. Greenlund, S. Daniels, G. Nichol, et al. "Defining and Setting National Goals for Cardiovascular Health Promotion and Disease Reduction: The American Heart Association's Strategic Impact Goal through 2020 and Beyond." *Circulation* 121, no. 4 (2010): 586–613. https://www.ahajournals.org/doi/10.1161/circulationaha.109.192703.

18. Havranek, E. P., M. S. Mujahid, D. A. Barr, I. V. Blair, M. S. Cohen, S. Cruz-Flores, G. Davey-Smith, C. R. Dennison-Himmelfarb, M. S. Lauer, et al. "Social Determinants of Risk and Outcomes for Cardiovascular Disease: A Scientific Statement from the American Heart Association." *Circulation* 132, no. 9 (2015): 873–898. https://www.ahajournals.org/doi/10.1161/cir.0000000000000228.

19. Banks, J., M. Marmot, Z. Oldfield, and J. P. Smith. "Disease and Disadvantage in the United States and in England." *JAMA* 295, no. 17 (2006): 2037–2045. https://jamanetwork.com/journals/jama/fullarticle/202788.

20. Lukachko, A., M. L. Hatzenbuehler, and K. M. Keyes. "Structural Racism and Myocardial Infarction in the United States." *Soc Sci Med* 103 (2014): 42–50. https://doi.org/10.1016/j.socscimed.2013.07.021.

21. Diez Roux, A. V. "Neighborhoods and Health: What Do We Know? What Should We Do?" *Am J Public Health* 106, no. 3 (2016): 430–431. https://www.ncbi.nlm.nih.gov/pmc/articles/PMC4815954/.

22. Rosengren, A., S. V. Subramanian, S. Islam, C. K. Chow, A. Avezum, K. Kazmi, K. Sliwa, M. Zubaid, S. Rangarajan, et al. "Education and Risk for Acute Myocardial Infarction in 52 High, Middle and Low-Income Countries: INTERHEART Case-Control Study." *Heart* 95, no. 24 (2009): 2014–2022. https://heart.bmj.com/content/95/24/2014.

23. Jones, D. W., L. E. Chambless, A. R. Folsom, G. Heiss, R. G. Hutchinson, A. R. Sharrett, M. Szklo, and H. A. Taylor. "Risk Factors for Coronary Heart Disease in African Americans: The Atherosclerosis Risk in Communities Study, 1987–1997." *Arch Intern Med* 162, no. 22 (2002): 2565–2571. https://jamanetwork.com/journals/jamainternalmedicine/fullarticle/754803.

24. Pearson, T. A., T. L. Bazzarre, S. R. Daniels, J. M. Fair, S. P. Fortmann, B. A. Franklin, L. B. Goldstein, Y. Hong, G. A. Mensah, et al. "American Heart Association Guide for Improving Cardiovascular Health at the Community Level: A Statement for Public Health Practitioners, Healthcare Providers, and Health Policy Makers from the American Heart Association Expert Panel on Population and Prevention Science." *Circulation* 107, no. 4 (2003): 645–651. https://www.ahajournals.org/doi/10.1161/01.cir.0000054482.38437.13.

25. CDC. "Million Hearts: Strategies to Reduce the Prevalence of Leading Cardiovascu-

lar Disease Risk Factors—United States, 2011." *MMWR Morb Mortal Wkly Rep* 60, no. 36 (2011): 1248–1251.

26. Krumholz, H. M., S. L. Normand, and Y. Wang. "Trends in Hospitalizations and Outcomes for Acute Cardiovascular Disease and Stroke, 1999–2011." *Circulation* 130, no. 12 (2014): 966–975. https://www.ncbi.nlm.nih.gov/pmc/articles/PMC4171056/.

27. Spatz, E. S., A. L. Beckman, Y. Wang, N. R. Desai, and H. M. Krumholz. "Geographic Variation in Trends and Disparities in Acute Myocardial Infarction Hospitalization and Mortality by Income Levels, 1999–2013." *JAMA Cardiol* 1, no. 3 (2016): 255–265. https://jamanetwork.com/journals/jamacardiology/fullarticle/2521458.

28. Kershaw, K. N., T. L. Osypuk, D. P. Do, P. J. De Chavez, and A. V. Diez Roux. "Neighborhood-Level Racial/Ethnic Residential Segregation and Incident Cardiovascular Disease: The Multi-Ethnic Study of Atherosclerosis." *Circulation* 131, no. 2 (2015): 141–148. https://www.ahajournals.org/doi/10.1161/circulationaha.114.011345.

29. "Exploring Racial Segregation and Income Inequality." *PD&R Edge*, n.d. https://www.huduser.gov/portal/pdredge/pdr_edge_research_032212.html.

30. Colantonio, L. D., C. M. Gamboa, J. S. Richman, E. B. Levitan, E. Z. Soliman, G. Howard, and M. M. Safford. "Black-White Differences in Incident Fatal, Nonfatal, and Total Coronary Heart Disease." *Circulation* 136, no. 2 (2017): 152–166. https://www.ahajournals.org/doi/10.1161/CIRCULATIONAHA.116.025848#.

31. Arnett, D. K., R. S. Blumenthal, M. A. Albert, A. B. Buroker, Z. D. Goldberger, E. J. Hahn, C. D. Himmelfarb, A. Khera, D. Lloyd-Jones, et al. "2019 ACC/AHA Guideline on the Primary Prevention of Cardiovascular Disease: Executive Summary: A Report of the American College of Cardiology/American Heart Association Task Force on Clinical Practice Guidelines." *J Am Coll Cardiol* 74, no. 10 (2019): 1376–1414. https://www.ahajournals.org/doi/10.1161/CIR.0000000000000677.

32. Billioux, A., K. Verlander, S. Anthony, and D. Alley. "Standardized Screening for Health-Related Social Needs in Clinical Settings: The Accountable Health Communities Screening Tool." National Academy of Medicine, May 30, 2017. Accessed July 26, 2021. https://nam.edu/standardized-screening-for-health-related-social-needs-in-clinical-settings-the-accountable-health-communities-screening-tool/.

33. Moran, K. E., M. J. Ommerborn, C. T. Blackshear, M. Sims, and C. R. Clark. "Financial Stress and Risk of Coronary Heart Disease in the Jackson Heart Study." *Am J Prev Med* 56, no. 2 (2019): 224–231. https://doi.org/10.1016/j.amepre.2018.09.022.

34. Shikany, J. M., M. M. Safford, P. K. Newby, R. W. Durant, T. M. Brown, and S. E. Judd. "Southern Dietary Pattern Is Associated With Hazard of Acute Coronary Heart Disease in the Reasons for Geographic and Racial Differences in Stroke (REGARDS) Study." *Circulation* 132, no. 9 (2015): 804–814. https://www.ahajournals.org/doi/10.1161/circulationaha.114.014421.

35. C. Huang, J. Huang, Y. Tian, X. Yang, and D. Gu. "Sugar Sweetened Beverages Consumption and Risk of Coronary Heart Disease: A Meta-Analysis of Prospective Studies." *Atherosclerosis* 234, no. 1 (2014): 11–16. https://doi.org/10.1016/j.atherosclerosis.2014.01.037.

36. O'Connor, G. T., H. B. Quinton, N. D. Traven, L. D. Ramunno, T. A. Dodds, T. A. Marciniak, and J. E. Wennberg. "Geographic Variation in the Treatment of Acute Myocar-

dial Infarction: The Cooperative Cardiovascular Project." *JAMA* 281, no. 7 (1999): 627–633. https://jamanetwork.com/journals/jama/article-abstract/188789.

37. Waring, M. E., R. H. McManus, J. S. Saczynski, M. D. Anatchkova, D. D. McManus, R. S. Devereaux, R. J. Goldberg, J. J. Allison, C. I. Kiefe, et al. "Transitions, Risks, and Actions in Coronary Events—Center for Outcomes Research and Education (TRACE-CORE): Design and Rationale." *Circ Cardiovasc Qual Outcomes* 5, no. 5 (2012): e44–50. https://www.ahajournals.org/doi/10.1161/circoutcomes.112.965418.

38. Goldberg, R. J., J. M. Gore, D. D. McManus, R. McManus, M. Tisminetzky, D. Lessard, J. H. Gurwitz, D. C. Parish, J. Allison, et al. "Race and Place Differences in Patients Hospitalized with an Acute Coronary Syndrome: Is There Double Jeopardy? Findings from TRACE-CORE." *Prev Med Rep* 6 (2017): 1–8. https://doi.org/10.1016/j.pmedr.2017.01.010.

39. Rathore, S. S., F. A. Masoudi, E. P. Havranek, and H. M. Krumholz. "Regional Variations in Racial Differences in the Treatment of Elderly Patients Hospitalized with Acute Myocardial Infarction." *Am J Med* 117, no. 11 (2004): 811–822. https://www.amjmed.com/article/S0002-9343(04)00539-X/fulltext.

40. Eastwood, J. A., B. D. Johnson, T. Rutledge, V. Bittner, K. S. Whittaker, D. S. Krantz, C. E. Cornell, W. Eteiba, E. Handberg et al. "Anginal Symptoms, Coronary Artery Disease, and Adverse Outcomes in Black and White Women: The NHLBI-Sponsored Women's Ischemia Syndrome Evaluation (WISE) Study." *Journal of Women's Health* 22, no. 9 (2013): 724–732. https://doi.org/10.1089/jwh.2012.4031.

41. Summers, R. L., G. J. Cooper, F. B. Carlton, M. E. Andrews, and J. C. Kolb. "Prevalence of Atypical Chest Pain Descriptions in a Population from the Southern United States." *Am J Med Sci* 318, no. 3 (1999): 142–145. https://doi.org/10.1097/00000441-199909000-00008.

42. Blackston, J. W., M. M. Safford, M. T. Mefford, E. Freeze, G. Howard, V. J. Howard, D. C. Naftel, T. M. Brown, and E. V. Levitan. "Cardiovascular Disease Events and Mortality after Myocardial Infarction among Black and White Adults: REGARDS Study." *Circ Cardiovasc Qual Outcomes* 13, no. 12 (2020): e006683. https://www.ahajournals.org/doi/10.1161/CIRCOUTCOMES.120.006683.

43. Drozda, J., Jr., J. V. Messer, J. Spertus, B. Abramowitz, K. Alexander, C. T. Beam, R. O. Bonow, J. S. Burkiewicz, M. Crouch, et al. "ACCF/AHA/AMA-PCPI 2011 Performance Measures for Adults with Coronary Artery Disease and Hypertension: A Report of the American College of Cardiology Foundation/American Heart Association Task Force on Performance Measures and the American Medical Association-Physician Consortium for Performance Improvement." *J Am Coll Cardiol* 58, no. 3 (2011): 316–336. https://www.sciencedirect.com/science/article/pii/S0735109711014872?via%3Dihub.

44. Ommerborn, M. J., C. T. Blackshear, D. A. Hickson, M. E. Griswold, J. Kwatra, L. Djoussé, and C. R. Clark. "Ideal Cardiovascular Health and Incident Cardiovascular Events: The Jackson Heart Study." *Am J Prev Med* 51, no. 4 (2016): 502–506. https://www.ajpmonline.org/article/S0749-3797(16)30251-3/fulltext.

45. Lauffenburger, J. C., J. G. Robinson, C. Oramasionwu, and G. Fang. "Racial/Ethnic and Gender Gaps in the Use of and Adherence to Evidence-Based Preventive Therapies among Elderly Medicare Part D Beneficiaries after Acute Myocardial Infarction." *Circulation* 129, no. 7 (2014): 754–763. https://www.ahajournals.org/doi/10.1161/circulationaha.113.002658.

46. Martin, B. J., T. Hauer, R. Arena, L. D. Austford, P. D. Galbraith, A. M. Lewin, M. L. Knudtson, W. A. Ghali, J. A. Stone, et al. "Cardiac Rehabilitation Attendance and Outcomes in Coronary Artery Disease Patients." *Circulation* 126, no. 6 (2012): 677–687. https://www.ahajournals.org/doi/10.1161/circulationaha.111.066738.

47. Ritchey, M. D., S. Maresh, J. McNeely, T. Shaffer, S. L. Jackson, S. J. Keteyian, C. A. Brawner, M. A. Whooley, T. Chang, et al. "Tracking Cardiac Rehabilitation Participation and Completion among Medicare Beneficiaries to Inform the Efforts of a National Initiative." *Circ Cardiovasc Qual Outcomes* 13, no. 1 (2020): e005902. https://www.ahajournals.org/doi/10.1161/CIRCOUTCOMES.119.005902.

48. Fang, J., C. Ayala, C. Luncheon, M. Ritchey, and F. Loustalot. "Use of Outpatient Cardiac Rehabilitation among Heart Attack Survivors—20 States and the District of Columbia, 2013 and Four States, 2015." *MMWR Morb Mortal Wkly Rep* 66, no. 33 (2017): 869–873. https://www.cdc.gov/mmwr/volumes/66/wr/mm6633a1.htm.

49. Li, S., G. C. Fonarow, K. Mukamal, R. A. Matsouaka, A. D. Devore, and D. L. Bhattet. "Sex and Racial Disparities in Cardiac Rehabilitation Referral at Hospital Discharge and Gaps in Long-Term Mortality." *J Am Heart Assoc* 2018;7, no. 8 (2018). https://www.ahajournals.org/doi/10.1161/jaha.117.008088.

9

Chronic Kidney Disease and End-Stage Kidney Disease

JASMINE T. WASHINGTON, MD,

RACHEL B. FISSELL, MD,

KERRI L. CAVANAUGH, MD, MHS,

and EBELE M. UMEUKEJE, MD, MPH

Chronic Kidney Disease Burden in the United States

In December 2019, more than 37 million Americans (an estimated nearly 15% of the US population) were living with chronic kidney disease (CKD) (Cain et al. 2019; CDC 2020; Flessner et al. 2009; Obialo et al. 2005; Ozieh et al. 2017; United States Renal Data System 2020). About 18% of African Americans are affected (CDC 2020; Cain et al. 2019; Flessner et al. 2009; Obialo et al. 2005; Ozieh et al. 2017; United States Renal Data System 2020). Nearly 90% of all Americans with CKD are unaware that they have the condition (Cain et al. 2019; CDC 2020; Flessner et al. 2009; Obialo et al. 2005; Ozieh et al. 2017; United States Renal Data System 2020). By the end of 2018, more than 750,000 Americans were affected by end-stage kidney disease (ESKD; also known as end-stage renal disease, ESRD), more than 550,000 persons were receiving dialysis, and almost 250,000 patients were living with kidney transplants (United States Renal Data System 2020). More than 35% of those receiving maintenance dialysis for ESKD are African American (Umeukeje and Young 2019). Over the last two decades, the dramatic increase in CKD and ESKD burden in the United States has outpaced that of other diseases, including diabetes, cardiovascular disease, and chronic lung disease. CKD burden disproportionately affects residents of the southern United States (fig. 9.1) (Bowe et al. 2018).

CKD is defined as an estimated glomerular filtration rate of less than 60 ml/min/1.73m^2 (Kidney Disease Improving Global Outcomes 2013). By this definition, CKD has resulted in nearly 60% more deaths in 2016 than in 2002; nearly 2 million healthy life years have been lost (Bowe et al. 2018). Each year since 2000, more people have died of kidney disease than have succumbed

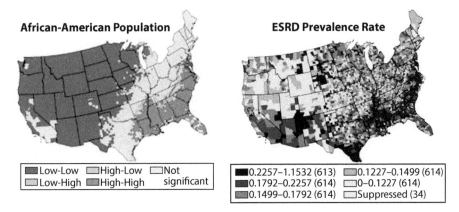

Figure 9.1. Spatial modeling of African American population and ESKD prevalence in the continental United States, 2006–2015. Reprinted from F. Bilgel, "Spatial Distribution of Inequalities in End-Stage Renal Disease in the United States," *Spatial and Spatio-temporal Epidemiology* 30 (2019): 1-1, with permission from Elsevier.

to breast or prostate cancer in the United States (National Institute of Diabetes and Digestive and Kidney Diseases 2020). CKD is independently associated with mortality and confers increased risk of death in connection with other chronic medical diseases such as diabetes and hypertension (fig. 9.2) (Bowe et al. 2018). In some areas of the southern United States, CKD disability-adjusted life year rates were more than 2 times that seen in other US regions (Bowe et al. 2018). Data from the Medical Expenditure Panel Survey Household Component Data (which is funded by the Agency for Healthcare Research and Quality) shows that CKD development is more likely among southern US residents and among African Americans than it is for other ethnic groups (Ozieh et al. 2017). The disproportionate CKD burden on residents of the southern United States, particularly on African Americans, is a concern.

Health Care Expenditures on CKD in the United States

Unadjusted health care expenditures for individuals with CKD are seven times higher than they are for individuals without CKD. Data for 2022 to 2011 shows that for persons with CKD, the expenditure is $38,000 per person; for those who do not have CKD, the cost is $5,500 per person (Ozieh et al. 2017). The cost of caring for Americans with CKD, including dialysis,

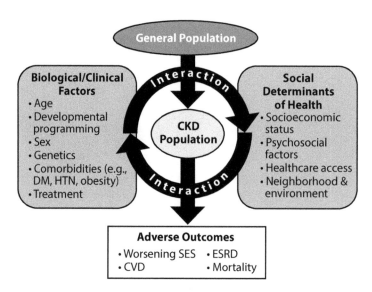

Figure 9.2. Theoretical model depicting the effect of social determinants of health and clinical/biological factors on CKD risk and clinical outcomes. Reprinted and adapted from J. M. Norton, M. M. Moxey-Mims, P. W. Eggers, A. S. Narva, R. A. Star, P. L. Kimmel, and G. P. Rodgers, "Social Determinants of Racial Disparities in CKD," *Journal of the American Society of Nephrology* 27, no. 9 (2016): 2576–2595, with permission.

amounts to tens of billions of dollars yearly (Afkarian et al. 2016). According to United States Renal Data System data, the cost of ESKD-related care totaled nearly $50 billion in Medicare expenditures in 2018 (United States Renal Data System 2020). This data also showed that the care of Americans with CKD, excluding those with ESKD, amounted to more than $80 billion of total Medicare fee-for-service spending (CDC 2020; United States Renal Data System 2020). Patients with CKD often have comorbidities, including diabetes, that drive up health care costs further (United States Renal Data System 2020). Diabetes, the leading cause of CKD in the United States, disproportionately affects minorities including African Americans (CDC 2020).

The Role of Genetics in Increasing CKD Risk

The discovery of a relationship between apolipoprotein L1 gene (APOL1) polymorphisms and nondiabetic ESKD established the role of genetics in ESKD-related disparities (Freedman et al. 2018; Norton et al. 2016;

Umeukeje and Young 2019). APOL1 high-risk variants (G1, G2) are found almost exclusively in those with sub-Saharan African ancestry. G1 and G2 variants confer survival benefit by decreasing the severity of Trypanosoma parasitic infections that cause African sleeping sickness, or trypanosomiasis (Freedman et al. 2018; Norton et al. 2016; Umeukeje and Young 2019). The presence of two APOL1 high-risk variants also confers a 7-fold to nearly 30-fold increase in the risk of kidney dysfunction in African Americans (Bock et al. 2019; Freedman et al. 2018; Ma et al. 2016). The kidney dysfunction conferred by APOL1 high-risk variants presents as primary focal segmental glomerulosclerosis, collapsing glomerulopathy, and other nondiabetic forms of kidney disease (Bock et al. 2019; Freedman et al. 2018; Ma et al. 2016). The presence of both APOL1 high-risk variant alleles, which are found in about 13% of African Americans, is associated with increased proteinuria, a 15% increased risk of CKD development, more rapid kidney function decline, greater risk of progression to ESKD, and dialysis initiation at a much younger age than is seen in whites (Freedman et al. 2018; Harding et al. 2017; Tzur et al. 2012; Umeukeje and Young 2019). APOL1 high-risk alleles are associated with a survival advantage in observational studies of patients receiving dialysis (Ma et al. 2016). However, African Americans with both high-risk alleles tend to start dialysis at an earlier age with fewer medical comorbidities than most dialysis patients, so this observation may be related to selection bias (Ma et al. 2016).

Clinical testing for APOL1 is still in its infancy, and no screening guidelines are available for clinicians. The ethics of genetic testing are complex and the clinical implications of the results are uncertain. Past events, such as the Tuskegee Study of Untreated Syphilis in African American men, have understandably led to a legacy of mistrust within the African American community. The views of the African American community regarding APOL1 genetic testing are crucial. Regional differences in the African American community's opinions regarding APOL1 genetic screening may exist. Data from a study in which two of three sites were located in the southern United States (Nashville, Tennessee and Jackson, Mississippi) show that in the context of kidney transplantation (Umeukeje et al. 2019), African Americans unanimously support the testing of deceased donor kidneys and almost unanimously support offering testing to living donors. Views related to mandatory living donor testing were divergent; only 73% agreed with testing (Umeukeje et al. 2019). Support for APOL1 testing in routine clinical care seemed closely related to its clinical application; study participants reported some suspicion about unintended harm from testing (Umeukeje et al. 2019).

Kidney Disease Risk among African Americans Living in the Southern United States

Access to Care as a Risk Factor

CKD patients with early nephrology referral have improved health outcomes (Norton et al. 2016). However, African Americans with CKD have delayed referral to nephrology compared to whites with CKD; African Americans are 2.6 times more likely to not be referred (Navaneethan et al. 2010; Norton et al. 2016). The probability of receiving any pre-ESKD nephrology care is less than 30% in the southern United States, compared to a probability of 35 to 40% in other regions (Yan et al. 2015). African Americans have lower rates of pre-ESKD care than whites do; 24% of African Americans less than 65 years old and 29% of African Americans greater than 65 years old receive nephrology care, compared to 29% and 31% of whites in those same age groups, respectively (Yan et al. 2015).

Comorbidities Increase CKD Risk

A multitude of complex factors affect risk for CKD development and disease progression (fig. 9.3) (Norton et al. 2016). For many health conditions, including CKD, African Americans experience earlier disease onset, higher rates of severe disease, and worse clinical outcomes than other ethnicities (Oates et al. 2017; Williams et al. 2010). African Americans have a higher prevalence of additional comorbidities that adds complexity to their care (Oates et al. 2017). Residents of southern states have more than twice the CKD burden than elsewhere in the United States (Bowe et al. 2018). CKD and cardiovascular disease are more prevalent in the southern United States than in other regions, and African Americans are disproportionately affected (Oates et al. 2017). CKD alone confers excess risk for cardiovascular mortality (Afkarian et al. 2016; Yan et al. 2015). Figure 9.3 shows the spatial distribution of several CKD risk factors in the United States; many are heavily concentrated in the southern United States. Multiple African American cohorts from the southern United States exhibit rates of hypertension of nearly 60%, rates of diabetes of roughly 20%, rates of metabolic syndrome of roughly 40%, and rates of CKD of 20% (Figure 9.3) (Flessner et al. 2009;

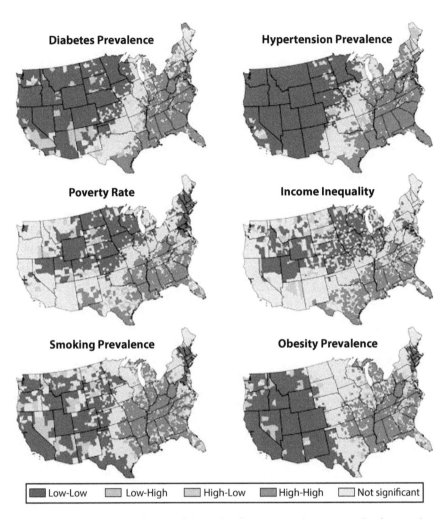

Figure 9.3. Spatial modeling of CKD risk factor prevalence rates in the continental United States, 2006–2015. Reprinted from F. Bilgel, "Spatial Distribution of Inequalities in End-Stage Renal Disease in the United States," *Spatial and Spatio-temporal Epidemiology* 30 (2019): 1-1, with permission from Elsevier.

Pike et al. 2019). This can yield a 7-fold increased risk of cardiovascular events and mortality among those with CKD alone and up to 13.4-fold increased risk for those with CKD and diabetes compared to individuals without either diagnosis (Afkarian et al. 2016; Yan et al. 2015).

African American residents of the southern United States have an increased risk of advanced kidney disease and higher CKD prevalence rates than southern whites (CDC 2020; Gatwood et al. 2018; Norton et al. 2016). In fact, African Americans have higher CKD prevalence rates at every CKD stage than other ethnic groups, and the risks grow as CKD advances (Norton et al. 2016; United States Renal Data System 2020). African Americans with CKD also suffer from higher mortality at every stage of disease than whites do (Lipworth et al. 2012; Norton et al. 2016; Plantinga et al. 2013; Peralta et al. 2011).

Albuminuria is a known risk factor for more rapid progression of CKD to ESKD. African Americans develop albuminuria earlier in life and are more likely to have albuminuria than whites even with preserved kidney filtration (estimated glomerular filtration rate greater than 90 ml/min/1.73m^2). This predisposes African Americans to greater CKD risk (McClellan et al. 2011; United States Renal Data System 2020). Even African Americans with normal kidney function at baseline without albuminuria have a greater risk of developing advanced CKD and faster disease progression over their lifetime (Gatwood et al. 2018; Norton et al. 2016; Peralta et al. 2011). This relationship persists even with adjustment for age, gender, income, education, and baseline kidney function (Peralta et al. 2011). The fact that this relationship is most pronounced in patients with normal kidney function (Peralta et al. 2011) suggests that disparities begin before any detectable clinical evidence of kidney disease is present.

Diabetes Mellitus

Diabetic nephropathy is the leading cause of CKD and constitutes 30 to 40% of CKD in the United States (Gatwood et al. 2018; Hebert et al. 2010; National Institute of Diabetes and Digestive and Kidney Diseases 2020; Wang et al. 2014). Diabetes prevalence in African Americans is consistently more than 13%; the corresponding figure for whites is 7.5% (Gatwood et al. 2018; Hebert et al. 2010; National Institute of Diabetes and Digestive and Kidney Diseases 2020; Wang et al. 2014). African Americans are 1.7 times more likely to be diagnosed with diabetes and 2.5 times more likely to develop ESKD from diabetes than whites (Afkarian et al. 2016). Using northeastern US veterans as a reference, one study showed that residents of all other US regions had increased CKD probability prior to or at the time of diabetes diagnosis (Gatwood et al. 2018). Southern residents had a 15% greater probability of CKD, which was among the highest (Gatwood et al. 2018). In the same study, CKD prevalence in African Americans in the southern United

States was among the highest, ranging from 26.6% to 45.3% (Gatwood et al. 2018).

In a cohort of African Americans in the southern United States, even CKD stage 1–2 from diabetes was associated with an up to 4% greater risk for cardiovascular disease than whites and up to 3% greater risk of stroke than whites after adjustment for sociodemographic factors and access to medical resources (Wang et al. 2014). African Americans living in the southern United States, especially in low-income rural areas, are even more disproportionately affected by CKD and diabetes (Afkarian et al. 2016). In one southern cohort study of African Americans, 16% of African Americans with low income were diagnosed with CKD and 25% were diagnosed with diabetes (Afkarian et al. 2016). The proportion of these diagnoses in upper-middle-class or wealthy African Americans was 6% for CKD and 14% for diabetes (Afkarian et al. 2016). The deleterious effects of diabetes and CKD are additive. Compared to those with diabetes or CKD alone, African Americans living in the southern United States with diabetes and CKD have a 3.3-fold increased risk of stroke, a 6.2-fold increased risk of heart disease, and a 6.4-fold increased risk of mortality from cardiovascular disease (Afkarian et al. 2016; Wang et al. 2014). As the incidence and prevalence of those affected with diabetes continue to rise in the United States, so do CKD incidence rates caused by this disease (CDC 2020).

Hypertension

CKD secondary to diabetes or hypertension is up to 12 times more prevalent in African Americans than it is in whites (Norton et al. 2016). The fact that diabetes and hypertension are more prevalent in the southern United States poses a greater threat of CKD development and progression to ESKD in African Americans living in those states than it does for whites (fig. 9.3) (Lipworth et al. 2012; Plantinga et al. 2013). Hypertension occurs more frequently and tends to be more severe in African Americans than it does in whites (Hughson et al. 2006; Lipworth et al. 2012; Seedat 1999; Selassie et al. 2011;). African Americans who are prehypertensive (blood pressures ranging systolic 120–139 mmHg or diastolic 80–89 mmHg), even in the absence of overt hypertension, have more adverse cardiovascular outcomes compared to whites living in the southern United States (Selassie et al. 2011). African Americans also have a 35% greater risk of rapid progression from prehypertension to hypertension even after adjusting for age, sex, and other comorbidities such as obesity, diabetes, and CKD (Selassie et al. 2011). This progression occurred in 50% after a median of 1.7 years in African Americans and a median of 2.7 years in whites (Selassie et al. 2011). CKD secondary to hypertension is also 5 times greater in African Americans living in the southern United States than in whites (Hughson et al. 2006).

Systemic Lupus Erythematosus and Lupus Nephritis

Lupus nephritis is one of the most severe complications of systemic lupus erythematosus (SLE), affecting 20 to 80% with SLE in childhood and up to 60% of adults with SLE (Costenbader et al. 2011; Hiraki et al. 2012; Plantinga et al. 2016). It can progress to ESKD within 15 years of diagnosis in 10 to 30% of people, even with aggressive treatment (Costenbader et al. 2011; Plantinga et al. 2016). The absolute lupus-related ESKD incidence rate has been greater in African Americans than whites since the late 1990s and has been rising steadily in recent years (Costenbader et al. 2011; Feldman et al. 2013; Hiraki et al. 2012; Ward and Studenski 1990;). African Americans have up to 6 to 7 times greater standardized lupus-related ESKD incidence rates than other ethnic groups in the United States (Costenbader et al. 2011; Feldman et al. 2013; Hiraki et al. 2012; Plantinga et al. 2016; Ward and Studenski 1990). In 2006, residents of the southern United States had standardized lupus-related ESKD incidence rates of 5.13 per million population per year, 1.5 times greater than any other US region, and these incidence rates continue to rise yearly (Costenbader et al. 2011). Increased mortality risk has been demonstrated among patients with SLE who have lower educational attainment, who have fewer financial resources, and who lack social support. African Americans in the southern United States are overrepresented in this population (Feldman et al. 2013; Hiraki et al. 2012; Plantinga et al. 2016; Ward and Studenski 1990). African Americans have increased risk of treatment-resistant disease and disease relapse in SLE (Gibson et al. 2009). Despite therapeutic advances in lupus nephritis from 1995 to 2006, one study showed no improvement in clinical outcomes for African Americans living in the southern United States who were diagnosed with SLE (Costenbader et al. 2011).

Other Types of Kidney Diseases

African Americans are at higher risk of focal segmental glomerulosclerosis than other racial groups, likely due to their risk related to APOL1

(O'Shaughnessy et al. 2017). Other glomerular diseases such as IgA nephropathy and glomerulonephritis associated with anti-neutrophil cytoplasmic antibodies are less prevalent in African American cohorts in the southern United States (O'Shaughnessy et al. 2017). Several shared risk factors for disease development and progression in heart failure and CKD have led to their increasing incidence and prevalence (Hebert et al. 2010). A recent study showed that African Americans have a 20 times greater risk of incident heart failure than whites before age 50 (Williams et al. 2010). CKD related to heart failure was seen in up to 1 in 4 patients in a recent southern cohort, and the prevalence was higher for African Americans than it was for other ethnic groups (Hebert et al. 2010). The southern United States is called the Stone Belt due to the high prevalence of kidney stone disease that is largely driven by the predominance of risk factors, including diabetes and obesity, in this region (Hsi et al. 2018). US stone disease prevalence has risen from 5.2% in 1988 to 1994 to 8.8% in 2007 to 2010 (Hsi et al. 2018). Although other ethnic groups have greater overall incidence of stone disease (Hsi et al. 2018), rates in African Americans rose 15% more in the period 1997 to 2012 than they did in other ethnic groups. This is a departure from historical data (Hsi et al. 2018; Tasian et al. 2016).

ESKD and Treatment Approaches

ESKD refers to advanced CKD that requires either dialysis or kidney transplantation for survival. African Americans are disproportionately affected by ESKD; they constitute roughly 15% of the US population but more than 30% of those with ESKD (Fan et al. 2007; Harding et al. 2017; Norton et al. 2016; Patzer et al. 2019). African Americans are more than 3.5 times more likely than whites to develop ESKD (Bergman et al. 1996; Hall et al. 2016; Harding et al. 2017; National Institute of Diabetes and Digestive and Kidney Diseases 2020; Norton et al. 2016; McClellan et al. 2011). In 2018, the unadjusted incidence of ESKD in the southern United States was 430 to 470 cases per million, a rate that is greater than in any other US region (Bragg-Gresham et al. 2020; Plantinga et al. 2013; Srinivas 2014; United States Renal Data System 2020).

Trends in Dialysis Modalities

African Americans living in the southern United States account for up to two-thirds of the ESKD population receiving dialysis (Patzer, Plantinga et al. 2014). Studies have shown that urban counties with high percentages of African American residents also have dialysis facilities that treat patients who received the lowest rates of pre-ESKD care (Fan et al. 2007; Hao et al. 2015). Less nephrology-specific care prior to dialysis may contribute to less community knowledge about treatment options such as dialysis vascular access creation, or peritoneal dialysis (PD), fewer conversations about available options, and less shared decision-making among African Americans. These factors may contribute to lower fistula prevalence rates for hemodialysis seen in African American patients and may lead to higher risk for infection-related complications and adverse outcomes (Hopson et al. 2008; Norton et al. 2016).

At the end of 2018, more than 80% of US patients on home dialysis were treated with PD. Nearly 70,000 dialysis patients were receiving PD, representing about 12.5% of the US dialysis population (United States Renal Data System 2020). US government programs, including Medicare, have recently increased financial incentives for providers to encourage PD use because it is cost effective and provides a better quality of life for some patients than hemodialysis (Wang et al. 2010). However, PD is less available in the southern United States (Wang et al. 2010), and African Americans in the southern United States are up to 56% less likely than whites to use home dialysis (Barker-Cummings et al. 1995; Harding et al. 2017; Norton et al. 2016; United States Renal Data System 2020). Data shows that 5.1% of African Americans with ESKD are treated with PD compared to 8.1% of whites with ESKD (United States Renal Data System 2020; Harding et al. 2017). US dialysis facility data from 2007 indicates that 4.7 to 5.9% of patients with ESKD in the southern United States are treated with PD, one of the lowest rates in the country (Patzer, Plantinga et al. 2014; United States Renal Data System 2020). Areas with a higher prevalence of African Americans with ESKD provide fewer PD services, which makes this modality less readily available (Kazley et al. 2014). The US government's recent focus on home therapies through the Advancing American Kidney Health Initiative may expand access and perhaps improve equitable provision of dialysis options for African Americans in the southern United States (United States Department of Health and Human Services 2019).

Kidney Transplantation

Southern states have the lowest number of kidney transplantation centers despite the disproportionate ESKD burden in this region (Patzer and Pastan 2014; Patzer, Plantinga et al. 2014). Because the supply of donor organs is limited, ESKD patients are more often managed with dialysis than with organ transplantation (Barker-Cummings et al. 1995). At the end of 2018, about 230,000 people in the United States had functioning kidney transplants, representing about 30% of those living with ESKD (United States Renal Data System 2020). About 21% of African Americans with ESKD have received a kidney transplant compared to 33% of ESKD patients from other ethnic groups (United States Renal Data System 2020). Kidney transplantation is the most cost-effective method of managing ESKD, and it provides improved health outcomes and a better quality of life regardless of the stage of the baseline kidney disease etiology (Costenbader et al. 2011; Ayanian et al. 1999).

In the southern United States, the rate is 2.3 to 3.3 kidney transplants per 100 patient years in ESKD patients receiving dialysis. This is among the lowest kidney transplant rates in the nation (Patzer Plantinga et al. 2014; Patzer Plantinga et al. 2014; United States Renal Data System 2020). About 10% of ESKD patients in the United States receive preemptive kidney transplants before requiring dialysis, but this practice is less common among African Americans, including those residing in the southern United States (Patzer et al. 2020). African Americans are also less likely than whites to receive adequate information about transplant options, be referred for transplant evaluations, complete transplant evaluations once referred, be deemed transplant candidates, be placed on transplant waiting lists once referred and evaluated, and be transplanted (Barker-Cummings et al. 1995; Norton et al. 2016; Patzer et al. 2012a, 2012b; Patzer et al. 2019). Impoverished African Americans in the southern United States are 70% less likely than whites to be listed for a kidney transplant (Patzer et al. 2009; Patzer et al. 2012a). Among African Americans listed for transplantation, wait times are longer, recipients are more likely to receive expanded-criteria donor kidneys (kidneys from older donors or donors with higher risk comorbidities prior to death, including hepatitis C), and waitlisted patients are less likely to receive a donor kidney (Barker-Cummings et al. 1995; Norton et al. 2016).

After organ transplantation, African Americans have a higher risk than whites of graft dysfunction and failure regardless of the type of donor kidney received (Barker-Cummings et al. 1995; Norton et al. 2016). Kidneys from deceased donors with APOL1 high-risk genotypes have twice the likelihood of graft failure by six years after transplant than donor kidneys that do not have this genotype (Freedman et al. 2018; Umeukeje and Young 2019). Interestingly, African Americans who themselves have APOL1 high-risk genotypes who receive kidney transplants that are not of the high-risk genotype do not have a shorter graft lifespan (Freedman et al. 2018; Umeukeje and Young 2019). There is ongoing discussion about the need to screen for APOL1 high-risk variants in living donors (Umeukeje and Young 2019). Screening may have unintentional consequences, such as insurance denials, emotional distress, lack of treatment for CKD specific to this genetic variant, and unknown prognosis regarding whether those with APOL1 high-risk genetic predisposition will actually develop CKD in their lifetimes. These potential downstream effects contribute to hesitation about making APOL1 screening a standard requirement in the kidney transplant evaluation process (Umeukeje and Young 2019).

Causes of CKD Disparities Seen in African Americans in the Southern United States

Social and Institutional Issues that Affect Access to Care

POVERTY AND EDUCATION

Poverty, which is significantly more prevalent in the southern United States than in other regions, is associated with poorer health outcomes (fig. 9.4A) (Hebert et al. 2010; Patzer and Pastan 2014). Analyses from the United States Census Bureau show a sizable wealth disparity in the South and greater poverty in the southern states than in other regions (fig. 9.3) (Rodriguez, Hotchkiss, and O'Hare 2013). African Americans in the southern United States have the lowest annual income and highest unemployment rates in the nation (fig. 9.3) (Oates et al. 2017). Low income has been associated with lower rates of pre-ESKD care (Bilgel 2019). Even among patients receiving pre-ESKD care, the presence of a higher percentage of African American residents increased the odds that patients would receive the lowest rates of care (Hao et al. 2015). African Americans who have reduced financial resources or who have completed less than a high school education have higher prevalence rates of more advanced CKD (Norton et al. 2016; Oates et al. 2017). The association between increased risk of advanced CKD, fewer financial resources, and lower educational attainment is seen more consistently in African Americans in the southern United States (Norton et al. 2016). A recent study of a southern cohort showed disparities in health behaviors by education and disparities by chronic diseases by income. This

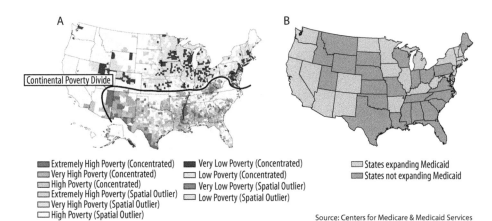

Figure 9.4. (A) County-level poverty concentrated areas depicting the continental poverty divide. (B) Medicaid expansion under the Affordable Care Act in the continental United States, 2014. Reprinted from R. E. Patzer and S. O. Pastan, "Kidney Transplant Access in the Southeast: View from the Bottom," *American Journal of Transplantation*. 2014;14, no. 7 (2014): 1499–1505. https://doi.org/10.1111/ajt.12748, with permission.

suggests that educational attainment may affect disease onset due to effect on lifestyles and behaviors and that income may have a stronger effect on disease progression (Oates et al. 2017).

FOOD INSECURITY AND NUTRITION BEHAVIORS

Dietary choices of residents of the southern United States are among the least healthy in the nation (Oates et al. 2017). African Americans who live in the southern United States have worse health behaviors than other ethnic groups (Norton et al. 2016; Oates et al. 2017). For example, African Americans in the southern United States have lower rates of fruit and vegetable consumption than other ethnic groups (Norton et al. 2016; Oates et al. 2017). Combined with a more sedentary lifestyle, these behaviors also lead to increased risk of obesity (Norton et al. 2016). The (Dietary Approaches to Stop Hypertension) DASH diet, which is rich in fruits and vegetables, improves blood pressure control in African Americans with and without CKD, even in the absence of strict adherence or direct sodium restriction (Tyson et al. 2019). The DASH diet also reduces the risk of CKD development and the rates of kidney function decline in those with pre-existing CKD (Tyson et al. 2019). Studies in southern cohorts of African Americans also noted a decreased risk of incident ESKD in those with diabetes who adhered to a low-protein diet (Malhotra et al. 2016). The fact that high dietary acid levels in diets high in protein but low in fruits and vegetables are associated with an increased risk of CKD adversely affects African Americans in the southern United States (Banerjee et al. 2018). Access to pricier but lower-quality foods with limited healthy food options in impoverished areas leads to poorer nutrition, and African Americans are disproportionately affected since they constitute a higher percentage of residents in these areas (Banerjee et al. 2018; Williams et al. 2010).

RACISM

Race relations have shaped US culture and the health of those targeted (Williams and Mohammed 2013). African Americans face various forms of discrimination in nearly all areas of their lives, which ultimately contribute to adverse effects on their physical and economic health (Ayanian et al. 1999). Racial discrimination causes health care inequity and leads to decreases in access to care and worse clinical outcomes (Williams and Mohammed 2013). Studies have shown that for African Americans, lifetime residence in the southern United States seemed to contribute to higher crude ESKD incidence rates, which was statistically significant when fully adjusted and combined with race (Plantinga et al. 2013). Efforts to improve health outcomes and access to care in marginalized groups must rapidly escalate to close gaps and eliminate health disparities in the United States (Williams and Mohammed 2013).

Health Care Institutional Issues That Affect Access to Care
PROVIDER AWARENESS, ATTITUDES, AND PERCEPTIONS

Medical providers and staff in dialysis units in the southern United States can play a major role in facilitating referrals for transplant evaluations and may represent an initial step in improving kidney transplant access in African Americans with ESKD (Browne et al. 2016; Lipford et al. 2018). However, a recent study found fewer than 20% of dialysis providers in facilities with lower transplant wait-listing rates knew about disparities in access to kidney transplant (Kim et al. 2018; Lipford et al. 2018). This knowledge gap is an area where provider and staff training and educational interventions might address disparities (Kim et al. 2018; Lipford et al. 2018). African Americans in the southern United States feel that they receive less information about managing kidney disease from their nephrologists and harbor more medical mistrust than do southern whites (Ayanian et al. 1999). Some researchers have suggested that racial concordance between African Americans patients and medical providers would support confidence in therapeutic relationships and provide clinical benefits (Tapolyai et al. 2010). However, the fact that African American physicians constitute only about 4% of the US physician and trainee work force (Norton et al. 2016) makes this challenging to implement in the near term. Therefore, it is imperative for medical providers to foster trust and build therapeutic relationships with African American patients through effective communication, timely referral to subspeciality care in nephrology, and increased patient education about the risks of CKD development and progression (Hao et al. 2015; Harding et al. 2017).

HEALTH INSURANCE

Access to health insurance facilitates access to preventive care and decreases disparities in care (Courtemanche et al. 2018; Schold et al. 2011; Umeukeje et al. 2018). Yet African Americans have some of the lowest rates of health insurance in the United States (Norton et al. 2016; Williams et al. 2010). Residents of the southern United States have lower rates of health insurance coverage than residents of other areas in the United States, and African Americans are most affected. This may be a primary contributor to the lack of pre-ESKD care (Bilgel 2019; Gatwood et al. 2018; Yan et al. 2015). Lack of preventative medical care associates with CKD and ESKD development and may account for up to 10% of disparities seen between African Americans and whites (Norton et al. 2016). The increased disease prevalence and severity that contribute to disparities may be related to the greater burden of chronic disease and greater delays in seeking medical care in this population (Gibson et al. 2009).

The Affordable Care Act of 2010 provided US states with additional federal funding to expand Medicaid coverage for low-income uninsured citizens. A 2018 study compared one-year mortality outcomes in patients with incident ESKD initiated on dialysis in states that expanded Medicaid to states that did not do so in the period 2011 to 2017. It found that patients with insurance coverage in Medicaid expansion states increased and one-year mortality declined from 6.9% before Medicaid expansion to 6.1% after Medicaid expansion in this population (Erickson, Ho, and Winkelmayer 2018).

This amounted to an 8.5% mortality reduction for patients in Medicaid expansion states and suggests that survival benefits could be even greater in African Americans (Erickson, Ho, and Winkelmayer 2018). This data compares to a 7.0% mortality decline before Medicaid expansion and a 6.8% decline after Medicaid expansion in non-Medicaid expansion states that was not statistically significant. Figure 9.4B shows Medicaid expansion in the continental United States in 2014. Even though a growing number of US states have elected to expand Medicaid since that time, the highest concentration of non-Medicaid expansion states is in the southern United States as of 2021 (Kaiser Family Foundation 2021).

Patient-Related Issues That Affect Access to Care
CHILDHOOD DISEASES, FAMILY HISTORY, AND GENETICS

In the southern United States, low birth weight is seen more commonly in African American infants (Hughson et al. 2006; Norton et al. 2016). African Americans have a 2 to 3 times increased risk of having low birth weight babies than whites do (Hughson et al. 2006). Low birth weight and decreased fetal growth associates with abnormal kidney development in utero, leading to a decreased number of nephrons and a lower kidney mass (Lackland et al. 2000; Norton et al. 2016). Low birth weight has been shown to associate with increased risk of CKD and ESKD in adulthood (Lackland et al. 2000). The combination of low birth weight and adulthood obesity increases the risk for the development of hypertension and heart disease (Hughson et al. 2006; Norton et al. 2016; Patzer and Pastan 2014). It is thought that low birth weight may be a plausible surrogate for and a reflection of lower socioeconomic status, which also predisposes individuals to an increased risk of CKD (Lackland et al. 2000).

LIFESTYLES AND BEHAVIORS

Lack of physical activity has been implicated as a major contributor to increased CKD development and progression in African Americans (Pike et al. 2019). The driver of lower rates of physical activity is unclear. Among African American patients in the southern United States with normal kidney function, physical activity was protective in lowering CKD and ESKD risk (Pike et al. 2019). This highlights the importance of preventive care and early screening in this population by increasing awareness of kidney disease risk factors and mitigating their adverse effects in order to prevent the disease or alter its course (CDC 2020).

SMOKING

An estimated 43% of Americans are current or former smokers (CDC 2020; Hall et al. 2016). While African Americans are less likely than whites to smoke, 40% of African Americans are current or former smokers and nearly 25% are current smokers (Hall et al. 2016). The southern United States has a higher number of current smokers than other areas of the country, and African American men in this region make up the highest percentage of current smokers among the subgroups (fig. 9.3) (Hall et al. 2016; Oates et al. 2017). In addition to metabolizing by-products of cigarette smoke such as nicotine (which is linked to kidney hyperfiltration) differently than other ethnic groups, African Americans tend to prefer menthol cigarettes, which have higher levels of trace elements associated with the development of kidney injury (Oates et al. 2017). Studies of African Americans living in the southern United States show a dose-dependent association between smoking and CKD progression even after adjustment for other risk factors that tend to coexist in smokers, including medical comorbidities such as diabetes and hypertension, level of physical activity, age, and educational attainment (Hall et al. 2016). It has been postulated that the greater CKD development and progression seen in African Americans in the southern United States may relate to synergy between several risk factors, including smoking, diabetes, and hypertension (Oates et al. 2017).

OBESITY

The obesity epidemic in the United States is not a new story. Obesity prevalence rates are up to 48% in African Americans compared to 33% in whites, predisposing African Americans to an increased risk of metabolic syndrome (Bruce et al. 2013; Norton et al. 2016; Pike et al. 2019). Metabolic syndrome is a group of risk factors for diabetes and heart disease that includes hypertension, elevated blood glucose, an abnormal lipid panel, and abdominal obesity (Mendy et al. 2014). Nearly 45% of African American women in the southern United States are classified as obese and have low rates of physical activity (Norton et al. 2016). Although obesity rates are higher in African American women, nearly 40% of African American men over the age of 40 are obese (Bruce et al. 2013). African American communities in the southern United States often have less access to and consume less healthy food because they live in or near food deserts (Norton et al. 2016; Pike et al. 2019). This predisposes them to increased obesity prevalence, sedentary lifestyles, diabetes, and hypertension, all of which increase the risk of CKD (Norton et al. 2016; Selassie et al. 2011). Obesity alone also increases the risk of CKD (Bruce et al. 2013; Patzer and Pastan 2014; Selassie et al. 2011; Bruce et al. 2013) even in the absence of other medical comorbidities (Bruce et al. 2013). In a study of children living in the southern United States, associations between childhood obesity and hypertension led to an increased risk of future ESKD, an effect that was noted especially in African Americans (Pike et al. 2019). Another southern cohort study showed that both overweight and obesity in early adulthood is associated with a risk of ESKD and that the correlation is stronger in African Americans than in other ethnic groups (Akwo et al. 2015). Among African Americans in the southern United States, hyperglycemia, hypertriglyceridemia, and obesity were the highest risk factors for CKD, confirming the effects of metabolic syndrome in CKD development and the importance of obesity management in preventing CKD development and progression (Cain et al. 2019; Mendy et al. 2014; Norton et al. 2016).

Psychosocial Factors

STRESS

Few studies have explored a potential association between the risk of CKD development and psychosocial factors, but this warrants evaluation, especially among African Americans (Cain et al. 2019; Norton et al. 2016). Allostatic load and repeated stressors such as institutional and interpersonal racism, mistrust of medical providers, and discrimination cause harmful health effects, including increased risk of CKD, in African Americans (Norton et al. 2016). Actual or perceived racism may exacerbate maternal-fetal stress and lead to a cascade of events that culminates in low nephron numbers and an increase in CKD risk and CKD risk factors (Cain et al. 2019). In a cohort of African Americans in the southern United States, higher stress triggered by the disparity between personal goals and attained goals was associated with 1.5 times increased CKD risk compared with those who experienced less stress even when the data were adjusted for factors such as age, sex, socioeconomic status, and comorbidities (Norton et al. 2016; Oates et al. 2017; Williams et al. 2010).

DEPRESSION

Data for depression in CKD patients varies across studies (Oates et al. 2017). A recent study that compared southern and non-southern US residents showed that African Americans experienced fewer depressive symptoms than other ethnic groups (Williams et al. 2010). Another study reports that African Americans experience lower current and lifetime depression but are more likely to experience untreated, persistent, severe, and disabling disease (Fischer et al. 2010). Advanced CKD is associated with increased depressive symptoms, especially in impoverished and unemployed African Americans (Norton et al. 2016). Symptoms of advanced CKD such as uremia can mask depression in routine screening (Fischer et al. 2010). Depressive symptoms commonly persist due to undertreatment in African American patients with CKD and ESKD (Fischer et al. 2010). It is commonly reported that people with CKD experience depressive symptoms before ESKD develops; the prevalence rate for African Americans is more than 1 in 4 (Kazley et al. 2014; Tapolyai et al. 2010).

NONADHERENCE

African Americans have a lower likelihood of adherence to disease-modifying therapies for CKD and dialysis treatment regimens for ESKD (Tapolyai et al. 2010). One study found that nonadherence among southern African Americans receiving dialysis was common. More than 85% of study participants shortened their dialysis sessions each month and nearly 30% missed one session a month (Tapolyai et al. 2010). Missed dialysis treatments lead to higher hospitalizations and greater morbidity and mortality (Flessner et al. 2009; Norton et al. 2016). Causes vary widely and can include transportation difficulty, scheduling, and mental health disorders (Kazley et al. 2014; Locke et al. 2015). Nonadherence in African American patients can also stem from denial, lack of kidney disease education on the scope and implications of this disease, financial challenges (Umeukeje et al. 2018), and medical mistrust that can lead to deliberate avoidance of medical care (Umeukeje et al. 2020). Solutions to this negative spiral exist. Shared decision-making and encouraging patient autonomy can improve the patient-physician relationship and support better adherence to medical therapy (Bock et al. 2019; Hao et al. 2015).

Interventions and Future Directions

Studies that show a higher risk of CKD development and rapid progression to ESKD in African Americans in the southern United States than in other ethnic groups emphasize the need for early preventive care (Harding et al. 2017; Norton et al. 2016) and timely referrals to nephrology specialists (Lipworth et al. 2012; Seedat 1999; Selassie et al. 2011). Careful but aggressive blood pressure control to less than 120/80 mmHg could reduce racial disparities in hypertension and CKD incidence (Yan et al. 2015). Enhanced patient-physician relationships may promote patient engagement and lead to improved adherence and outcomes (Patzer Gander et al. 2014). Strategic alliances between kidney transplantation centers and dialysis units in addition to supplemental staff education about racial disparities could help increase dialysis treatment adherence and kidney transplantation rates (Hao et al. 2015; McClellan et al. 2011). Social support for CKD patients, especially in African American faith communities, can support patient satisfaction with their care, better quality of life, adherence to medical therapy, a reduction in hospitalizations, and a decline in depressive symptoms (Patzer et al. 2019). Given the role of spiritual influences in health and lifestyle choices for African Americans in the southern United States, interventions that incorporate houses of worship as safe spaces may be particularly effective in promoting disease awareness (United States Department of Health and Human Services 2019; United States Renal Data System 2020). Efforts to diversify the nephrology workforce are also necessary (Norton et al. 2016). Culturally appropriate educational interventions related to modifying risk factors for kidney disease can provide a foundation that enables African Americans to actively engage in their care and reduce CKD incidence and progression within their community (United States Department of Health and Human Services 2019).

The Affordable Care Act of 2010 and the 2019 Advancing Kidney Health Initiative have brought new attention to CKD and the need to improve access to care (Rodriguez, Hotchkiss, and O'Hare 2013). The United States is uniquely and historically positioned to implement institutional policy changes to address the many factors that contribute to health care disparities that disproportionately affect African Americans (Rodriguez, Hotchkiss, and O'Hare 2013).

REFERENCES

Afkarian, Maryam, Ronit Katz, Nisha Bansal, Adolfo Correa, Bryan Kestenbaum, Jonathan Himmelfarb, Ian H. de Boer, and Bessie Young. 2016. "Diabetes, Kidney Disease, and Cardiovascular Outcomes in the Jackson Heart Study." *Clinical Journal of the American Society of Nephrology* 11 (8): 1384–1391. https://doi.org/10.2215/CJN.13111215.

Akwo, Elvis A., Kerri L. Cavanaugh, Talat Alp Ikizler, William J. Blot, and Loren Lipworth. 2015. "Increased Body Mass Index May Be Associated with Greater Risk of End-Stage Renal Disease in Whites Compared to Blacks: A Nested Case-Control Study." *BMC Nutrition* 1 (24): 1–18. https://doi.org/10.1186/s40795-015-0022-x.

Ayanian, J., P. Cleary, J. Weissman, and A. Epstein. 1999. "The Effect of Patients' Preferences on Racial Differences in Access to Renal Transplantation." *New England Journal of Medicine* 341 (22): 1661–1669. https://doi.org/10.1056/NEJM199911253412206.

Banerjee, Tanushree, Katherine Tucker, Michael Griswold, Sharon B. Wyatt, Jane Harman, Bessie Young, Herman Taylor, and Neil R. Powe. 2018. "Dietary Potential Renal Acid Load and Risk of Albuminuria and Reduced Kidney Function in the Jackson Heart Study." *Journal of Renal Nutrition* 28 (4): 251–258. https://doi.org/10.1053/j.jrn.2017.12.008.

Barker-Cummings, Christie, William McClellan, J. Michael Soucie, and Jenna Krisher. 1995. "Ethnic Differences in the Use of Peritoneal Dialysis as Initial Treatment for End-Stage Renal Disease." *JAMA* 274: 1858–1862.

Bergman, Suzanne, Beverly O. Key, Katharine A. Kirk, David G. Warnock, and Stephen G. Rostand. 1996. "Kidney Disease in the First-Degree Relatives of African-Americans with Hypertensive End-Stage Renal Disease Index Cases." *American Journal of Kidney Diseases* 27 (3): 341–346. https://doi.org/10.1016/s0272-6386(96)90356-x.

Bilgel, Fırat. 2019. "Spatial Distribution of Inequalities in End-Stage Renal Disease in the United States." *Spatial and Spatio-Temporal Epidemiology* 30 (August): 1–17. https://doi.org/10.1016/j.sste.2019.100282.

Bock, Fabian, Thomas G. Stewart, Cassianne Robinson-Cohen, Jennifer Morse, Edmond K. Kabagambe, Kerri L. Cavanaugh, Kelly A. Birdwell, Adriana M. Hung, Khaled Abdel-Kader, et al. 2019. "Racial Disparities in End-Stage Renal Disease in a High-Risk Population: The Southern Community Cohort Study." *BMC Nephrology* 20 (1): 1–10. https://doi.org/10.1186/s12882-019-1502-z.

Bowe, Benjamin, Yan Xie, Tingting Li, Ali H. Mokdad, Hong Xian, Yan, Geetha Maddukuri, and Ziyad Al-Aly. 2018. "Changes in the US Burden of Chronic Kidney Disease from 2002 to 2016: An Analysis of the Global Burden of Disease Study." *JAMA Network Open* 1 (7): 1–16. https://doi.org/10.1001/jamanetworkopen.2018.4412.

Bragg-Gresham, Jennifer, Hal Morgenstern, Vahakn Shahinian, Bruce Robinson, Kevin Abbott, and Rajiv Saran. 2020. "An Analysis of Hot Spots of ESRD in the United States: Potential Presence of CKD of Unknown Origin in the USA?" *Clinical Nephrology* 93 (1): S113–S119. https://doi.org/10.5414/CNP92S120.

Browne, Teri, Rachel E. Patzer, Jennifer Gander, M. Ahinee Amamoo, Jenna Krisher, Leigh-ann Sauls, and Stephen Pastan. 2016. "Kidney Transplant Referral Practices in South-eastern Dialysis Units." *Clinical Transplantation* 30 (4): 365–371. https://doi.org/10.1111/ctr.12693.

Bruce, Marino A., Bettina M. Beech, Errol D. Crook, Mario Sims, Derek M. Griffith, Sean L. Simpson, Jamy Ard, and Keith C. Norris. 2013. "Sex, Weight Status, and Chronic Kidney Disease among African Americans: The Jackson Heart Study." *Journal of Investigative Medicine* 61 (4): 701–707. https://doi.org/10.2310/JIM.0b013e3182880bf5.

Cain, Loretta R., LáShauntá S. Glover, Bessie Young, and Mario Sims. 2019. "Goal-Striving Stress Is Associated with Chronic Kidney Disease among Participants in the Jackson Heart Study." *Journal of Racial and Ethnic Health Disparities* 6 (1): 64–69. https://doi.org/10.1007/s40615-018-0499-5.

CDC (Centers for Disease Control and Prevention). 2020. "Chronic Kidney Disease (CKD). Surveillance System in the United States." https://nccd.cdc.gov/ckd/default.aspx.

Costenbader, Karen H., Amrita Desai, Graciela S. Alarcón, Linda T. Hiraki, Tamara Shaykev-ich, M. Alan Brookhart, Elena Massarotti, Bing Lu, Daniel H. Solomon, and Wolfgang C. Winkelmayer. 2011. "Trends in the Incidence, Demographics, and Outcomes of End-Stage Renal Disease Due to Lupus Nephritis in the US from 1995 to 2006." *Arthritis and Rheumatism* 63 (6): 1681–188. https://doi.org/10.1002/art.30293.

Courtemanche, Charles, James Marton, Benjamin Ukert, Aaron Yelowitz, and Daniela Za-pata. 2018. "Effects of the Affordable Care Act on Health Care Access and Self-Assessed Health after 3 Years." *INQUIRY: The Journal of Health Care Organization, Provision, and Financing* 55 (January): 1–10. https://doi.org/10.1177/0046958018796361.

Erickson, Kevin F., Vivian Ho, and Wolfgang C. Winkelmayer. 2018. "Did Medicaid Expan-sion Reduce Mortality among Patients Initiating Dialysis for Irreversible Kidney Fail-ure?" *JAMA* 320 (21): 2206–2208. https://doi.org/10.1001/jama.2018.14291.

Fan, Z. J., Daniel T. Lackland, Stuart R. Lipsitz, Joyce S. Nicholas, Brent M. Egan, W. Tim Garvey, and Florence N. Hutchison. 2007. "Geographical Patterns of End-Stage Renal Disease Incidence and Risk Factors in Rural and Urban Areas of South Carolina." *Health and Place* 13 (1): 179–187. https://doi.org/10.1016/j.healthplace.2005.12.002.

Feldman, Candace H., Linda T. Hiraki, Jun Liu, Michael A. Fischer, Daniel H. Solomon, Graciela S. Alarcõn, Wolfgang C. Winkelmayer, and Karen H. Costenbader. 2013. "Epi-demiology and Sociodemographics of Systemic Lupus Erythematosus and Lupus Ne-phritis among US Adults with Medicaid Coverage, 2000–2004." *Arthritis and Rheuma-tism* 65 (3): 753–763. https://doi.org/10.1002/art.37795.

Fischer, Michael J., Paul L. Kimmel, Tom Greene, Jennifer J. Gassman, Xuelei Wang, Debo-rah H. Brooks, Jeanne Charleston, Donna Dowie, Denyse Thornley-Brown, et al. 2010. "Sociodemographic Factors Contribute to the Depressive Affect among African Ameri-cans with Chronic Kidney Disease." *Kidney International* 77 (11): 1010–1019. https://doi.org/10.1038/ki.2010.38.

Flessner, Michael F., Sharon B. Wyatt, Ermeg L. Akylbekova, Sean Coady, Tibor Fulop, Fred-erick Lee, Herman A. Taylor, and Errol Crook. 2009. "Prevalence and Awareness of CKD among African Americans: The Jackson Heart Study." *American Journal of Kidney Dis-eases* 53 (2): 238–247. https://doi.org/10.1053/j.ajkd.2008.08.035.

Freedman, Barry I., Sophie Limou, Lijun Ma, and Jeffrey B. Kopp. 2018. "APOL1-Associated Nephropathy: A Key Contributor to Racial Disparities in CKD." *American Journal of Kidney Diseases* 72 (5): 1–20. https://doi.org/10.1053/j.ajkd.2018.06.020.

Gatwood, Justin, Marie Chisholm-Burns, Robert Davis, Fridtjof Thomas, Praveen Potukuchi, Adriana Hung, and Csaba P. Kovesdy. 2018. "Evidence of Chronic Kidney Disease in Veterans with Incident Diabetes Mellitus." *PLOS ONE* 13 (2): 1–13. https://doi.org/10.1371/journal.pone.0192712.

Gibson, Keisha L., Debbie S. Gipson, Susan A. Massengill, Mary Anne Dooley, William A. Primack, Maria A. Ferris, and Susan L. Hogan. 2009. "Predictors of Relapse and End Stage Kidney Disease in Proliferative Lupus Nephritis: Focus on Children, Adolescents, and Young Adults." *Clinical Journal of the American Society of Nephrology* 4 (12): 1962–1967. https://doi.org/10.2215/CJN.00490109.

Hall, Michael E., Wei Wang, Victoria Okhomina, Mohit Agarwal, John E. Hall, Albert W. Dreisbach, Luis A. Juncos, Michael D. Winniford, Thomas J. Payne, et al. 2016. "Cigarette Smoking and Chronic Kidney Disease in African Americans in the Jackson Heart Study." *Journal of the American Heart Association* 5 (6): 1–6. https://doi.org/10.1161/JAHA.116.003280.

Hao, Hua, Brendan P. Lovasik, Stephen O. Pastan, Howard H. Chang, Ritam Chowdhury, and Rachel E. Patzer. 2015. "Geographic Variation and Neighborhood Factors Are Associated with Low Rates of Pre-End-Stage Renal Disease Nephrology Care." *Kidney International* 88 (3): 614–621. https://doi.org/10.1038/ki.2015.118.

Harding, Kimberly, Tesfaye B. Mersha, Fern J. Webb, Joseph A. Vassalotti, and Susanne B. Nicholas. 2017. "Current State and Future Trends to Optimize the Care of African Americans with End-Stage Renal Disease." *American Journal of Nephrology* 46 (2): 156–164. https://doi.org/10.1159/000479479.

Hebert, Kathy, Andre Dias, Maria Carolina Delgado, Emiliana Franco, Leonardo Tamariz, Dylan Steen, Patrick Trahan, Brittny Major, and Lee M. Arcement. 2010. "Epidemiology and Survival of the Five Stages of Chronic Kidney Disease in a Systolic Heart Failure Population." *European Journal of Heart Failure* 12 (8): 861–865. https://doi.org/10.1093/eurjhf/hfq077.

Hiraki, Linda T., Candace H. Feldman, Jun Liu, Graciela S. Alarcón, Michael A. Fischer, Wolfgang C. Winkelmayer, and Karen H. Costenbader. 2012. "Prevalence, Incidence, and Demographics of Systemic Lupus Erythematosus and Lupus Nephritis From 2000 to 2004 Among Children in the US Medicaid Beneficiary Population." *Arthritis and Rheumatism* 64 (8): 2669–2676. https://doi.org/10.1002/art.34472.

Hopson, Sari, Diane Frankenfield, Michael Rocco, and William McClellan. 2008. "Variability in Reasons for Hemodialysis Catheter Use by Race, Sex, and Geography: Findings From the ESRD Clinical Performance Measures Project." *American Journal of Kidney Diseases* 52 (4): 753–760. https://doi.org/10.1053/j.ajkd.2008.04.007.

Hsi, Ryan S., Edmond K. Kabagambe, Xiang Shu, Xijing Han, Nicole L. Miller, and Loren Lipworth. 2018. "Race- and Sex-Related Differences in Nephrolithiasis Risk among Blacks and Whites in the Southern Community Cohort Study." *Urology* 118 (August): 36–42. https://doi.org/10.1016/j.urology.2018.04.036.

Hughson, M. D., R. Douglas-Denton, J. F. Bertram, and W. E. Hoy. 2006. "Hypertension,

Glomerular Number, and Birth Weight in African Americans and White Subjects in the Southeastern United States." *Kidney International* 69 (4): 671–678. https://doi.org/10.1038/sj.ki.5000041.

Kaiser Family Foundation. 2021. "Status of State Medicaid Expansion Decisions: Interactive Map." https://www.kff.org/medicaid/issue-brief/status-of-state-medicaid-expansion-decisions-interactive-map/.

Kazley, Abby S, Emily E. Johnson, Kit N. Simpson, Kenneth D. Chavin, and Prabhakar Baliga. 2014. "Health Care Provider Perception of Chronic Kidney Disease: Knowledge and Behavior among African American Patients." *BMC Nephrology* 15 (1): 1–15. http://www.biomedcentral.com/1471-2369/15/112.

Kidney Disease Improving Global Outcomes. 2013. "KDIGO 2012 Clinical Practice Guideline for the Evaluation and Management of Chronic Kidney Disease." *Kidney International Supplements* 3 (1): 1–150. https://kdigo.org/wp-content/uploads/2017/02/KDIGO_2012_CKD_GL.pdf.

Kim, Joyce J., Mohua Basu, Laura Plantinga, Stephen O. Pastan, Sumit Mohan, Kayla Smith, Taylor Melanson, Cam Escoffery, and Rachel E. Patzer. 2018. "Awareness of Racial Disparities in Kidney Transplantation among Health Care Providers in Dialysis Facilities." *Clinical Journal of the American Society of Nephrology* 13 (5): 772–781. https://doi.org/10.2215/CJN.09920917.

Lackland, Daniel T., Holly E. Bendall, Clive Osmond, Brent M. Egan, and David J. P. Barker. 2000. "Low Birth Weights Contribute to the High Rates of Early-Onset Chronic Renal Failure in the Southeastern United States." *Archives of Internal Medicine* 160 (10): 1472–1476. https://doi.org/10.1001/archinte.160.10.1472.

Lipford, Kristie J., Laura McPherson, Reem Hamoda, Teri Browne, Jennifer C. Gander, Stephen O. Pastan, and Rachel E. Patzer. 2018. "Dialysis Facility Staff Perceptions of Racial, Gender, and Age Disparities in Access to Renal Transplantation." *BMC Nephrology* 19 (1): 1–11. https://doi.org/10.1186/s12882-017-0800-6.

Lipworth, Loren, Michael T. Mumma, Kerri L. Cavanaugh, Todd L. Edwards, T. Alp Ikizler, Robert E. Tarone, Joseph K. McLaughlin, and William J. Blot. 2012. "Incidence and Predictors of End Stage Renal Disease among Low-Income Blacks and Whites." *PLOS ONE* 7 (10): 1–7.

Locke, Jayme E., Haiyan Qu, Richard Shewchuk, Roslyn B. Mannon, Robert Gaston, Dorry L. Segev, Elinor C. Mannon, and Michelle Y. Martin. 2015. "Identification of Strategies to Facilitate Organ Donation among African Americans Using the Nominal Group Technique." *Clinical Journal of the American Society of Nephrology* 10 (2): 286–293. https://doi.org/10.2215/CJN.05770614.

Ma, Lijun, Carl D. Langefeld, Mary E. Comeau, Jason A. Bonomo, Michael V. Rocco, John M. Burkart, Jasmin Divers, Nicholette D. Palmer, Pamela J. Hicks, et al. 2016. "APOL1 Renal-Risk Genotypes Associate with Longer Hemodialysis Survival in Prevalent Nondiabetic African American Patients with End-Stage Renal Disease." *Kidney International* 90 (2): 389–395. https://doi.org/10.1016/j.kint.2016.02.032.

Malhotra, R., K. L. Cavanaugh, W. J. Blot, T. A. Ikizler, L. Lipworth, and E. K. Kabagambe. 2016. "Higher Protein Intake Is Associated with Increased Risk for Incident End-Stage Renal Disease among Blacks with Diabetes in the Southern Community Cohort Study."

Nutrition, Metabolism and Cardiovascular Diseases 26 (12): 1079–1087. https://doi.org/10 .1016/j.numecd.2016.07.009.

McClellan, William M., David G. Warnock, Suzanne Judd, Paul Muntner, Reshma Kewalra- mani, Mary Cushman, Leslie A. McClure, Britt B. Newsome, and George Howard. 2011. "Albuminuria and Racial Disparities in the Risk for ESRD." *Journal of the American Soci- ety of Nephrology* 22 (9): 1721–1728. https://doi.org/10.1681/ASN.2010101085.

Mendy, Vincent L., Mario J. Azevedo, Daniel F. Sarpong, Sylvia E. Rosas, Olugbemiga T. Ekundayo, Jung Hye Sung, Azad R. Bhuiyan, Brenda C. Jenkins, and Clifton Addison. 2014. "The Association between Individual and Combined Components of Metabolic Syndrome and Chronic Kidney Disease among African Americans: The Jackson Heart Study." *PLOS ONE* 9 (7): 1–7. https://doi.org/10.1371/journal.pone.0101610.

National Institute of Diabetes and Digestive and Kidney Diseases. 2020. "Kidney Disease Statistics for the United States." https://www.niddk.nih.gov/health-information/health -statistics/kidney-disease.

Navaneethan, S. D., P. Kandula, V. Jeevanantham, J. V. Nally, and S. E. Liebman. 2010. "Re- ferral Patterns of Primary Care Physicians for Chronic Kidney Disease in General Pop- ulation and Geriatric Patients." *Clinical Nephrology* 73 (4): 260–267.

Norton, Jenna M., Marva M. Moxey-Mims, Paul W. Eggers, Andrew S. Narva, Robert A. Star, Paul L. Kimmel, and Griffin P. Rodgers. 2016. "Social Determinants of Racial Dis- parities in CKD." *Journal of the American Society of Nephrology* 27 (9): 2576–2595. https:// doi.org/10.1681/ASN.2016010027.

Oates, Gabriela R., Bradford E. Jackson, Edward E. Partridge, Karan P. Singh, Mona N. Fouad, and Sejong Bae. 2017. "Sociodemographic Patterns of Chronic Disease: How the Mid-South Region Compares to the Rest of the Country." *American Journal of Preven- tive Medicine* 52 (1): S31–S39. https://doi.org/10.1016/j.amepre.2016.09.004.

Obialo, Chamberlain I., Elizabeth O. Ofili, Alexander Quarshie, and Phyllis C. Martin. 2005. "Ultralate Referral and Presentation for Renal Replacement Therapy: Socioeconomic Implications." *American Journal of Kidney Diseases* 46 (5): 891–886. https://doi.org/10 .1053/j.ajkd.2005.08.003.

O'Shaughnessy, Michelle M., Susan L. Hogan, Caroline J. Poulton, Ronald J. Falk, Harsha- ran K. Singh, Volker Nickeleit, and J. Charles Jennette. 2017. "Temporal and Demo- graphic Trends in Glomerular Disease Epidemiology in the Southeastern United States, 1986–2015." *Clinical Journal of the American Society of Nephrology* 12 (4): 614–623. https:// doi.org/10.2215/CJN.10871016.

Ozieh, Mukoso N., Kinfe G. Bishu, Clara E. Dismuke, and Leonard E. Egede. 2017. "Trends in Healthcare Expenditure in United States Adults with Chronic Kidney Disease: 2002– 2011." *BMC Health Services Research* 17 (1): 1–9. https://doi.org/10.1186/s12913-017-2303-3.

Patzer, R. E., and S. O. Pastan. 2014. "Kidney Transplant Access in the Southeast: View from the Bottom." *American Journal of Transplantation* 14 (7): 1499–1505. https://doi.org/10 .1111/ajt.12748.

Patzer, R. E., L. Plantinga, J. Krisher, and S. O. Pastan. 2014. "Dialysis Facility and Network Factors Associated with Low Kidney Transplantation Rates among United States Dial- ysis Facilities." *American Journal of Transplantation* 14 (7): 1562–1572. https://doi.org /10.1111/ajt.12749.

Patzer, Rachel E., Sandra Amaral, Haimanot Wasse, Nataliya Volkova, David Kleinbaum, and William M. McClellan. 2009. "Neighborhood Poverty and Racial Disparities in Kidney Transplant Waitlisting." *Journal of the American Society of Nephrology* 20 (6): 1333–1340. https://doi.org/10.1681/ASN.2008030335.

Patzer, Rachel E., Jennifer Gander, Leighann Sauls, M. Ahinee Amamoo, Jenna Krisher, Laura L. Mulloy, Eric Gibney, Teri Browne, Laura Plantinga, and Stephen O. Pastan. 2014. "The RaDIANT Community Study Protocol: Community-Based Participatory Research for Reducing Disparities in Access to Kidney Transplantation." *BMC Nephrology* 15 (1): 1–12. https://doi.org/10.1186/1471-2369-15-171.

Patzer, Rachel E., Laura McPherson, Nakeva Redmond, Derek DuBay, Carlos Zayas, Erica Hartmann, Laura Mulloy, Jennie Perryman, Stephen Pastan, and Kimberly Jacob Arriola. 2019. "A Culturally Sensitive Web-Based Intervention to Improve Living Donor Kidney Transplant among African Americans." *Kidney International Reports* 4 (9): 1285–1295. https://doi.org/10.1016/j.ekir.2019.05.771.

Patzer, Rachel E., Laura McPherson, Zhensheng Wang, Laura C. Plantinga, Sudeshna Paul, Matthew Ellis, Derek A. DuBay, Joshua Wolf, Amber Reeves-Daniel, et al. 2020. "Dialysis Facility Referral and Start of Evaluation for Kidney Transplantation among Patients Treated with Dialysis in the Southeastern United States." *American Journal of Transplantation* 20 (8): 2113–2125. https://doi.org/10.1111/ajt.15791.

Patzer, Rachel E., Jennie P. Perryman, Stephen Pastan, Sandra Amaral, Julie A. Gazmararian, Mitch Klein, Nancy Kutner, and William M. McClellan. 2012a. "Impact of a Patient Education Program on Disparities in Kidney Transplant Evaluation." *Clinical Journal of the American Society of Nephrology* 7 (4): 648–655. https://doi.org/10.2215/CJN.10071011.

Patzer, R. E., J. P. Perryman, J. D. Schrager, S. Pastan, S. Amaral, J. A. Gazmararian, M. Klein, N. Kutner, and W. M. McClellan. 2012a. "The Role of Race and Poverty on Steps to Kidney Transplantation in the Southeastern United States." *American Journal of Transplantation* 12 (2): 358–368. https://doi.org/10.1111/j.1600-6143.2011.03927.x.

Peralta, Carmen A., Ronit Katz, Ian DeBoer, Joachim Ix, Mark Sarnak, Holly Kramer, David Siscovick, Steven Shea, Moyses Szklo, and Michael Shlipak. 2011. "Racial and Ethnic Differences in Kidney Function Decline among Persons without Chronic Kidney Disease." *Journal of the American Society of Nephrology* 22 (7): 1327–1334. https://doi.org/10.1681/ASN.2010090960.

Pike, Mindy, Jacob Taylor, Edmond Kabagambe, Thomas G. Stewart, Cassianne Robinson-Cohen, Jennifer Morse, Elvis Akwo, Khaled Abdel-Kader, Edward D. Siew, et al. 2019. "The Association of Exercise and Sedentary Behaviours with Incident End-Stage Renal Disease: The Southern Community Cohort Study." *BMJ Open* 9 (8): 1–9. https://doi.org/10.1136/bmjopen-2019-030661.

Plantinga, Laura, Virginia J. Howard, Suzanne Judd, Paul Muntner, Rikki Tanner, Dana Rizk, Daniel T. Lackland, David G. Warnock, George Howard, and William M. McClellan. 2013. "Association of Duration of Residence in the Southeastern United States with Chronic Kidney Disease May Differ by Race: The REasons for Geographic and Racial Differences in Stroke (REGARDS). Cohort Study." *International Journal of Health Geographics* 12 (March): 1–12. https://doi.org/10.1186/1476-072X-12-17.

Plantinga, Laura, S. Sam Lim, Rachel Patzer, William McClellan, Michael Kramer, Mitchel Klein, Stephen Pastan, Caroline Gordon, Charles Helmick, and Cristina Drenkard. 2016. "Incidence of End-Stage Renal Disease among Newly Diagnosed Systemic Lupus Erythematosus Patients: The Georgia Lupus Registry." *Arthritis Care & Research* 68 (3): 357–365. https://doi.org/10.1002/acr.22685.

Rodriguez, Rudolph A., John R. Hotchkiss, and Ann M. O'Hare. 2013. "Geographic Information Systems and Chronic Kidney Disease: Racial Disparities, Rural Residence and Forecasting." *Journal of Nephrology* 26 (1): 3–15. https://doi.org/10.5301/jn.5000225.

Schold, Jesse D., Jon A. Gregg, Jeffrey S. Harman, Allyson G. Hall, Pamela R. Patton, and Herwig Ulf Meier-Kriesche. 2011. "Barriers to Evaluation and Wait Listing for Kidney Transplantation." *Clinical Journal of the American Society of Nephrology* 6 (7): 1760–1767. https://doi.org/10.2215/CJN.08620910.

Seedat, Y. K. 1999. "Improvement in Treatment of Hypertension Has Not Reduced Incidence of End-Stage Renal Disease." *Journal of Human Hypertension* 13: 747–751. https://doi.org/10.1038/sj.jhh.1000911.

Selassie, Anbesaw, C. Shaun Wagner, Marilyn L. Laken, M. Lafrance Ferguson, Keith C. Ferdinand, and Brent M. Egan. 2011. "Progression Is Accelerated From Prehypertension to Hypertension in Blacks." *Hypertension* 58 (4): 579–587. https://doi.org/10.1161/HYPERTENSIONAHA.111.177410.

Srinivas, T. R. 2014. "Kidney Transplant Access in the Southeastern United States: The Need for a Top-Down Transformation." *American Journal of Transplantation* 14 (7): 1506–1511. https://doi.org/10.1111/ajt.12747.

Tapolyai, Mihály, Tibor Fülöp, Aşkin Uysal, Zsolt Lengvárszky, Tibor Szarvas, Kathleen Ballard, and Neville R Dossabhoy. 2010. "Regional Differences in Nonadherence to Dialysis among Southern Dialysis Patients: A Comparative Cross-Sectional Study to the Dialysis Outcomes and Practice Patterns Study." *American Journal of the Medical Sciences* 339 (6): 516–518. https://doi.org/10.1097/MAJ.0b013e3181d94f7a.

Tasian, Gregory E., Michelle E. Ross, Lihai Song, David J. Sas, Ron Keren, Michelle R. Denburg, David I. Chu, Lawrence Copelovitch, Christopher S. Saigal, and Susan L. Furth. 2016. "Annual Incidence of Nephrolithiasis among Children and Adults in South Carolina from 1997 to 2012." *Clinical Journal of the American Society of Nephrology* 11 (3): 488–496. https://doi.org/10.2215/CJN.07610715.

Tyson, Crystal C., Clemontina A. Davenport, Pao Hwa Lin, Julia J. Scialla, Rasheeda Hall, Clarissa J. Diamantidis, Joseph Lunyera, Nrupen Bhavsar, Casey M. Rebholz, et al. 2019. "DASH Diet and Blood Pressure among Black Americans with and without CKD: The Jackson Heart Study." *American Journal of Hypertension* 32 (10): 975–982. https://doi.org/10.1093/ajh/hpz090.

Tzur, Shay, Saharon Rosset, Karl Skorecki, and Walter G. Wasser. 2012. "APOL1 Allelic Variants Are Associated with Lower Age of Dialysis Initiation and Thereby Increased Dialysis Vintage in African and Hispanic Americans with Non-Diabetic End-Stage Kidney Disease." *Nephrology Dialysis Transplantation* 27 (4): 1498–1505. https://doi.org/10.1093/ndt/gfr796.

Umeukeje, Ebele M., Rabia Osman, Arie L. Nettles, Kenneth A. Wallston, and Kerri L. Cavanaugh. 2020. "Provider Attitudes and Support of Patients' Autonomy for Phosphate Binder Medication Adherence in ESRD." *Journal of Patient Experience* 7 (5): 708–712. https://doi.org/10.1177/2374373519883502.

Umeukeje, Ebele M., Marcus G. Wild, Saugar Maripuri, Teresa Davidson, Margaret Rutherford, Khaled Abdel-Kader, Julia Lewis, Consuelo H. Wilkins, and Kerri Cavanaugh. 2018. "Black Americans' Perspectives of Barriers and Facilitators of Community Screening for Kidney Disease." *Clinical Journal of the American Society of Nephrology* 13 (4): 551–559. https://doi.org/10.2215/CJN.07580717.

Umeukeje, Ebele M., and Bessie A. Young. 2019. "Genetics and ESKD Disparities in African Americans." *American Journal of Kidney Diseases* 74 (6): 811–821. https://doi.org/10.1053/j.ajkd.2019.06.006.

Umeukeje, Ebele M., Bessie A. Young, Stephanie M. Fullerton, Kerri Cavanaugh, Delia Owens, James G. Wilson, Wylie Burke, and Erika Blacksher. 2019. "You Are Just Now Telling Us About This? African American Perspectives of Testing for Genetic Susceptibility to Kidney Disease." *Journal of the American Society of Nephrology* 30 (4): 526–530. https://doi.org/10.1681/ASN.2018111091.

United States Department of Health and Human Services. 2019. "Advancing American Kidney Health." https://aspe.hhs.gov/pdf-report/advancing-american-kidney-health.

United States Renal Data System. 2020. "USRDS Annual Data Report: Epidemiology of Kidney Disease in the United States." https://adr.usrds.org/2020.

Wang, Virginia, Shoou Yih D. Lee, Uptal D. Patel, Bryan J. Weiner, Thomas C. Ricketts, and Morris Weinberger. 2010. "Geographic and Temporal Trends in Peritoneal Dialysis Services in the United States between 1995 and 2003." *American Journal of Kidney Diseases* 55 (6): 1079–1087. https://doi.org/10.1053/j.ajkd.2010.01.022.

Wang, Yujie, Peter T. Katzmarzyk, Ronald Horswell, Wenhui Zhao, Jolene Johnson, and Gang Hu. 2014. "Kidney Function and the Risk of Cardiovascular Disease in Patients with Type 2 Diabetes." *Kidney International* 85 (5): 1192–1199. https://doi.org/10.1038/ki.2013.396.

Ward, Michael M., and Stephanie Studenski. 1990. "Clinical Manifestations of Systemic Lupus Erythematosus Identification of Racial and Socioeconomic Influences." *Archives of Internal Medicine* 150 (4): 849–853.

Williams, David R., and Selina A. Mohammed. 2013. "Racism and Health II: A Needed Research Agenda for Effective Interventions." *American Behavioral Scientist* 57 (8): 1200–1226.

Williams, David R., Selina A. Mohammed, Jacinta Leavell, and Chiquita Collins. 2010. "Race, Socioeconomic Status, and Health: Complexities, Ongoing Challenges, and Research Opportunities." *Annals of the New York Academy of Sciences* 1186: 69–101. https://doi.org/10.1111/j.1749-6632.2009.05339.x.

Yan, Guofen, Alfred K. Cheung, Tom Greene, Alison J. Yu, M. Norman Oliver, Wei Yu, Jennie Z. Ma, and Keith C. Norris. 2015. "Interstate Variation in Receipt of Nephrologist Care in US Patients Approaching ESRD: Race, Age, and State Characteristics." *Clinical Journal of the American Society of Nephrology* 10 (11): 1979–1788. https://doi.org/10.2215/CJN.02800315.

10

Diabetes

MARIANNE K. WILSON, MD,

AUNDREA E. LOFTLEY, MD,

KELLY J. HUNT, PhD,

CAROLYN M. JENKINS, DrPH, MSN, MS, RN, RD, LD, FAAN,

and KATHIE L. HERMAYER, MD, MS

Diabetes is a disease that causes hyperglycemia due to absolute or relative insulin deficiency. The Centers for Disease Control and Prevention (CDC) lists diabetes as the seventh highest cause of death in the United States. The annual costs of diabetes are high; in 2017, the estimated annual cost of diabetes, including direct and indirect costs, was $327 billion (American Diabetes Association 2018, 917). Studies have demonstrated that African Americans are at particularly higher risk for type 2 diabetes and its complications. This is cause for concern given the morbidity and mortality of diabetes. This chapter will address data regarding the incidence and complications of diabetes among African Americans, factors contributing to this increased risk, and the research that is currently being done to help lower the diabetes burden.

Classification and Diagnostic Criteria

Diabetes is classified as type 1 diabetes, type 2 diabetes, gestational diabetes, or other causes of diabetes, including monogenic diabetes syndromes, drug-induced diabetes, and pancreatic diabetes (in the context of pancreatitis or cystic fibrosis). Type 2 diabetes accounts for 90–95% of all diabetes cases (CDC 2020b, 1). Diagnostic criteria for diabetes include fasting plasma glucose $\geq$ 126 mg/dL (7.0 mmol/L), two-hour post-prandial glucose $\geq$ 200 mg/dL (11.1 mmol/L) during 75 g oral glucose tolerance test, hemoglobin A1C $\geq$ 6.5% (48 mmol/mol), or random plasma glucose $\geq$ 200 mg/dL (11.1 mmol/L) with symptoms of hyperglycemia or hyperglycemic crisis (American Diabetes Association 2020a).

Risk Factors for Diabetes in African Americans in the Southern United States

Historically, African Americans have been recognized as a population with a higher risk for diabetes, largely due to their increased risk of type 2 diabetes (Marshall 2005, 734). In 2020, the CDC estimated the prevalence of diabetes to be 13.3% in Black non-Hispanic American adults and 9.4% in white, non-Hispanic American adults (CDC 2020b, 2). While type 2 diabetes accounts for the overwhelming majority of diabetes cases and is more common in Black non-Hispanic American adults, type 1 diabetes is more common in white non-Hispanic American adults than in Black non-Hispanic American adults.

In the southern US states, diabetes and rates of complications and hospitalizations in African Americans are higher than in most other areas of the US. In the early 20th century, many of the southern states had significantly higher levels of diabetes than many of the other states. In 2011, Barker and colleagues identified portions of Alabama, Arkansas, Florida, Georgia, Kentucky, Louisiana, North Carolina, Ohio, Pennsylvania, South Carolina, Tennessee, Texas, Virginia, and West Virginia and the entire state of Mississippi as the Diabetes Belt, a geographic area with higher rates of diabetes, particularly among African Americans (Barker et al. 2011, 436–437). The prevalence of diabetes in the Diabetes Belt was 11.7% (95% CI = 11.4%, 12.0%) while prevalence in the remainder of the United States was 8.5% (95% CI = 8.3%, 8.6%). The authors attributed the reasons for the increased prevalence to a sedentary lifestyle and obesity and to the high percentage of African Americans living in the area (Barker et al. 2011, 438).

In 2017, the hospitalization rates for uncontrolled diabetes (both with and without complications) among African Americans was more than two to three times the rate of non-Hispanic whites and some of the highest rates were in the South. Additionally, incidence rates for diagnosis of end-stage renal disease related to diabetes was approximately three times higher than that of non-Hispanic whites and was significantly higher than those of any other racial group in the South (Agency for Healthcare Research and Quality 2021). Furthermore, blood pressure control (130/80 mm Hg) for African Americans aged 40 years and over with diabetes is significantly lower than that of other groups; fewer than 40% of African Americans in this group have controlled blood pressure (Agency for Healthcare Research and Quality 2021).

Why is there a higher risk for diabetes in African Americans? The reasons for the increased incidence of type 2 diabetes in African Americans include genetic, environmental, and behavioral issues. Factors such as poor diet, physical inactivity, high levels of stress, poor health literacy, inadequate access to health care, low socioeconomic status, and obesity contribute to this risk.

Genetic Risk

Family history of diabetes is a known risk factor for type 2 diabetes. Data from the 1999–2002 National Health and Nutrition Examination Survey suggests a five-fold increase in the risk of diabetes among individuals who have a first-degree relative with diabetes (Annis et al. 2005, 1). Various theories have been proposed regarding the increased genetic risk of diabetes for African Americans. The "thrifty gene" theory implies that a survival advantage developed for excessive storage of fat during times of famine in individuals of African descent. Once food became plentiful, this survival advantage led to an increased incidence of obesity, thus increasing the risk for insulin resistance and type 2 diabetes (Dagogo-Jack 2003, 779–780; Marshall 2005, 734). Currently, genome-wide association studies are trying to identify loci related to type 2 diabetes. Because the majority of genome-wide association studies focused on diabetes have been completed in individuals of European descent, fewer loci have been identified for African Americans with type 2 diabetes than for individuals of European descent, illustrating the need for further genetic research in type 2 diabetes in African Americans (Ng 2015, 2, 6).

Lifestyle Risk Factors

Lifestyle risk factors such as poor diet and lack of physical activity are associated with the development of type 2 diabetes. Physical activity has shown to reduce the risk of developing non-insulin-dependent diabetes (Helmrich et al. 1991, 147). This is why the American Diabetes Association recommends 150 minutes of exercise per week among individuals with pre-diabetes or individuals at high risk for diabetes (Colberg et al. 2016, 2066). Information from the 2018 National Health Interview Survey through the CDC indicated that only 46.2% of African Americans engage in regular physical activity, defined as more than 150 minutes per week or more than 75 minutes per week of vigorous activity, compared to 57.6% of white Americans (HealthyPeople.gov 2020, 3). A healthy diet is also important for lowering the risk of developing type 2 diabetes. Access to healthy foods in grocery stores is needed. Food insecurity also contributes to poor diet. Estimates from United States Census Bureau survey data from over 37,000 households in 2018 showed that 11.1% of US households struggled with food insecurity, or a lack of access to affordable and nutritious food (Coleman-Jensen et al. 2019, 2, 6). African Americans have a higher burden of food insecurity than the national average; this Census Bureau information estimated that 21.2% of households with non-Hispanic Black individuals struggled with food insecurity (Coleman-Jensen et al. 2019, 14). Diabetes that is likely related to poor nutrition has been found to be more prevalent among individuals with food insecurity (Eicher-Miller 2020, 4).

Psychosocial Risk Factors

Many psychosocial factors influence diabetes outcomes, such as anxiety, depression, lack of social support, and levels of diabetes distress. Depression is a known risk factor for diabetes; and 25% of individuals with diabetes have depressive disorders or symptoms (Young-Hyman et al. 2016, 2133). Social support is valuable in diabetes care. Studies have demonstrated higher mortality rates among patients with diabetes who have low social support (Ciechanowski et al. 2010, 539–541; Zhang et al. 2007, 273–279). Diabetes-related distress stems from concerns about lack of support and limited access to care (Wardian and Sun 2014, 2). Elevated levels of diabetes-related distress are linked to poorer glycemic control and higher hemoglobin A1C (Aikens 2012, 2476–2477; Fisher et al. 2012, 259–263).

Another factor that likely contributes to the observed racial disparities in diabetes outcomes is allostatic load, or the physiological consequence of consistent exposure to environmental (including social) stressors. The endogenous consequences of this exposure include increased levels of cortisol and other hormone levels that have detrimental impacts on health, quality of life, and life expectancy (Duru et al. 2012, 89–90). The poor health outcomes among African Americans, particularly those of lower socioeconomic status, may be in part explained by allostatic load. This concept is a larger reflection of stress that has accumulated over many centuries and is deeply rooted in the African American experience.

Health Literacy

Health literacy refers to possession of the reading and mathematical skills needed to effectively navigate the health care system (Council on Scientific Affairs 1999). This type of literacy is important for understanding how to take medications, following instructions from physicians, reading prescription labels, understanding when to seek medical attention, and knowing what abnormal blood glucose readings mean. Health literacy has also been found to improve adherence to diabetes therapy (Osborn et al. 2011, 1). Schillinger, et al. (2002, 475) reported that lower health literacy was associated with higher hemoglobin A1C after adjusting for pharmacotherapy, socioeconomic status, social support, duration of diabetes, and depression. Individuals with lower health literacy in this study had a twofold increase in poorly controlled diabetes. Some studies have suggested increased rates of low health literacy among African Americans. Spears, Guidry, and Harvey (2018, 55), who conducted a survey among middle-class African Americans, found that 70.2% of survey participants could not correctly recognize all of the risks for developing type 2 diabetes. Another study found that African Americans have less understanding of type 2 diabetes than white Americans (Ledford, Seehusen, and Crawford 2019, 1).

Access to Health Care

Access to health care is important in diabetes care. Frequent visits with providers are needed to monitor glycemic control and screen for many diabetes-related conditions. When individuals are diagnosed with pre-diabetes, lifestyle interventions can be made to prevent or slow the development of type 2 diabetes. The fact that more African Americans than other racial groups lack health care insurance affects their access to care and their ability to afford the medications needed to manage diabetes. In 2019, 9.6% of African Americans were uninsured, compared to 5.2% of white Americans (Keisler-Starkey and Bunch 2020, 6).

Socioeconomic Status

Low socioeconomic status is a risk factor for diabetes. Studies have shown an inverse relationship between income level and incidence of diabetes. Data from the 1999–2004 National Health and Nutrition Examination Survey found that neighborhoods with higher poverty levels had a higher prevalence of diabetes. This study also found that neighborhoods consisting of predominantly African Americans had higher incidences of diabetes than largely white neighborhoods (Gaskin et al. 2014, 2147). Why does an individual living in a lower-income neighborhood have an increased risk of diabetes?

Poorer neighborhoods are less likely to have access to healthy foods. Neighborhoods are considered to be food deserts when they are far from grocery stores or access to healthy foods. In poorer neighborhoods, residents may get less physical activity because of the decreased walkability of the neighborhood. Evidence suggests that living in a walkable neighborhood decreases the odds of being overweight or obese (Gaskin et al. 2014, 2151–2152). Access to health care and health literacy are also correlated with socioeconomic status: lower socioeconomic status is associated with lower access to health care and lower health literacy.

Obesity

Obesity, which occurs at a high rate among African Americans, is a risk factor for diabetes. Data from the 2017–2018 National Health and Nutrition Examination Survey shows that obesity rates are rising in the United States. Non-Hispanic Blacks (49.6%) have the highest rate of obesity; the statistic for non-Hispanic whites is 42.2% and for Hispanic adults is 44.8% (Hales et al. 2020, 2).

Pre-Diabetes and Prevention of Progression to Diabetes

Type 2 diabetes is a chronic disease with significant associated complications and an increased risk of mortality. Studies demonstrate that even tight control of hyperglycemia in individuals with type 2 diabetes does not reduce the associated complications and increased risk of mortality to non-disease levels. Prevention of diabetes is essential for reducing the incidence of complications of diabetes, including increased mortality.

Individuals with pre-diabetes have abnormal glucose levels that are not high enough to be classified as diabetes. Criteria for diagnosis of pre-diabetes includes hemoglobin A1C between 5.7 and 6.4%, impaired fasting glucose (between 100 and 125 mg/dL), or impaired glucose tolerance (two-hour glucose between 140 and 199 mg/dL during 75 g oral glucose tolerance test). Because pre-diabetes increases the risk of developing type 2 diabetes, it is recommended that patients with pre-diabetes have annual screenings for diabetes (American Diabetes Association 2020b, S32). Estimates from the 2013–2016 National Health and Nutrition Examination Survey indicate that the prevalence of pre-diabetes is higher among Black non-Hispanic Americans (36.6%) than among white non-Hispanic Americans (31%) (CDC 2020b, 17).

Several studies have demonstrated the benefit of lifestyle interventions in preventing the development of type 2 diabetes. The Diabetes Prevention Program provides clear evidence that lifestyle changes and pharmacotherapy can reduce the risk of developing type 2 diabetes among individuals with pre-diabetes. This trial followed 3,234 individuals with impaired fasting glucose and impaired glucose tolerance over three years. It assigned patients to either a placebo group, a group that received 850 mg of metformin twice daily, or to an intensive lifestyle modification program that included a goal of 7% weight loss and a physical activity program of 150 minutes of moderate-intensity exercise each week. The lifestyle intervention group had a reduced incidence of type 2 diabetes of 58% compared to the placebo group and the metformin group had a 31% reduction compared to the placebo group. Notably, 19.9% of trial participants were African American; these participants experienced a 61% reduction in the risk of developing type 2 diabetes with lifestyle interventions and a 44% reduction with metformin (Knowler et al. 2002, 1, 17). This evidence has led the American Diabetes Association to recommend loss of 7% of initial body weight and 150 minutes of weekly exercise for patients with pre-diabetes. The American Diabetes Association also recommends consideration of metformin therapy for patients with pre-diabetes, especially in patients with a body mass index ≥ 35 kg/m^2 in patients less than 60 years old and in women with a history of gestational diabetes mellitus (American Diabetes Association 2020b, S34).

Treatment of Diabetes

Type 1 Diabetes

Because type 1 diabetes is caused by insulin deficiency secondary to autoimmune pancreatic beta cell destruction, insulin therapy is necessary for treatment. Insulin therapy for patients with type 1 diabetes includes both basal insulin and prandial insulin. Basal insulins are intermediate acting or long acting. Neutral protamine hagedorn is an intermediate-acting basal insulin that is dosed twice daily in most patients. Long-acting basal insulin preparations include glargine, detemir and degludec. Short-acting insulin preparations used for prandial coverage include regular insulin and the rapidly acting insulin analogs, which include lispro, aspart, and glulisine. Individuals with type 1 diabetes usually require 50% of their total daily dose of insulin to be delivered as basal insulin and 50% as prandial insulin. Usual total daily insulin doses for patient range from 0.4–1.0 units/kg/day (American Diabetes Association 2020c, S98–S99). Patients receive their insulin either by daily subcutaneous injections or by continuous subcutaneous insulin infusion.

Type 2 Diabetes

Type 2 diabetes is characterized by insulin resistance and a decrease in pancreatic beta cell insulin secretion. Initial therapy for type 2 diabetes includes lifestyle changes such as diet changes, weight loss, and an exercise regimen in addition to metformin therapy unless contraindications to metformin are present such as estimated glomerular filtration rate of < 30 mL/minute/1.73 m^2. Metformin falls into the class of medications know as biguanides, which act by improving insulin sensitivity, decreasing the absorption of glucose by the intestines, and lowering hepatic glucose production. While some patients can be treated with metformin monotherapy, most individuals progress to the need for additional pharmacotherapy.

When an individual has not met the target hemoglobin A1C, other diabetes medications are added to metformin. Many factors are taken into consideration when choosing the next medication, including cost, adverse side effects, and other medical comorbidities, including atherosclerotic cardiovascular disease, heart failure and chronic kidney disease. Other classes of anti-diabetes medications include glucagon-like peptide 1 (GLP-1) receptor agonists, dipeptidyl peptidase 4 (DPP-4) inhibitors, sodium-glucose cotransporter 2 (SGLT2) inhibitors, thiazolidinediones, and sulfonylureas. Often patients with type 2 diabetes may go on to need insulin therapy in addition to non-insulin therapies (American Diabetes Association 2020c, S100–S104).

GLP-1 RECEPTOR AGONISTS AND DPP-4 INHIBITORS

GLP-1 receptor agonists and DPP-4 inhibitors act by increasing the levels of glucagon-like peptide 1 and glucose-dependent insulinotropic polypeptide, which lead to increased insulin secretion in response to food, reduced gastric emptying, reduced glucagon secretion, and increased satiety. GLP-1 agonists are analogs of GLP-1, while DPP-4 inhibitors inhibit DPP-4, the enzyme that degrades GLP-1, leading to longer action of endogenous GLP-1. GLP-1 agonists have been shown to reduce cardiovascular events, thus making it a good choice among patients with known atherosclerotic cardiovascular disease. In addition, patients often lose weight with GLP-1 agonists, making that a good option for patients because weight loss improves insulin resistance (Melmed et al. 2016, 1430).

SGLT2 INHIBITORS

SGLT2 inhibitors act on the sodium-glucose cotransporter in the renal glomeruli, decreasing glucose reabsorption, and causing glycosuria, which leads to decreased plasma glucose levels. This class of medications has been shown to benefit patients with heart failure and diabetic kidney disease, making it a good choice in this subset of patients. In addition, two of the SGLT2 inhibitors, empagliflozin and canagliflozin, have also been shown to benefit patients with atherosclerotic cardiovascular disease (American Diabetes Association 2020c, S101; Melmed et al. 2016, 1431).

THIAZOLIDINEDIONES

Thiazolidinediones are insulin sensitizers that work by activating nuclear transcription factor peroxisome proliferator-activated receptor gamma. These medications have been shown to increase the risk of heart failure, so they are not recommended in patients with known heart failure (Melmed et al. 2016, 1427).

SULFONYLUREAS

Sulfonylureas are older medications that increase insulin release from the pancreatic beta cells by binding to ATP-sensitive potassium channels. Their main benefit is their low cost. Sulfonylureas are associated with weight gain and the risk of hypoglycemia (Melmed et al. 2016, 1428).

Racial Disparities among Treatment for Diabetes

Unfortunately, there is much data to suggest that racial disparities exist in the preventive care and treatment of diabetes in African Americans. Treatment of diabetes should not be different for African Americans and non-African Americans. One study looked at over 1.9 million US Medicare claims in the years 1997–1999 to investigate the completion of three quality measures among patients with diabetes: testing of hemoglobin A1C, eye examinations, and lipid panel. Lower rates of these quality measures were seen in African Americans, individuals < 65 years of age, individuals with lower socioeconomic status, and individuals that had ≤ 5 outpatient visits per year (Arday et al. 2002, 2232). Another study looked at 2008 Medical Expenditure Panel Survey data, which showed similar results: lower rates of eye exam, diabetic foot exam, and at least two hemoglobin A1C tests among African

Americans (Pu and Chewning 2013, 793). Additional studies have demonstrated a lower quality of care in management of diabetes among minority populations, including African Americans (Lanting et al. 2005, 2280). Studies have also shown consistently poor glycemic control and higher hemoglobin A1C values in African Americans than in non-Hispanic whites (Campbell et al. 2012, 5; Hunt et al. 2020, 2460). There is also some data to suggest that African Americans may have less intensification of their diabetes regimen. One study reports that African Americans take fewer oral medications for type 2 diabetes than white Americans even though their glycemic control is worse (Schectman et al. 2002, 1015–1018).

Annual screening for complications of diabetes is recommended to help prevent the development or slow the progression of diabetes-related disease. Educating health care providers about the potentially lower quality of diabetes care delivered to African Americans should empower them to improve these metrics with the goal of reducing the morbidity and mortality of diabetes among this group. Systems should be in place to monitor goals of diabetes care. Because better glycemic control is associated with fewer complications, strategies should be implemented to improve glycemic management among African Americans.

Studies of Tight Glycemic Control

While studies have shown that glycemic control to near normal values reduces the risk of microvascular complications of diabetes, randomized controlled studies of type 2 diabetes focused on macrovascular outcomes did not indicate that tight glycemic control was related to a reduction in macrovascular outcomes (Duckworth et al. 2009, 129; Gerstein et al. 2008, 2549; Patel et al. 2008, 2560). The Diabetes Control and Complications Trial study of 1982–1993 followed 1,441 patients with type 1 diabetes in order to compare intensive insulin therapy with conventional therapy. The intensive therapy group had a 35–76% reduction in microvascular disease compared to the group that received conventional therapy (Nathan 2014, 9). These reduced rates of microvascular disease in the intensive group persisted in follow-up studies (Lachin et al. 2000, 381). The UK Prospective Diabetes Study of 1977–1997 followed over 3,800 patients with type 2 diabetes. The intensive treatment group had a 25% reduction in microvascular disease (Lancet 1998, 837). This evidence suggests that having good glycemic control is important for preventing microvascular complications, including diabetic retinopathy, nephropathy, and neuropathy. In contrast, the Veteran Affairs Diabetes Trial, the Action to Control Cardiovascular Risk in Diabetes trial, and the ADVANCE trial indicated that tight glycemic control was not associated with reduced macrovascular endpoints or reduced mortality (Duckworth et al. 2009, 129; Gerstein et al. 2008, 2549; Patel et al. 2008, 2560).

Complications of Diabetes

Complications of diabetes include both microvascular complications such as retinopathy, nephropathy, and neuropathy and macrovascular complications such as ischemic heart disease, peripheral vascular disease, and cerebrovascular disease. Hyperglycemia and diabetes-related diseases contribute to many hospital admissions. In addition, diabetes is associated with worse outcomes among patients infected with COVID-19.

Microvascular Complications of Diabetes

Diabetic retinopathy has an estimated prevalence of 35.4% worldwide (Solomon et al. 2017, 412). Based on 2005–2008 data from the National Health and Nutrition Examination Survey, its prevalence in the United States is estimated to be 28.5% (Zhang et al. 2010, 2). Among adults aged 20–74 years in developed countries, diabetic retinopathy is considered the most common etiology for new-onset blindness. Recommendations for screening for diabetic retinopathy include an initial dilated eye exam five years after diagnosis of type 1 diabetes and at the time of diagnosis of type 2 diabetes and then continued dilated eye exams every one to two years (Solomon et al. 2017, 414).

Diabetic nephropathy develops in 20–40% of patients with diabetes. It is the most common cause of end-stage renal disease in the United States (American Diabetes Association 2020e, S136). Recommendations for screening include checking the urine albumin-to-creatine ratio and estimated glomerular filtration rate each year in patients with type 2 diabetes and in patients who have had type 1 diabetes for ≥ 5 years.

Diabetic neuropathy is a broad group of neuropathies that includes peripheral neuropathy, autonomic neuropathy, gastrointestinal neuropathies such as gastroparesis, and genitourinary disturbances that include erectile dysfunction. It is recommended that patients with type 2 diabetes and patients who have had type 1 diabetes for at least five years be evaluated annually for peripheral neuropathy. The potential complications of diabetic neuropathy include foot ulcers and amputations (American Diabetes Association 2020e, S143–S145).

Macrovascular Complications of Diabetes

Atherosclerotic cardiovascular disease includes coronary artery disease, cerebrovascular disease, and peripheral vascular disease. It is the primary cause of mortality among people with diabetes. This disease is estimated to cost $37.3 billion dollars every year (American Diabetes Association 2020d, S111). Important goals in preventing and managing atherosclerotic cardiovascular disease include managing blood pressure, managing lipid levels, smoking cessation, prescribing anti-platelet medications, and using particular medications for type 2 diabetes such as GLP-1 receptor agonists and SGLT2 inhibitors in individuals with known cardiovascular disease.

Complications of Diabetes in African Americans

Research shows that African Americans have higher rates of microvascular complications, especially diabetic retinopathy and diabetic kidney disease leading to end-stage renal disease. Diabetic retinopathy rates are higher among African Americans than among non-Hispanic white Americans. One study suggests that the prevalence among non-Hispanic Black Americans is 38.8 %, compared to 26.4% in non-Hispanic white Americans. The same study also found higher rates of vision-threatening retinopathy among African Americans than among non-Hispanic white Americans (9.3% versus 3.2%) (Zhang et al. 2010, 2). Both clinical and nonclinical factors likely contribute to this increased risk. Studies have shown that hypertension and poorly controlled diabetes increase the risk of new-onset diabetic retinopathy and the progression of existing diabetic retinopathy (Adler et al. 2000, 412; Klein et al. 1988, 2864). Reduced access to eye care and delays in seeking eye care may contribute to the increased prevalence of retinopathy. Delay in establishing with an eye care provider may be related to low referral rate by physicians for eye exams, financial issues, and poor patient knowledge about diabetic eye disease (Baker 2003, 114–115). Medicare Part B covers ophthalmology care for patients with diabetes. Claims from 2017 for patients with diabetes showed that overall only 54.1% of patients with diabetes had had an eye exam. This statistic was racially disparate: only 48.9% of African Americans had received an eye exam, but 55.6% of white non-Hispanic Americans had had an eye exam (Lundeen et al. 2019, 1).

All-cause end-stage renal disease is also higher among African Americans than among white Americans. In 2018, the rate of end-stage renal disease was recorded as 834.1 per million people in African Americans, compared to 312.7 cases per million people among white Americans (USRDS 2020, fig. 1.4). Studies have also demonstrated a higher risk of end-stage renal disease secondary to diabetes among African Americans than among white Americans (Shen et al. 2019, 1).

Race-based estimates of glomerular filtration rate have led to disparities in the prevalence and treatment of chronic kidney disease. The current calculations for glomerular filtration rate differ based on race (Black and non-Black). The glomerular filtration rate calculations for African Americans are higher than those of whites; this may delay the diagnosis and effective treatment of chronic kidney disease in African Americans. This also has detrimental consequences with regard to timely consideration and candidacy for renal transplantation (Franks and Scott 2020, 1–10). In order to avoid inequities in health outcomes, race should not be considered a biological construct. The National Kidney Foundation and the American Society of Nephrology are compiling a task force to reevaluate the historical practice of using race while estimating glomerular filtration rate. The objective is to determine how race-based adjustments in glomerular filtration rate impact the diagnosis and treatment of patients who are at risk for and have kidney disease (National Kidney Foundation and American Society of Nephrology 2020).

Macrovascular complications have also been found to be higher in African Americans. Diabetes greatly increases the risk of having an amputation. Medicare claims from 1996–1997 showed that rates of major amputations were 3.83 per 1,000 in individuals with diabetes compared to 0.38 per 1,000 in individuals who did not have diabetes (Wrobel, Mayfield, and Reiber 2001, 860). Medicare data from 2007–2011 shows higher rates of amputations among African Americans than among non-African Americans (5.5 per 1,000 versus 1.9 per 1,000) (Newhall et al. 2016, 1). African Americans are less likely to undergo revascularization to try to save a limb prior to amputation (Holman et al. 2011, 1).

Hospitalizations for Diabetes-Related Conditions in African Americans

Studies have been done to examine hospitalizations for individuals with diabetes. There appears to be higher rates of hospital readmissions for diabetes-related conditions among African Americans. Information from the 1999 HCUP State Inpatient Databases, including data from 2 southern states Tennessee and Virginia, demonstrated higher 180-day readmission rates among African Americans with diabetes on Medicare compared to white non-Hispanic African Americans (30.7% versus 27.9%) (Jiang et al. 2005, 1565). More recent data from 2009 to 2014 showed higher rates of 30-day all-cause readmission to hospitals among Black Americans compared to white non-Hispanic Americans, at 12.2% versus 10.2%. In this study, lower socioeconomic status with income < $40,000 yearly increased readmission risk in African Americans (Rodriguez-Gutierrez et al. 2019, 3).There also appears to be a higher incidence of hyperglycemia and hospital related complications among African Americans compared to white Americans (Fayfman et al. 2016, 1–2). Average per person health care expenditures attributed to diabetes are also higher for the Black, non-Hispanic ($10,470) population compared to the white non-Hispanic population ($9,800) due to higher use of emergency care and hospital outpatient care (American Diabetes Association 2018, 923).

COVID-19 and Diabetes

Another complication of diabetes is worse outcomes in cases of COVID-19. As of December 2020, there have been over 17 million cases in the United States and over 316,000 deaths attributed to COVID-19 (Fayfman et al. 2016, 1–2). Diabetes appears to place individuals with COVID-19 at higher risk for severe complications. Various studies quote an 14–32% increase in rates of severe or critical illness (Singh et al. 2020, 304). As diabetes incidence is increased among African Americans, this poses a significant risk to Black Americans in the context of the continued increase in the number of cases of COVID-19. Studies have also shown that African Americans are more likely to get COVID-19 and to have higher fatality rates (Yancy 2020, 1891).

Social Determinants of Health That Affect Diabetes Care

The U.S. Department of Health and Human Services ([2020]) lists five major categories of the social determinants of health: "economic stability, education access and equality, health care access and equality, neighborhood and built environment, and social and community context." All of these factors influence diabetes care.

Economic factors that contribute to an individual's health include access to healthy foods, access to health care, medication costs, and access to transportation to medical visits. Access to healthy foods is important both for preventing the development of diabetes and for promoting weight loss, which is known to improve insulin resistance and diabetes. Anti-diabetic medications can be costly and if an individual cannot afford particular medications, then suboptimal care may be delivered. For example, the GLP-1 receptor agonists are the recommended second line after metformin in patients with type 2 diabetes and atherosclerotic cardiovascular disease. However, these medications are very expensive; some estimates range from $744 to $1,106 per 30-day supply, making it cost prohibitive for most patients without insurance (American Diabetes Association 2020c, S106). In addition, insulin prices in the United States have steadily increased over the years; cash prices range from $250 to $645 for long-acting insulins (Fralick and Kesselheim 2019, 1794).

Education influences a person's understanding of diabetes. Individuals with lower education levels are more likely to have poorer health literacy. This influences diabetes outcomes and is associated with less adherence to treatment regimens (Osborn et al. 2011, 1).

Access to health care is necessary for the best outcomes in diabetes care. Annual screening for neuropathy, nephropathy, and hyperlipidemia and annual or biennial screening for retinopathy is recommended for early diagnosis of any diabetes-related disease. Monitoring of hemoglobin A1C monitoring is necessary, and pharmacotherapy should be intensified if a patient's hemoglobin A1C is above the goal. If an individual does not have access to health care, then poorer diabetes outcomes will likely occur. Telehealth is an option for individuals who live a great distance from medical care. However, the fact that individuals need access to a computer or a smartphone in order to access telehealth creates barriers for individuals without access to technology.

A person's neighborhood can provide a safe place for physical activity and access to healthy foods, which helps reduce the risk of obesity, which increases the risk of type 2 diabetes. However, unsafe environments can lead to stress and depression, putting an individual at higher risk for diabetes (Young-Hyman et al. 2016, 2133).

Social support is known to be very important in diabetes care. Patients with more social support have better diabetes outcomes (Ciechanowski et al. 2010, 539; Zhang et al. 2007, 273).

Systems in Process and Strategies to Help with Diabetes Mellitus Management

National Diabetes Prevention Program

In 2010, the CDC created the National Diabetes Prevention Program with the goal of reduction the incidence of diabetes in the United States. Individuals at risk for type 2 diabetes are eligible for participation, which includes a one-year lifestyle program to promote healthy diet and physical activity that is modeled after the Diabetes Prevention Program trial. Ways of promoting lifestyle changes include in-person and online classes. Currently, there are National Diabetes Prevention Program programs in all 50 states and the District of Columbia. By 2019, over 324,000 individuals were enrolled (Ritchie, Baucom, and Sauder 2020, 2949–2950).

Improving Access to Care: Telehealth, Telemedicine, and Use of Technology

Telehealth uses technology to deliver health care virtually; telemedicine practices medicine virtually via technology. Telemedicine has been an effective way for physicians to care for individuals with diabetes. Telehealth has been useful for other health care services, such as remote retinal screenings for diabetic retinopathy (McDonnell 2018, 1–5). If a patient is unable to see an ophthalmologist, a remote retinal screening test can be done locally at the office of the patient's primary care physician. Telehealth is also a feasible option for diabetes education. One study evaluated telehealth services for diabetes education that offered a one-year diabetes education program using videoconferencing in a primarily African American population. Individuals who participated in the telehealth services had improved LDL cholesterol and reductions in hemoglobin A1C than individuals who did not participate (Davis et al. 2010, 1712). Telehealth and telemedicine have the potential to improve access to care, especially in remote areas where health care options may be limited.

Technology such as continuous glucose monitors have become increasingly valuable in the management of type 1 diabetes and patients with type 2 diabetes who are being treated with insulin therapy. Many studies have shown improvements in hemoglobin A1C, less hypoglycemia, and increased time in goal blood sugar range when a continuous glucose monitor is integrated in the patient's care (Beck et al. 2017, 365; Kruger et al. 2019, 5S). The fact that patients can share their glucose data remotely with providers so they can review and help guide treatment decisions can further enhance the role of telemedicine in improving diabetes care.

Education and Motivation Initiatives

Strategies that focus on diabetes education and improving self-efficacy are necessary for improving diabetes outcomes. Diabetes education has been shown to reduce hospital admissions and readmissions, lower rates of diabetes complications, and lower hemoglobin A1C values by up to 1% in patients with type 2 diabetes (Powers et al. 2015, 1323). The American Diabetes Association recommends that patients with new-onset diabetes receive diabetes education. However, in 2011–2012, the CDC found that only 6.8% of privately insured patients who were diagnosed with diabetes received diabetes education during the first year after diagnosis (Li et al. 2014, 1046). Thus, our health care system needs to improve its provision of diabetes education to patients. Paying attention to one's educational attainment is also necessary when providing diabetes education. Rothman et al. (2004, 263–271), who evaluated literacy levels among patients with poorly controlled type 2 diabetes (hemoglobin A1C $\geq$ 8), found that 55% of patients with type 2 diabetes had a $\leq$ sixth grade literacy level. Their diabetes management program tailored diabetes education to each individual's literacy level by using techniques that improve understanding in individuals with lower literacy. After a six-month follow-up period, both the high and low literacy groups had similar improvements in hemoglobin A1C. This illustrates the importance of identifying individuals with lower literacy levels and using low-literacy-level educational material.

Motivating patients to be engaged in their diabetes care and promoting self-efficacy is important. Diabetes self-management is an essential aspect of diabetes care because physicians ask patients to do many things: take medications, self-monitor blood glucose levels, eat a healthy diet, and exercise regularly. Self-efficacy, or a person's confidence in their ability to bring about change, leads to better compliance with a regimen of medications, diet, and exercise (Nelson, McFarland, and Reiber 2007, 442). Self-efficacy has also been associated with lower diabetes distress, which is associated with better glycemic control (Aikens 2012, 2476–2477; Fisher et al. 2012, 263).

Smalls et al. (2015, 177–178) performed a systemic review of community-based initiatives to improve glycemia among African Americans. In this review, various community-based interventions lowered hemoglobin A1C using strategies such as group counseling, supervised exercise, dieticians, community health care workers, and mobile device software.

Future Directions

Diabetes has significant rates of mortality and morbidity with potential serious complications. Data has shown an increased incidence of type 2 diabetes, increased rates of diabetic complications, and poorer glycemic control among African Americans, and that racial disparities exist in the treatment of diabetes. Thus, a focus on improving lifestyles, preventing diabetes, and controlling complications for African Americans is needed across the United States and specifically in the South. Healthier lifestyles, healthier communities with access to healthy foods, environments that encourage physical activities, and stress reduction have the potential to increase diabetes prevention and control of blood glucose and blood pressure for those with diabetes. Although a number of programs focus on diabetes prevention and control such as the CDC's Diabetes Control and Prevention programs, few have been evaluated for their effects on racial disparities related to diabetes in African Americans, and those that have been evaluated show less successful outcomes for African Americans. For example, the National Diabetes Prevention Program reported that fewer African Americans than non-African Americans participated in and completed the program and that African American participants lost less weight and had less overall success in preventing diabetes than non-Hispanic whites (Ely et al. 2017, 1334, 1338). Medicare and other programs focused on improving diabetes care and management also show poorer outcomes for African Americans than non-Hispanic whites. Thus, more research that includes African American input during planning and implementation is needed to improve both prevention of diabetes among African Americans and care for diabetic African American patients. Additionally, successful programs that work in small areas need to be carefully assessed to identify factors that affect success and then carefully examined to identify factors that led to success for African American participants. Armed with the information garnered from such analysis, government and nongovernment programs can work together to disseminate and implement these programs in other communities to increase prevention, improve care, and increase the outcomes that are critically needed in order to improve the health of African Americans, particularly in the southern United States. We know how to prevent and control many of problems related to diabetes, but much more work is needed to translate this into action for African Americans and to assess why current knowledge and practices are not effective for many southern African Americans.

REFERENCES

Adler, A. I., I. M. Stratton, H. A. Neil, J. S. Yudkin, D. R. Matthews, C. A. Cull, A. D. Wright, R. C. Turner, and R. R. Holman. 2000. "Association of Systolic Blood Pressure with Macrovascular and Microvascular Complications of Type 2 Diabetes (UKPDS 36): Prospective Observational Study." *BMJ* 321 (7258): 412–419. https://doi.org/10.1136/bmj.321.7258.412.

Agency for Healthcare Research and Quality. 2021. *National Healthcare Quality and Disparities Report*. Rockville, MD: Agency for Healthcare Research and Quality. https://www.ahrq.gov/research/findings/nhqrdr/nhqdr21/index.html.

Aikens, J. E. 2012. "Prospective Associations between Emotional Distress and Poor Outcomes in Type 2 Diabetes." *Diabetes Care* 35 (12): 2472–2478. https://doi.org/10.2337/dc12-0181.

American Diabetes Association. 2018. "Economic Costs of Diabetes in the U.S. in 2017." 2018. *Diabetes Care* 41 (5): 917–928. https://doi.org/10.2337/dci18-0007.

———. 2020a. "2. Classification and Diagnosis of Diabetes: Standards of Medical Care in Diabetes—2020." *Diabetes Care* 43 (suppl. 1): S14–s31. https://doi.org/10.2337/dc20-S002.

———. 2020b. "3. Prevention or Delay of Type 2 Diabetes: Standards of Medical Care in Diabetes—2020." *Diabetes Care* 43 (suppl. 1): S32–s36. https://doi.org/10.2337/dc20-S003.

———. 2020c. "9. Pharmacologic Approaches to Glycemic Treatment: Standards of Medical Care in Diabetes—2020." *Diabetes Care* 43 (suppl. 1): S98–s110. https://doi.org/10.2337/dc20-S009.

———. 2020d. "10. Cardiovascular Disease and Risk Management: Standards of Medical Care in Diabetes—2020." *Diabetes Care* 43 (suppl. 1): S111–s134. https://doi.org/10.2337/dc20-S010.

———. 2020e. "11. Microvascular Complications and Foot Care: Standards of Medical Care in Diabetes—2020." 2020. *Diabetes Care* 43 (suppl. 1): S135–s151. https://doi.org/10.2337/dc20-S011.

Annis, A. M., M. S. Caulder, M. L. Cook, and D. Duquette. 2005. "Family History, Diabetes, and Other Demographic and Risk Factors among Participants of the National Health and Nutrition Examination Survey 1999–2002." *Prev Chronic Dis* 2 (2): A19.

Arday, D. R., B. B. Fleming, D. K. Keller, P. W. Pendergrass, R. J. Vaughn, J. M. Turpin, and D. A. Nicewander. 2002. "Variation in Diabetes Care among States: Do Patient Characteristics Matter?" *Diabetes Care* 25 (12): 2230–2237. https://doi.org/10.2337/diacare.25.12.2230.

Baker, R. S. 2003. "Diabetic Retinopathy in African Americans: Vision Impairment, Prevalence, Incidence, and Risk Factors." *Int Ophthalmol Clin* 43 (4): 105–122. https://doi.org/10.1097/00004397-200343040-00011.

Barker, L. E, K. A. Kirtland, E. W. Gregg, L. S. Geiss, and T. J. Thompson. 2011. "Geographic

Distribution of Diagnosed Diabetes in the U.S.: A Diabetes Belt." *Am J Prev Med* 40 (4): 434–439. https://doi.org/10.1016/j.amepre.2010.12.019.

Beck, R. W., T. D. Riddlesworth, K. Ruedy, A. Ahmann, S. Haller, D. Kruger, J. B. McGill, W. Polonsky, D. Price, S. Aronoff, R. Aronson, E. Toschi, C. Kollman, and R. Bergenstal. 2017. "Continuous Glucose Monitoring versus Usual Care in Patients with Type 2 Diabetes Receiving Multiple Daily Insulin Injections: A Randomized Trial." *Ann Intern Med* 167 (6): 365–374. https://doi.org/10.7326/m16-2855.

Campbell, J. A., R. J. Walker, B. L. Smalls, and L. E. Egede. 2012. "Glucose Control in Diabetes: The Impact of Racial Differences on Monitoring and Outcomes." *Endocrine* 42 (3): 471–482. https://doi.org/10.1007/s12020-012-9744-6.

CDC. 2020a. "CDC COVID Data Tracker." Last modified December 21, 2020. Accessed December 22, 2020. https://covid.cdc.gov/covid-data-tracker/#cases_casesper100klast7 days.

———. 2020b. *National Diabetes Statistics Report 2020: Estimates of Diabetes and Its Burden in the United States*. https://www.cdc.gov/diabetes/pdfs/data/statistics/national -diabetes-statistics-report.pdf.

Ciechanowski, P., J. Russo, W. J. Katon, E. H. Lin, E. Ludman, S. Heckbert, M. Von Korff, L. H. Williams, and B. A. Young. 2010. "Relationship Styles and Mortality in Patients with Diabetes." *Diabetes Care* 33 (3): 539–44. https://doi.org/10.2337/dc09-1298.

Colberg, S. R., R. J. Sigal, J. E. Yardley, M. C. Riddell, D. W. Dunstan, P. C. Dempsey, E. S. Horton, K. Castorino, and D. F. Tate. 2016. "Physical Activity/Exercise and Diabetes: A Position Statement of the American Diabetes Association." *Diabetes Care* 39 (11): 2065–2079. https://doi.org/10.2337/dc16-1728.

Coleman-Jensen, A., M. P. Rabbitt, C. A. Gregory, and A. Singh. 2019. *Household Food Security in the United States in 2018*. United States Department of Agriculture, Economic Research Service Report 270. Washington, DC: United States Department of Agriculture. https://www.ers.usda.gov/webdocs/publications/94849/err-270.pdf?v=590.1.

Council on Scientific Affairs. 1999. "Health Literacy: Report of the Council on Scientific Affairs." *JAMA* 281 (6): 552–557.

Dagogo-Jack, S. 2003. "Ethnic Disparities in Type 2 Diabetes: Pathophysiology and Implications for Prevention and Management." *J Natl Med Assoc* 95 (9): 774, 779–789.

Davis, R. M., A. D. Hitch, M. M. Salaam, W. H. Herman, I. E. Zimmer-Galler, and E. J. Mayer-Davis. 2010. "TeleHealth Improves Diabetes Self-Management in an Underserved Community: Diabetes TeleCare." *Diabetes Care* 33 (8): 1712–1717. https://doi.org/10.2337 /dc09-1919.

Duckworth, W., C. Abraira, T. Moritz, D. Reda, N. Emanuele, P. D. Reaven, F. J. Zieve, J. Marks, S. N. Davis, R. Hayward, S. R. Warren, S. Goldman, M. McCarren, M. E. Vitek, W. G. Henderson, G. D. Huang, and VADT Investigators. 2009. "Glucose Control and Vascular Complications in Veterans with Type 2 Diabetes." *N Engl J Med*. 360 (2): 129–139. https://doi.org/10.1056/NEJMoa0808431.

Duru, O. K., N. T. Harawa, D. Kermah, and K. C. Norris. 2012. "Allostatic Load Burden and Racial Disparities in Mortality." *J Natl Med Assoc* 104 (1–2): 89–95. https://doi.org/10 .1016/S0027-9684(15)30120-6.

Eicher-Miller, H. A. 2020. "A Review of the Food Security, Diet and Health Outcomes of

Food Pantry Clients and the Potential for Their Improvement through Food Pantry Interventions in the United States." *Physiol Behav* 220: 112871. https://doi.org/10.1016/j.physbeh.2020.112871.

Ely, E. K., S. M. Gruss, E. T. Luman, E. W. Gregg, M. K. Ali, K. Nhim, D. B. Rolka and A. L. Albright. 2017. "A National Effort to Prevent Type 2 Diabetes: Participant-Level Evaluation of CDC's National Diabetes Prevention Program." *Diabetes Care* 40 (10): 1331–1341. https://doi.org/10.2337/dc16-2099.

Fayfman, M., P. Vellanki, A. S. Alexopoulos, L. Buehler, L. Zhao, D. Smiley, S. Haw, J. Weaver, F. J. Pasquel, and G. E. Umpierrez. 2016. "Report on Racial Disparities in Hospitalized Patients with Hyperglycemia and Diabetes." *J Clin Endocrinol Metab* 101 (3): 1144–50. https://doi.org/10.1210/jc.2015-3220.

Fisher, L., D. M. Hessler, W. H. Polonsky, and J. Mullan. 2012. "When Is Diabetes Distress Clinically Meaningful? Establishing Cut Points for the Diabetes Distress Scale." *Diabetes Care* 35 (2): 259–264. https://doi.org/10.2337/dc11-1572.

Fralick, M., and A. S. Kesselheim. 2019. "The U.S. Insulin Crisis—Rationing a Lifesaving Medication Discovered in the 1920s." *N Engl J Med* 381 (19): 1793–1795. https://doi.org/10.1056/NEJMp1909402.

Franks, C. E. and M. G. Scott. 2020. "On the Basis of Race: The Utility of a Race Factor in Estimating Glomerular Filtration." *J Appl Lab Med* 6 (1): 155–166. https://doi.org/10.1093/jalm/jfaa128.

Gaskin, D. J., R. J. Thorpe Jr., E. E. McGinty, K. Bower, C. Rohde, J. H. Young, T. A. LaVeist, and L. Dubay. 2014. "Disparities in Diabetes: The Nexus of Race, Poverty, and Place." *Am J Public Health* 104 (11): 2147–155. https://doi.org/10.2105/ajph.2013.301420.

Gerstein, H. C., M. E. Miller, R. P. Byington, D. C. Goff Jr., J. T. Bigger, J. B. Buse, W. C. Cushman, S. Genuth, F. Ismail-Beigi, R. H. Grimm Jr., J. L. Probstfield, D. G. Simons-Morton, and W. T. Friedewald. 2008. "Effects of Intensive Glucose Lowering in Type 2 Diabetes." *N Engl J Med* 358 (24): 2545–2559. https://doi.org/10.1056/NEJMoa0802743.

Hales, C. M, M. D. Carroll, C. D. Fryar, and C. L. Ogden. 2020. *Prevalence of Obesity and Severe Obesity among Adults: United States, 2017–2018.* NCHS Data Brief no. 360. https://www.cdc.gov/nchs/data/databriefs/db360-h.pdf.

HealthyPeople.gov. 2020. "Adults Engaging in Regular Physical Activity—Light or Moderate for 150+ Minutes/Week or Vigorous for 75+ Minutes/Week (Age Adjusted, Percent, 18+ Years) By Race/Ethnicity." https://www.healthypeople.gov/2020/topics-objectives/topic/physical-activity/national-snapshot.

Helmrich, S. P., D. R. Ragland, R. W. Leung, and R. S. Paffenbarger Jr. 1991. "Physical Activity and Reduced Occurrence of Non-Insulin-Dependent Diabetes Mellitus." *N Engl J Med* 325 (3): 147–152. https://doi.org/10.1056/nejm199107183250302.

Holman, K. H., P. K. Henke, J. B. Dimick, and J. D. Birkmeyer. 2011. "Racial Disparities in the Use of Revascularization before Leg Amputation in Medicare Patients." *J Vasc Surg* 54 (2): 420–426E1. https://doi.org/10.1016/j.jvs.2011.02.035.

Hunt, K. J., M. Davis, J. Pearce, J. Bian, M. F. Guagliardo, E. Moy, R. N. Axon, and B. Neelon. 2020. "Geographic and Racial/Ethnic Variation in Glycemic Control and Treatment in a National Sample of Veterans With Diabetes." *Diabetes Care* 43 (10): 2460–2468. https://doi.org/10.2337/dc20-0514.

Jiang, H. J., R. Andrews, D. Stryer, and B. Friedman. 2005. "Racial/Ethnic Disparities in Potentially Preventable Readmissions: The Case of Diabetes." *Am J Public Health* 95 (9): 1561–1567. https://doi.org/10.2105/ajph.2004.044222.

Keisler-Starkey, K., and L. N. Bunch 2020. "Health Insurance Coverage in the United States: 2019." https://www.census.gov/content/dam/Census/library/publications/2020/demo/p60-271.pdf.

Klein, R., B. E. Klein, S. E. Moss, M. D. Davis, and D. L. DeMets. 1988. "Glycosylated Hemoglobin Predicts the Incidence and Progression of Diabetic Retinopathy." *JAMA* 260 (19): 2864–2871.

Knowler, W. C., E. Barrett-Connor, S. E. Fowler, R. F. Hamman, J. M. Lachin, E. A. Walker, and D. M. Nathan. 2002. "Reduction in the Incidence of Type 2 Diabetes with Lifestyle Intervention or Metformin." *N Engl J Med* 346 (6): 393–403. https://doi.org/10.1056/NEJMoa012512.

Kruger, D. F., S. V. Edelman, D. A. Hinnen, and C. G. Parkin. 2019. "Reference Guide for Integrating Continuous Glucose Monitoring into Clinical Practice." *Diabetes Educ* 45 (suppl. 1): 3s–20s. https://doi.org/10.1177/0145721718818066.

Lachin, J. M., S. Genuth, P. Cleary, M. D. Davis, and D. M. Nathan. 2000. "Retinopathy and Nephropathy in Patients with Type 1 Diabetes Four Years after a Trial of Intensive Therapy." *N Engl J Med* 342 (6): 381–389. https://doi.org/10.1056/nejm200002103420603.

Lancet. 1998. "Intensive Blood-Glucose Control with Sulphonylureas or Insulin Compared with Conventional Treatment and Risk of Complications in Patients with Type 2 Diabetes (UKPDS 33). UK Prospective Diabetes Study (UKPDS) Group." *Lancet* 352 (9131): 837–853.

Lanting, L. C., I. M. Joung, J. P. Mackenbach, S. W. Lamberts, and A. H. Bootsma. 2005. "Ethnic Differences in Mortality, End-Stage Complications, and Quality of Care among Diabetic Patients: A Review." *Diabetes Care* 28 (9): 2280–2288. https://doi.org/10.2337/diacare.28.9.2280.

Ledford, C. J. W., D. A. Seehusen, and P. F. Crawford. 2019. "Geographic and Race/Ethnicity Differences in Patient Perceptions of Diabetes." *J Prim Care Community Health* 10: 2150132719845819. https://doi.org/10.1177/2150132719845819.

Li, R., S. S. Shrestha, R. Lipman, N. R. Burrows, L. E. Kolb, and S. Rutledge. 2014. "Diabetes Self-Management Education and Training among Privately Insured Persons with Newly Diagnosed Diabetes—United States, 2011–2012." *MMWR Morb Mortal Wkly Rep* 63 (46): 1045–1049.

Lundeen, E. A., J. Wittenborn, S. R. Benoit, and J. Saaddine. 2019. "Disparities in Receipt of Eye Exams among Medicare Part B Fee-for-Service Beneficiaries with Diabetes—United States, 2017." *MMWR Morb Mortal Wkly Rep* 68 (45): 1020–1023. https://doi.org/10.15585/mmwr.mm6845a3.

Marshall, M. C., Jr. 2005. "Diabetes in African Americans." *Postgrad Med J* 81 (962): 734–740. https://doi.org/10.1136/pgmj.2004.028274.

McDonnell, M. E. 2018. "Telemedicine in Complex Diabetes Management." *Curr Diab Rep* 18 (7): 42. https://doi.org/10.1007/s11892-018-1015-3.

Melmed, S., K. S. Polonsky, P. R. Larsen, and H. M. Kronenberg. 2016. *Williams Textbook of Endocrionlogy*. Philadelphia, PA: Elsevier.

Nathan, D. M. 2014. "The Diabetes Control and Complications Trial / Epidemiology of Diabetes Interventions and Complications Study at 30 Years: Overview." *Diabetes Care* 37 (1): 9–16. https://doi.org/10.2337/dc13-2112.

National Kidney Foundation and American Society of Nephrology. 2020. "Establishing a Task Force to Reassess the Inclusion of Race in Diagnosing Kidney Diseases." Accessed December 21, 2020. https://www.kidney.org/news/establishing-task-force-to-reassess-inclusion-race-diagnosing-kidney-diseases.

Nelson, K. M., L. McFarland, and G. Reiber. 2007. "Factors Influencing Disease Self-Management Veterans with Diabetes and Poor Glycemic Control." *J Gen Intern Med* 22 (4): 442–447. https://doi.org/10.1007/s11606-006-0053-8.

Newhall, K., E. Spangler, N. Dzebisashvili, D. C. Goodman, and P. Goodney. 2016. "Amputation Rates for Patients with Diabetes and Peripheral Arterial Disease: The Effects of Race and Region." *Ann Vasc Surg* 30: 292–298.e1. https://doi.org/10.1016/j.avsg.2015.07.040.

Ng, M. C. 2015. "Genetics of Type 2 Diabetes in African Americans." *Curr Diab Rep* 15 (10): 74. https://doi.org/10.1007/s11892-015-0651-0.

Osborn, C. Y., K. Cavanaugh, K. A. Wallston, S. Kripalani, T. A. Elasy, R. L. Rothman, and R. O. White. 2011. "Health Literacy Explains Racial Disparities in Diabetes Medication Adherence." *J Health Commun* 16 (suppl. 3): 268–278. https://doi.org/10.1080/10810730.2011.604388.

Patel, A., S. MacMahon, J. Chalmers, B. Neal, L. Billot, M. Woodward, M. Marre, M. Cooper, P. Glasziou, D. Grobbee, P. Hamet, S. Harrap, S. Heller, L. Liu, G. Mancia, C. E. Mogensen, C. Pan, N. Poulter, A. Rodgers, B. Williams, S. Bompoint, B. E. de Galan, R. Joshi, and F. Travert. 2008. "Intensive Blood Glucose Control and Vascular Outcomes in Patients with Type 2 Diabetes." *N Engl J Med.* 358 (24): 2560–2572. https://doi.org/10.1056/NEJMoa0802987.

Powers, M. A., J. Bardsley, M. Cypress, P. Duker, M. M. Funnell, A. H. Fischl, M. D. Maryniuk, L. Siminerio, and E. Vivian. 2015. "Diabetes Self-Management Education and Support in Type 2 Diabetes: A Joint Position Statement of the American Diabetes Association, the American Association of Diabetes Educators, and the Academy of Nutrition and Dietetics." *J Acad Nutr Diet* 115 (8): 1323–1334. https://doi.org/10.1016/j.jand.2015.05.012.

Pu, J., and B. Chewning. 2013. "Racial Difference in Diabetes Preventive Care." *Res Social Adm Pharm* 9 (6): 790–796. https://doi.org/10.1016/j.sapharm.2012.11.005.

Ritchie, N. D., K. J. W. Baucom, and K. A. Sauder. 2020. "Current Perspectives on the Impact of the National Diabetes Prevention Program: Building on Successes and Overcoming Challenges." *Diabetes Metab Syndr Obes* 13: 2949–2957. https://doi.org/10.2147/dmso.S218334.

Rodriguez-Gutierrez, R., J. Herrin, K. J. Lipska, V. M. Montori, N. D. Shah, and R. G. McCoy. 2019. "Racial and Ethnic Differences in 30-Day Hospital Readmissions among US Adults with Diabetes." *JAMA Netw Open* 2 (10): e1913249. https://doi.org/10.1001/jamanetworkopen.2019.13249.

Rothman, R., R. Malone, B. Bryant, C. Horlen, D. DeWalt, and M. Pignone. 2004. "The Relationship between Literacy and Glycemic Control in a Diabetes Disease-Management Program." *Diabetes Educ* 30 (2): 263–273. https://doi.org/10.1177/014572170403000219.

Schectman, J. M., M. M. Nadkarni, and J. D. Voss. 2002. "The Association between Diabetes Metabolic Control and Drug Adherence in an Indigent Population." *Diabetes Care* 25 (6): 1015–1021. https://doi.org/10.2337/diacare.25.6.1015.

Schillinger, D., K. Grumbach, J. Piette, F. Wang, D. Osmond, C. Daher, J. Palacios, G. D. Sullivan, and A. B. Bindman. 2002. "Association of Health Literacy with Diabetes Outcomes." *JAMA* 288 (4): 475–482. https://doi.org/10.1001/jama.288.4.475.

Shen, Y., L. Shi, E. Nauman, P. T. Katzmarzyk, E. G. Price-Haywood, P. Yin, A. N. Bazzano, S. Nigam, and G. Hu. 2019. "Race and Sex Differences in Rates of Diabetic Complications." *J Diabetes* 11 (6): 449–456. https://doi.org/10.1111/1753-0407.12869.

Singh, A. K., R. Gupta, A. Ghosh, and A. Misra. 2020. "Diabetes in COVID–19: Prevalence, Pathophysiology, Prognosis and Practical Considerations." *Diabetes Metab Syndr* 14 (4): 303–310. https://doi.org/10.1016/j.dsx.2020.04.004.

Smalls, B. L., R. J. Walker, H. S. Bonilha, J. A. Campbell, and L. E. Egede. 2015. "Community Interventions to Improve Glycemic Control in African Americans with Type 2 Diabetes: A Systemic Review." *Glob J Health Sci* 7 (5): 171–182. https://doi.org/10.5539/gjhs.v7n5p171.

Solomon, S. D., E. Chew, E. J. Duh, L. Sobrin, J. K. Sun, B. L. VanderBeek, C. C. Wykoff, and T. W. Gardner. 2017. "Diabetic Retinopathy: A Position Statement by the American Diabetes Association." *Diabetes Care* 40 (3): 412–418. https://doi.org/10.2337/dc16-2641.

Spears, E. C., J. J. Guidry, and I. S. Harvey. 2018. "Measuring Type 2 Diabetes Mellitus Knowledge and Perceptions of Risk in Middle-Class African Americans." *Health Educ Res* 33 (1): 55–63. https://doi.org/10.1093/her/cyx073.

U.S. Department of Health and Human Services, Office of Disease Prevention and Health Promotion. [2020]. "Social Determinants of Health." Accessed December 22, 2020 https://health.gov/healthypeople/objectives-and-data/social-determinants-health.

USRDS (United States Renal Data System). 2020. *End Stage Renal Disease.* Vol. 2 of *USRDS Annual Data Report: Epidemiology of Kidney Disease in the United States.* https://adr.usrds.org/2020.

Wardian, J., and F. Sun. 2014. "Factors Associated with Diabetes-Related Distress: Implications for Diabetes Self-Management." *Soc Work Health Care* 53 (4): 364–381. https://doi.org/10.1080/00981389.2014.884038.

Wrobel, J. S., J. A. Mayfield, and G. E. Reiber. 2001. "Geographic Variation of Lower-Extremity Major Amputation in Individuals with and without Diabetes in the Medicare Population." *Diabetes Care* 24 (5): 860–4. https://doi.org/10.2337/diacare.24.5.860.

Yancy, C. W. 2020. "COVID–19 and African Americans." *Jama* 323 (19): 1891–1892. https://doi.org/10.1001/jama.2020.6548.

Young-Hyman, D., M. de Groot, F. Hill-Briggs, J. S. Gonzalez, K. Hood, and M. Peyrot. 2016. "Psychosocial Care for People With Diabetes: A Position Statement of the American Diabetes Association." *Diabetes Care* 39 (12): 2126–2140. https://doi.org/10.2337/dc16-2053.

Zhang, X., S. L. Norris, E. W. Gregg, and G. Beckles. 2007. "Social Support and Mortality among Older Persons with Diabetes." *Diabetes Educ* 33 (2): 273–281. https://doi.org/10.1177/0145721707299265.

Zhang, X., J. B. Saaddine, C. F. Chou, M. F. Cotch, Y. J. Cheng, L. S. Geiss, E. W. Gregg, A. L. Albright, B. E. Klein, and R. Klein. 2010. "Prevalence of Diabetic Retinopathy in the United States, 2005–2008." *JAMA* 304 (6): 649–656. https://doi.org/10.1001/jama.2010 .1111.

11

Stroke

CAROLYN JENKINS, DrPH, MS, MSN, RD, RN, FAAN,
DANIEL LACKLAND, DrPH,
and BRUCE OVBIAGELE, MD, FRCP

About every 40 seconds someone in the United States has a stroke, and every four minutes someone dies from a stroke (CDC 2020; Virani et al. 2020). Stroke symptoms occur when there is loss of blood flow to a part of the brain that does not get the oxygen and other nutrients it needs to keep brain cells living. When stroke is not treated adequately, it can cause permanent problems and long-term disabilities or death. Stroke risks increase with each successive decade after the age of 55, but strokes can and do happen at any age. Hospitalization for stroke in the United States is the tenth most common reason for hospitalization. In 2018, the cost was $7.9 billion, or an average of $14,900 per stay (McDermott and Roemer 2021). This amount does not include the costs of rehabilitation and lost income for working individuals. Stroke is the fifth leading cause of death across the United States. The risk of first stroke or cerebrovascular accident is nearly twice as high for African American/Black men and women than it is for non-Hispanic whites; African Americans/Blacks have the highest rate of death due to stroke (Ingram and Montresor-Lopez 2015; Virani et al. 2020). Black men are 70% more likely to die of stroke than white men (US Department of Health and Human Services, Office of Minority Heath 2021). Stroke is the leading cause of serious long-term disability (Ingram and Montresor-Lopez 2015; Kochanek et al. 2019; Virani et al. 20201). Stroke reduces mobility in more than half of stroke survivors aged 65 and over (CDC 2021a; Kochanek et al. 2019; Schwamm et al. 2010).

African Americans, particularly those in the Deep South, are most affected by stroke. Multiple risks for stroke have been identified and progress is being made to improve stroke outcomes, but more research and resources are needed at the individual, family, system, community and national levels to increase quality of life, decrease risk factors, prevent and treat stroke, and improve stroke recovery and decrease stroke disabilities and death, especially in African Americans. This chapter presents a brief overview of the epidemiology of stroke and stroke risk factors; the social determinants of health associated with stroke; the medical/health care professional view of stroke risks, stroke diagnosis, stroke treatment, and stroke recovery and palliative care for stroke patients and their families; the systems in place to support prevention, treatment, recovery and/or palliative care and the role of individuals, families and communities in using systems for prevention and treatment of stroke; and the gaps in care and actions that are needed to prevent initial and secondary strokes. The focus of the chapter is African Americans living in the southeastern United States.

Epidemiology of Stroke Risk Factors and Stroke Prevalence and Death

It is unclear why African Americans have an increased risk of stroke, but more than two-thirds have one or more risks for stroke and 3–4% of African American adults have experienced one or more strokes (American Heart Association 2021). Data based on the US population show that while there has been a decrease in stroke incidence among Non-Hispanic whites over the past two decades, the incidence of stroke among African Americans has remained virtually the same (Kleindorfer et al. 2010). In addition, the prevalence of stroke incidence in the United States is projected to increase at a higher rate for racial and ethnic minorities than for non-Hispanic whites (Ovbiagele et al. 2013). Children with sickle cell may also have a stroke. The risk factors for stroke, the incidence of stroke, and stroke-related deaths are more common in African Americans, particularly those living in the southeastern United States. The known risks for stroke include:

— High blood pressure. Over half of African American adults (58.3% of males and 57.6% of females) have high blood pressure. This condition is defined as systolic pressure of 130 mm Hg or higher; diastolic pressure of 80 mm Hg or higher; requiring antihypertensive medicine; or being told twice by a physician or other professional that an individual has hypertension (American Heart Association 2021). It develops earlier in Black Americans and is often more severe for members of that group. Additionally, high blood pressure is more common in the South.

— Overweight and obesity. The American Heart Association reports that 69.9% of Black non-Hispanic males and 78.4% of Black non-Hispanic females are overweight or obese. Within that population, "69.9% of males and 78.4% of females were overweight or obese, 38.2% of males and 55.2% of females were obese, and 7.5% of males and 16.3% of females were extremely obese" (American Heart Association. 2021).

— Diabetes. Approximately 11.7% of Black non-Hispanic adults have diabetes and around 32% have pre-diabetes. Type 2 diabetes in youth for all individuals but especially for African Americans is growing (American Diabetes Association 2022). African Americans are more likely to have diabetes than non-Hispanic whites.

— High cholesterol. Nearly 30% of black Americans have high levels of LDL cholesterol. However, African American women had significantly higher HDL cholesterol (good cholesterol) than white women (52.6 vs. 47.5 mg/dL; $p = 0.019$) (Koval et al. 2010).

— Sickle cell anemia. This common genetic disorder in African Americans is a risk factor for stroke. An estimated 80,151 African Americans have the disease. Among African Americans with sickle cell anemia, 53% live in the South (Brousseau et al. 2010; Sedrak and Kondamudi 2021).

— Smoking. Over 15% of black adults smoke. Smoking increases their risk of stroke 6-fold. Even passive smoking nearly doubles the risk of stroke (Bonita et al. 1999).

— Eating too much salt. Research shows that African Americans may have a gene that greatly increases sensitivity to salt and its effects (Jackson 1991). Southern food is often high in sodium.

— Stress. African American adults face daily stressors that may increase risks for stroke (Booth et al. 2015). Other factors that have been identified as increasing risks of stroke include inflammation, including the inflammatory markers C-reactive protein and fibrogen (Kelly, Lemmens, and Tsivgoulis 2021 McDermott and Roemer 2021).

Stroke prevalence and stroke deaths nationally for African Americans and non-Hispanic whites are shown in tables 11.1–11.3. The data in these tables reveal that the national stroke prevalence is higher for non-Hispanic Black males and females. Data suggest that more than 25% of persons with

Table 11.1. Stroke prevalence and stroke deaths in the United States

	Males		Females	
	NH[1] White	NH Black	NH White	NH Black
Stroke prevalence 2013–2016[2]	2.4%	3.1%	2.5%	3.8%
Stroke deaths 2017[3]	45,078	8,566	64,960	10,522

Source: Adapted from "Heart Disease and Stroke Statistics, 2020 Updates: Chapter 14," *Circulation* 141 (2020): e379.
1. Non-Hispanic.
2. Age ≥ 20 years.
3. All ages.

Table 11.2. Diagnosed cases of stroke: Age-adjusted percentages of stroke among persons 18 years of age and over, 2018

	NH Black	NH White	NH Black : NH White Ratio
Men	3.2	3.1	1.0
Women	4.6	2.3	2.0
Total	4.0	2.7	1.5

Source: National Center for Health Statistics, "Summary Health Statistics: National Health Interview Survey: 2018," Table A-1a, CDC, 2019, https://ftp.cdc.gov/pub/Health_Statistics/NCHS /NHIS/SHS/2018_SHS_Table_A-1.pdf.

Table 11.3. Age-adjusted stroke death rates per 100,000, 2017

	NH Black	NH White	NH Black : NH White Ratio
Men	57.9	36.0	1.6
Women	48.3	26.0	1.3
Total	52.7	36.4	1.4

Source: Kenneth D. Kochanek, Sherry L. Murphy, Jiaquan Xu, and Elizabeth Arias, "Deaths: Final Data for 2017," *National Vital Statistics Report* 68, no. 9 (2019): Table 10, https://www.cdc .gov/nchs/data/nvsr/nvsr68/nvsr68_09-508.pdf.

stroke experience cognitive or language difficulties. Stroke deaths are higher for non-Hispanic black males and females than they are for non-Hispanic white males and females.

Geographical differences exist for stroke and stroke mortality. The Stroke Belt states, those with the higher rates, include Alabama, Arkansas, Georgia, Louisiana, Mississippi, North and South Carolinas, and Tennessee. To be defined as part of the Stroke Belt, a state must have either a stroke rate or a stroke death rate that is at least 10% above the national average. Since the 1940s, the overall average stroke mortality rate has been about 30% higher in the Stroke Belt than other areas of the United States. The stroke mortality rate in the "buckle" of the Stroke Belt (Georgia, North Carolina, and South Carolina) is about 40% higher than in other areas of the United States. When individuals live within the Stroke Belt for the first 20 years of their life, their risk of stroke increases.

As research progresses on the epidemiology of stroke risks, stroke morbidity, stroke recovery and stroke deaths, and the genetics and genomics of related factors affecting stroke, it is to be hoped that the data will lead us to improved methods of surveillance and outcomes. The outcomes include improved methods for prevention, early diagnosis and treatment, and rehabilitation and preventing deaths from stroke. We can then identify and learn about other factors that influence health and stroke outcomes and use this information to improve care and recovery.

Social Determinants of Health Associated with Stroke

One relatively new area of study is the social determinants of health associated with stroke prevention and outcomes related to stroke. These are defined as the conditions in the environments where people are born, live, learn, work, play, worship, and age that affect a wide range of health conditions, functioning, and quality-of-life outcomes and risks. Healthy People 2030 has grouped social determinants of health into five domains: social and community context, quality of a person's neighborhood and the built environment, economic stability, access to and quality of education, and access to and quality of health care. Social determinants of health have a major impact on people's health, levels of well-being or stress, and quality of life. They include the following issues:

- Safe housing, transportation, and neighborhoods
- Racism, discrimination, and violence
- Education, job opportunities, and income
- Access to basic needs, healthy foods, physical activity, and quality health care

Historical slavery has been found to be associated with modern-day stroke mortality in the southern Stroke Belt (Esenwa 2018). Esenwa and colleagues concluded that it is "likely that poverty, lack of geographical access to care, migration patterns, and a complex web of other socioeconomic factors, some of which left over from the era of slavery, are interacting to affect stroke mortality" (Esenwa 2018, 468), particularly in the southeastern

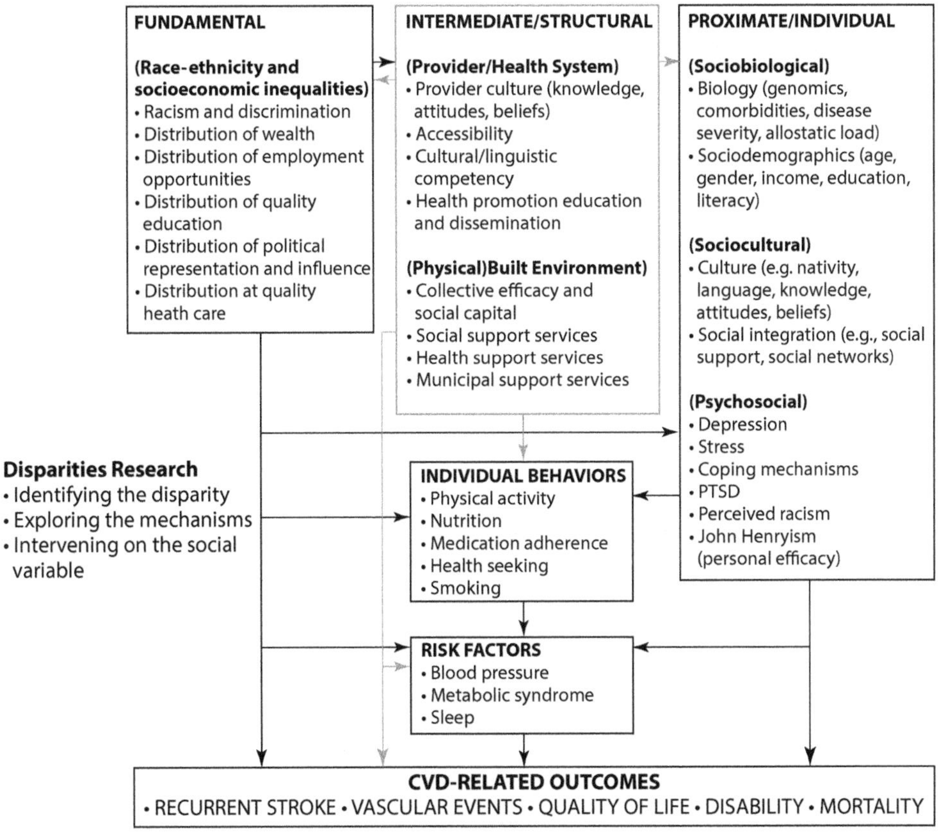

Figure 11.1. Proposed model for understanding the social determinants of health. Reproduced from Schulz and Northridge (2004) and modified with CVD-related outcomes in L. E. Skolarus, A. Sharrief, H. Gardener, C. Jenkins, and B. Boden-Albala, "Considerations in Addressing Social Determinants of Health to Reduce Racial/Ethnic Disparities in Stroke Outcomes in the United States," *Stroke* 51, no. 11 (2020): 3433–3439.

United States. However, little or no research has been done to document intervention methods and their effect on social determinants of health in order to address stroke prevalence, recovery from stroke, or death related to stroke. Figure 11.1 shows an example of a model that seeks to determine the social determinants of cardiovascular disease, which includes stroke (Skolarus 2020).

It is hoped that applying this model in research and practice settings can help identify intervening mechanisms for addressing the many disparities in health, stroke risk factors, stroke occurrences, hospitalization from stroke, recovery and deaths related to stroke. The Centers for Disease Control and Prevention offer a data set directory and suggested methods for addressing social determinants of health (CDC 2021b; Esenwa 2018). As we move forward to address the social determinants of health and their effect on stroke outcomes for African Americans, we must include African Americans from communities we study in the planning process, the development and implementation of interventions, and evaluations of the results.

Stroke Risks, Diagnosis and Treatment

Why Are Black Individuals at Higher Risk for Stroke?

Black and white differences in stroke occurrences were first recognized in the 1970s. At first, the differences were hypothesized to be mainly due to diabetes and high blood pressure (Howard 2013) or medical problems. However, the reasons are more complex and it is unclear why African Americans have an increased risk of stroke and death from stroke (Cruz-Flores et al. 2011). However, varied hypotheses posited include:

1. Differential impact of risk factors based on race such that presence of certain risk factors could have a greater impact, as has been shown for three-times-higher impact of elevated systolic blood pressure on stroke risk among Blacks than among whites (Howard et al. 2013).
2. Incomplete assessment of traditional risk factors and failure to capture crucial aspects such as duration of risk factors or fluctuations over time. Such practices could introduce confounding by failing to measure the full impact of a risk factor.
3. Novel risk factors such as psychosocial factors, environmental pollution, dietary factors, and inflammation that may relate to racially driven independent effects or interact with traditional risk factors to potentiate or attenuate impact on stroke risk.
4. Unconscious biases within health care systems and on the part of providers. (Ovbiagele 2020)

According to the American Stroke Association, over two-thirds of Black Americans have at least one risk factor for stroke. Black Americans have higher levels of overweight and obesity, high blood pressure, diabetes, high cholesterol, sickle cell anemia. In addition, over 1 in 10 Black Americans smoke, a practice that doubles the risk of stroke (American Stroke Association 2020). Black Americans also have significantly higher risks for second strokes than white Americans.

In addition to the more common risks, less common risks have been identified. However, little information exists on how these risks apply to African Americans. These risks include young adult survivors of preterm birth; the Swedish Birth and Swedish Death Registers identified this population as having an increased risk for both ischemic or hemorrhagic stroke (Dlamini and Jordan 2021). The risk increases by 3% for each week of lower gestation or prematurity. The age of the study cohort ranged from 25 to 43 years. Other researchers in the United States have identified health risks for stroke and other illnesses in adulthood that are associated with preterm births (Crump 2021). Using data from the Jackson Heart Study of African Americans, Bidulescu et al. (2013) found that adiponectin was directly associated with stroke for Black women. Lisabeth and Bushnell (2012) have identified an association of age at menopause and stroke risk. The younger the age of menopause, whether it occurs naturally or is the result of surgery, the higher the stroke risk. Estrogen administration, especially oral delivery, was also identified as increasing stroke risk in women. Lisabeth and Bushnell did not distinguish between white and Black women in their findings on early menopause and estrogen administration.

Health professionals and health researchers are relatively good at identifying and measuring risks. However, we must also focus on the causes of the risks, identifying new risks (such as genomic risks), and interventions for reducing stroke risks and improving the quality of life, especially in largely African American communities and populations. We must involve those affected by the risks when we plan interventions to decrease or eliminate the risks of stroke. Many studies have focused on identifying and reporting stroke risks for African Americans, but few have focused on decreasing those risks and even fewer report that researchers involved African American communities in plans to decrease risks. Much work remains to be done to identify, develop, and test a plan of action for decreasing stroke in Black women and men.

Signs of Stroke and Actions Needed When Stroke Occurs

The common signs and symptoms of a stroke include (1) numbness in face, arm leg, side; (2) confusion and trouble speaking; (3) trouble walking;

(4) sudden trouble seeing; and (5) sudden severe headache. This list is presented according to highest level of knowledge of signs and symptoms in the CDC's National Health Interview Survey for 2009, 2014 and 2017. Although fewer than 70% of survey participants recognized all five symptoms, most knew to call emergency medical support. These symptoms can occur any time but appear to be most common in midmorning to late morning. All research studies support the conclusion that stroke is least likely to occur in the late evening before midnight. The first action to take is to call 911 or an ambulance for transportation and assistance in reaching the nearest hospital, ideally a hospital that has a stroke center. The American Stroke Association and other groups use the term FAST to help people remember the major signs of stroke and the assessments they should make when they suspect someone is having a stroke.

- F is for face drooping: ask the person to smile and observe if the smile is drooping, uneven, or lopsided.
- A is for arm weakness: ask the person to raise both arms and observe if one arm is drifting down.
- S is for speech difficulty: ask the person to repeat a simple sentence and observe if the speech is slurred or if you are unable to understand the person.
- T is for time to call 911 for support in getting to a hospital as quickly as possible.

An estimated 60% or more of the US population lives within an hour of a certified stroke center, including most residents of the Deep South. People living in urban areas are usually closer to the hospitals with certified stroke centers, but even most rural residents in the South, live within 60 minutes of a certified stroke center. These centers have the services stroke patients need and experience in diagnosing and managing all types of strokes. The key is getting the stroke patient to the hospital and getting a stroke diagnosed as rapidly as possible.

Our research team conducted focus groups with African Americans with stroke living in rural communities in South Carolina on the topic of reducing the time from onset of stroke symptoms to arrival at the emergency department of the hospital. Some participants conveyed their concerns related to stroke and getting to the hospital. One participant described the choice their family made about transportation: "*I got to the hospital faster by having my daughter take me rather than calling an ambulance. It would have taken the ambulance more than 30 minutes to even get to my house! I could get to the hospital in 25 minutes!*" Another participant described the consequences for him of his wife's lack of knowledge about stroke onset:

> I got up and my arm and hand was numb and I told my wife that I thought I was having a stroke. She told me 'Oh, you just don't want to go to work today. You go to work and it will get better!' And I went to work and by the time I got there, my leg was numb and I could not get out of my truck. Instead, I just drove to the hospital and when I got to the hospital emergency room entrance, I just honked the horn, and they came out and got me.

After one year, the left leg and arm of this participant were still paralyzed. It was about 3 hours from the time he thought he was having a stroke until he arrived at the hospital. A third participant described the distress she experienced when the EMS team did not explain their process:

> My mother was having a stroke and I knew that it was a stroke. I called EMS (Emergency Medical Services ambulance) and they came in about 18 minutes. They put my mother on a stretcher and took her to the ambulance. Then they closed the door and sat in my driveway for about 15 minutes. I went out and beat on the door of the ambulance, but they would not open it. Finally, they left for the hospital. I could have put her in the car and taken her to the hospital in about 20 minutes! Next time, I will do it myself.

Qualitative interviews with the EMS staff revealed that only one ambulance was available and they had previously taken an accident victim to the hospital, then quickly cleaned the ambulance and driven to the patient's house. During the time they were in the driveway, they were sending EKG results and other vital signs of the patient to the emergency room physician and providing oxygen to the patient, who had coded in the ambulance. These actions enabled the emergency room physician to communicate with a university stroke center to design treatment and the transfer of the patient to the stroke center.

These are just a few of the examples of negative experiences that people with stroke, their caregivers, and health care staff experienced. Other participants shared other problems, but it was clear that some members of the community had had negative experiences. Thus, we must continue to work with our communities to teach them to recognize stroke symptoms, explore issues and take actions to improve stroke identification, and take actions to decrease transportation time to the hospital. Community members need to better understand the processes that identify potential stroke and what actions they should take to maximize the health of stroke patients.

Types of Stroke and Diagnosis

The 2021 Guideline for the Prevention of Stroke in Patients with Stroke and Transient Ischemic Attack describes the types and subtypes of strokes (Kleindorfer et al. 2021). Ischemic stroke, the most common type, accounts for an estimated 88% of all strokes. This type of stroke happens when blood flow to or in the brain is blocked by a blood clot that forms in the brain or travels from other parts of the body to the brain. Plaque, a fatty substance that builds up in an artery leading to the brain, may also block blood flow to certain parts of the brain.

Hemorrhagic strokes account for an estimated 12% of strokes. This type is caused by blood leaking out of the blood vessels into brain tissue (intracerebral hemorrhage) or blood leaking out of the blood vessels between the brain and the skull (subarachnoid). The blood vessel may be damaged from the aging process or from high blood pressure. Falls can also cause a tear in the blood vessel between the brain and the skull. Another type is the "ministroke," or transient ischemic stroke (TIA), which is formed when a blood clot or plaque temporally blocks blood flow in the brain and then quickly breaks loose and allows the blood to flow again. The symptoms are the same as those for an ischemic stroke, but the symptoms quickly pass and the person feels better as symptoms clear up. However, a TIA is a warning sign of a lasting ischemic stroke. Finally, although it is not common, it is possible to have a stroke with no recognized symptoms. Tests may show lesions in the brain that are evidence of damaged brain tissue. This problem increases the risk of a future stroke.

Further identification of the specific cause(s) of stroke is needed to improve prevention and treatment. For example, an ischemic stroke may be identified as lacunar (a type that accounts for approximately 23% of ischemic strokes) or non-lacunar (a type that accounts for 77% of ischemic strokes). Lacunar strokes are caused by diseased small vessels. Non-lacunar strokes are caused by blood clots that are formed in the heart (cardioembolic), in large blood vessels (a large artery), or in other parts of the body that are unknown (cryptogenic).

Methods for assessing and diagnosing the type of stroke are very important for locating the injury to the brain and planning the type of treatment. Other problems such as seizures, drug overdose, fainting, and migraine headaches must be ruled out. The health care provider needs to know what the symptoms are (lack of mental alertness; problems with speaking clearly or seeing clearly numbness or weakness in the face, arms, legs) and when the symptoms started. They also need access to other medical history and to conduct a physical exam that includes blood tests; tests for mental alertness, coordination and balance; and other tests. The types of tests (imaging and blood flow tests of the brain) that may be done to diagnose the stroke and identify the type of stroke include computed tomography (CT) scans and magnetic resonance imaging (MRI). These have been identified as the best diagnostic tests for strokes.

A CT scan can provide a clear view of the head tissues and blood vessels by using X-rays and computers to create multiple images of the head from various angles. It can easily show the size and location of any abnormalities in the brain, such as tumors or blood clots. It can also reveal infections, such as areas of the brain where the tissue is dying or dead due to loss of blood flow. CT scans are the most popular intervention when stroke is suspected because CT machines are available at most hospitals. Typically, a CT scan for potential stroke patients takes priority over other more routine problems, as the scan provides information that is needed for treatment design. An MRI uses magnetic fields, radiofrequency pulses, and computers to identify changes in the brain. Like a CT scan, an MRI for stroke takes multiple images of the inside of the head using sophisticated X-rays and computers. While a CT scan cannot reveal blockage of blood flow until several hours after the start of symptoms, an MRI can reveal brain damage within an hour of the onset of stroke symptoms. MRIs are also more accurate than CT scans because they are far more sensitive. They reveal all issues related to a stroke within the brain. MRIs are excellent at detecting even tiny abnormalities, which are often too small to be clearly seen in a CT scan. However, not all hospitals have MRI machines. While an MRI is excellent for getting highly detailed images of the inside of the head, it may not be the ideal choice in emergencies when rapid treatment is essential for reducing the potentially debilitating side effects of a stroke. Because it uses magnetic fields to create the image, it is not a viable option for people with metallic or electronic implants, such as pacemakers or shrapnel wounds. A head MRI is an excellent way to diagnose whether a stroke is ischemic or hemorrhagic, and it is also good for finding abnormalities in the skull and spinal cord.

Another test is the computed tomographic angiography. In this test, a special contrast dye is injected into a vein and images are taken of blood vessels to identify abnormalities such as an aneurysm. Other tests include magnetic resonance angiography, in which the blood vessels are imaged to locate a blocked artery or cerebral aneurysm, and cerebral angiography, in which special substances are injected into the bloodstream and X-rays are taken to produce a picture of blood flow through the vessels. This makes visible the size and location of blockages and can reveal aneurysms and malformed blood vessels.

CT scan and MRI of the heart can also help detect heart problems or blood clots that may have led to a stroke. Other possible tests include electrocardiogram (EKG) and an echocardiography. CT scans, MRIs, EKGs, X-rays, and echocardiography are not painful, but if contrast dyes are needed, the injection can be a bit uncomfortable. An MRI takes longer than other tests, and being enclosed the machine may be a challenge for people with claustrophobia. A discussion between the patient and the health care provider is needed before an MRI. Reading CT scans, MRIs, and EKGs requires skills. Some smaller hospitals that lack such expertise link with larger hospitals or university hospitals for support and recommendations that may include transfer of the patient for interventions. Time is critical for most stroke interventions, especially for clot-busting tPA treatment and for possible surgery interventions to remove a clot (when possible). Once the stroke-related problem is identified, the treatment plan becomes the major priority for rapid action.

African Americans experience all of the types of strokes but are most susceptible to hemorrhagic strokes. As with all stroke patients, it is most important to diagnose the type of stroke and the cause of the stroke, develop a treatment plan, rapidly implement the plan, share the treatment plan with the patient or their specified family member(s) for input and decision-making, and then tailor the plan to the individual patient. The guidelines for stroke care emphasize shared decision-making and tailoring for treatment, for preventing secondary stroke, and for maximizing recovery.

Stroke Treatment in the Hospital

A severe first or secondary stroke may lead to major complications, disabilities, or death. The differences in treatment and outcomes are often confusing for the patient and their family. While some older studies documented disparities in treatment, more recent studies do not document or report treatment disparities for African Americans, Schwamm and colleagues (2010, 1492) analyzed data from 1,181 hospitals across the United States that were participating in Get with the Guidelines stroke program. They reported that "Black patients with stroke received fewer evidence-based care processes than Hispanic or white patients." However, they noted that care had improved over time. Sacco and colleagues (2017), who examined racial differences in stroke care in Florida and Puerto Rico, found minimal or no differences for African Americans but reported that Hispanic patients received less care for strokes. More recent reports have identified no disparities in care of hospitalized African American stroke patients. However, African Americans have reported that they continue to be concerned about care in the hospital. Members of several focus groups reported that they were put in patient rooms "farther from the nurses desk" and got different or poorer quality care than whites, but others expressed that the care they received was excellent. All providers need to work with the patient and their family, and other health care professionals to ensure that all patients receive quality stroke care and comfort.

Stroke Rehabilitation and Recovery and Palliative Care

Rehabilitation from stroke and its complications should begin as soon as possible, usually within a day or two after stroke, and it should be individualized for each patient. While some people recover quickly, others may take longer. Many have long-term disabilities or even permanent problems that they learn to live with. Following discharge from an acute care hospital, rehabilitation from stroke is a major goal that is usually accomplished in rehabilitation facilities or in the stroke survivor's home. The Paul Coverdell National Acute Stroke Program at the Centers for Disease Control and Prevention has identified the more common challenges of stroke as:

- Paralysis (inability to move some parts of the body) or weakness or both on one side of the body

- Trouble with thinking, awareness, attention, learning, judgment, and memory
- Problems understanding or forming speech
- Trouble controlling or expressing emotions
- Numbness or strange sensations
- Pain in the hands and feet that worsens with movement and changes in temperature
- Trouble with chewing and swallowing
- Problems with bladder and bowel control
- Depression (CDC 2021a)

The goal is to use rehabilitation to help patients recover or learn to live with their disability and to prevent another stroke, as about one in four strokes are secondary strokes. It is extremely important to identify and treat the causes of stroke, including heart disease, high blood pressure, atrial fibrillation, elevated cholesterol, and diabetes (CDC 2021a).

Some patients who experience a stroke may prefer palliative care or hospice care over high-risk interventions. A review of the literature (from 2015 to 2021) related to palliative care after stroke revealed that most published research focused on palliative care needs, organization of palliative care for stroke, and shared decision-making between health care providers and patients and/or their families (Cowey et al. 2021). The review also found that racial disparities in access to palliative care after stroke were common. Another study identified the outcome measures needed for research on palliative care and end-of-life care after severe stroke as (listed in order of priority):

- Shared decision-making between professionals, the patient, and family members
- The degree of distress about fear of dying or living with severe disability the patient is feeling
- Whether the patient feels that they are being treated and valued as a person
- Perceptions of the quality and appropriateness of care provided on the part of the patient and/or their family
- The patient's ability to understand and respond to communication from others
- The amount of distress treatment for stroke causes the patient
- Amount of pain a patient has (Mason et al. 2020)

Much research is needed before guidelines are developed for palliative and end-of-life care for stroke patients. We also need research related to prevention, treatment, and recovery. Although we know a great deal, more research and more incorporation of research findings into care plans are needed. We need to translate current knowledge into actions that will increase prevention.

Actions Individuals and Families Can Take to Prevent Primary and Secondary Strokes

Many resources exist for helping individuals, families, and health care professionals learn more about stroke prevention, treatment, recovery, and living with stroke. The key is finding the right resources and implementing the actions that are needed. Ideally the hospital discharge coordinator or hospital staff will give the patient and their family a guide or list of resources with the discharge plan. The Centers for Disease Control and Prevention and the American Heart Association and its affiliated American Stroke Association have good resources and information about evidence-based practices for individuals and health care providers. Although the leading stroke organizations recognize that some stroke risk factors such as age, gender, race, family history, and previous stroke or transient ischemic attack cannot be controlled, up to 80% of strokes can be prevented by making lifestyle changes and managing medical conditions.

Individuals who take these steps can significantly reduce their risk of stroke:

- Eating more fruits and vegetables, especially fresh or frozen ones without added sugar, salt, and fats
- Reducing salt in the diet by avoiding or limiting salty foods and avoiding adding salt at the table
- Increasing physical activity, which can be done in ways that the person enjoys
- Quitting smoking (if a smoker) and avoiding secondary smoke from others who smoke.
- Losing excess body weight; even five to ten pounds helps
- Managing stress in ways that work for the individual

One of the most important actions a person can take is to work with a health care provider to ensure that blood pressure is controlled and to take the medications they have been prescribed for controlling risk factors. For health care professionals, the American Heart Association and American Stroke Association have developed evidence-based guidelines for preventing and controlling blood pressure and stroke risks that are updated regularly based on the latest research. These associations also fund research. Much research is funded by the National Institutes of Health (NIH), particularly the National Institute of Neurological Disorders and Stroke, other NIH Institutes, and the Agency for Healthcare Research and Quality. Private agencies are another source of research funding. Rehabilitation inpatient and outpatient agencies also provide guidelines for rehabilitation. The Centers for Disease Control and Prevention focuses on translating research and guidelines into action for individuals, communities, and states across the United States, particularly those with higher risks. But much more needs to be done if we are to continue to reduce the incidence of stroke for all Americans, particularly for African Americans living in the South.

In 2021, the American Stroke Association issued the "2021 Guideline for the Prevention of Stroke in Patients with Stroke and Transient Ischemic Attack" (Kleindorfer et al. 2021). One of the American Stroke Association's ten important messages is related to African Americans and social determinants of health: "Stroke survivors from historically under-resourced communities, including Black and Hispanic populations, may face social and economic difficulties, systemic racism and poor living conditions that contribute to ill health and make it difficult to make changes to prevent future strokes. Health care professionals should evaluate these factors when managing stroke risk to address gaps in care. Further research is needed to determine the best methods for reducing care gaps after stroke for vulnerable populations" (American Stroke Association 2021).

The challenges for all of us are improving optimal control of risk factors, improving the frequency and timeliness of proven interventions for acute stroke, and addressing gaps in the continuum of care for stroke patients. We must all work together to address these issues and tailor our approach to the problems African Americans who experience stroke face if we are to improve their outcomes. This is especially true for African Americans living in the Stroke Belt of the United States, who experience a higher incidence of stroke, more severe strokes than people in other parts of the country, and higher mortality from stroke.

REFERENCES

American Diabetes Association. 2022. "Statistics about Diabetes." Last modified February 4, 2022. Accessed July 27, 2021. https://www.diabetes.org/resources/statistics/statistics-about-diabetes.

American Heart Association. 2021. "2021 Heart Disease & Stroke Statistical Update Fact Sheet Black Race & Cardiovascular Diseases." https://professional.heart.org/-/media/PHD-Files-2/Science-News/2/2021-Heart-and-Stroke-Stat-Update/2021_Stat_Update_factsheet_Black_Race_and_CVD.pdf.

American Stroke Association. 2019. "Let's Talk about Black Americans and Stroke." Accessed July 23, 2021. https://www.stroke.org/-/media/stroke-files/lets-talk-about-stroke/prevention/lets-talk-about-black-americans-and-stroke-sheet.pdf?la=en.

———. 2021. "Guideline for the Prevention of Stroke and Transient Ischemic Attack, Top 10 Patient Messages." Accessed July 24, 2021. https://www.stroke.org/-/media/stroke-images/infographics/preventinganotherstroke2021-guidelines.pdf?la=en accessed.

Bidulescu, A., J. Liu, Z. Chen, D. A. Hickson, S. K. Musani, T. E. Samdarshi, E. R. Fox, H. A. Taylor, and G. H. Gibbons. 2013. "Associations of Adiponectin and Leptin with Incident Coronary Heart Disease and Ischemic Stroke in African Americans: The Jackson Heart Study." *Frontiers in Public Health* 1 (16). https://pubmed.ncbi.nlm.nih.gov/24350185/.

Bonita, R. J. Duncan, T. Truelsen, R. T. Jackson, and R. Beaglehole. 1999. "Passive Smoking as Well as Active Smoking Increases the Risk of Acute Stroke." *Tobacco Control* 8 (2): 156–160.

Booth, J., L. Connelly, M. Lawrence, C. Chalmers, S. Joice, C. Becker, and N. Dougall. 2015. "Evidence of Perceived Psychosocial Stress as a Risk Factor for Stroke in Adults: A Meta-Analysis." *BMC Neurology* 15 (1): 1–12.

Brousseau, D. C., J. A. Panepinto, M. Nimmer, and R. G. Hoffmann. 2010. "The Number of People with Sickle-Cell Disease in the United States: National and State Estimates." *American Journal of Hematology* 85 (1): 77–78.

CDC (Centers for Disease Control and Prevention). 2021a. "Recovering from Stroke." Last modified May 25, 2021. Accessed July 25, 2021. https://www.cdc.gov/stroke/recovery.htm.

———. 2021b. "Tools for Putting Social Determinants of Health into Action." Last reviewed October 14, 2021. https://www.cdc.gov/socialdeterminants/tools/index.htm.

Cowey, E., M. Schichtel, J. D. Cheyne, L. Tweedie, R. Lehman, R. Melifonwu, and G. E. Mead. 2021. "Palliative Care after Stroke: A Review." *International Journal of Stroke* 16 (6): 632–639.

Crump, C. 2021. "Adult Mortality after Preterm Birth—Time to Translate Findings Into Clinical Practice." *JAMA Network Open* 4 (1): e2033361. https://jamanetwork.com/journals/jamanetworkopen/fullarticle/2774714.

Cruz-Flores, S., A. Rabinstein, J. Biller, and M. S. Elkind. 2011. "Racial-Ethnic Disparities in Stroke Care: The American Experience." *Stroke* 42 (7), 2091–20116.

Dlamini, N., and L. C. Jordan. 2021. "Young Adult Survivors of Preterm Birth Are at Increased Risk of Stroke: The Missing Link." *Stroke* 52 (8): 2618–2620.

Esenwa, C., D. Ilunga Tshiswaka, M. Gebregziabher, and B. Ovbiagele. 2018. "Historical Slavery and Modern-Day Stroke Mortality in the United States Stroke Belt." *Stroke* 49 (2): 465–469.

Howard, G., D. T. Lackland, D. O. Kleindorfer, B. M. Kissela, C. S. Moy, S. E. Judd, M. M. Safford, M. Cushman, S. P. Glasser, et al. 2013. "Racial Differences in the Impact of Elevated Systolic Blood Pressure on Stroke Risk." *JAMA Internal Medicine* 173 (1): 46–51.

Howard, V. J. 2013. "Reasons Underlying Racial Differences in Stroke Incidence and Mortality." *Stroke* 44 (suppl. 6): S126–S128.

Ingram, D. D., and J. A. Montresor-Lopez. 2015. "Differences in Stroke Mortality Among Adults Aged 45 and Over: United States, 2010–2013." NCHS Data Brief No. 207. https://www.cdc.gov/nchs/products/databriefs/db207.htm.

Jackson, F. L. 1991. "An Evolutionary Perspective on Salt, Hypertension, and Human Genetic Variability." *Hypertension* 17(suppl. 1): I129.

Kelly, P. J., R. Lemmens, and G. Tsivgoulis. 2021. "Inflammation and Stroke Risk: A New Target for Prevention." *Stroke* 52 (8): 2697–2706.

Kleindorfer, D. O., J. Khoury, C. J. Moomaw, K. Alwell, D. Woo, M. L. Flaherty, P. Khatri, O. Adeoye, S. Ferioli, et al. 2010. "Stroke Incidence Is Decreasing in Whites but Not in Blacks: A Population-Based Estimate of Temporal Trends in Stroke Incidence from the Greater Cincinnati / Northern Kentucky Stroke Study." *Stroke* 41 (7): 1326–1331.

Kleindorfer, D. O., A. Towfighi, S. Chaturvedi, K. M. Cockroft, J. Gutierrez, D. Lombardi-Hill, H. Kamel, W. N. Kernan, S. J. Kittner, et al. 2021. "2021 Guideline for the Prevention of Stroke in Patients with Stroke and Transient Ischemic Attack: A Guideline From the American Heart Association / American Stroke Association." *Stroke* 52 (7). https://www.ahajournals.org/doi/10.1161/STR.0000000000000375.

Kochanek, K. D., S. L. Murphy, J. Xu, and E. Arias. 2019. "Deaths: Final Data for 2017." *National Vital Statistics Reports* 68 (9): 1–77. Accessed July 25, 2021. https://www.cdc.gov/nchs/data/nvsr/nvsr68/nvsr68_09-508.pdf.

Koval, K. W., T. L. Setji, E. Reyes, and A. Brown. 2010. "Higher High-Density Lipoprotein Cholesterol in African-American Women with Polycystic Ovary Syndrome Compared with Caucasian Counterparts." *Journal of Clinical Endocrinology and Metabolism* 95 (9): E49–E53. https://doi.org/10.1210/jc.2010-0074.

Lisabeth, L., and C. Bushnell. 2012. "Stroke Risk in Women: The Role of Menopause and Hormone Therapy." *Lancet Neurology* 11 (1): 82–91. https://doi.org/10.1016/S1474-4422(11)70269-1.

Mason, B., K. Boyd, F. Doubal, M. Barber, M. Brady, E. Cowey, A. Visvanathan, S. Lewis, K. Gallacher, et al. 2020. "Core Outcome Measures for Palliative and End-of-Life Research after Severe Stroke: Mixed-Method Delphi Study." *Stroke* 52 (11): 3507–3513.

McCabe, J. J., and Kelly, P. J. "Inflammation, Cholesterol, and Stroke Risk: Building Evidence for a Dual Target Strategy for Secondary Prevention." *Stroke* 52 (9). https://www.ahajournals.org/doi/10.1161/STROKEAHA.121.035676.

McDermott, K. W., and M. Roemer. 2021. "Most Frequent Principal Diagnoses for Inpatient Stays in U.S. Hospitals, 2018." AHRQ Statistical Brief #277. https://www.hcup-us.ahrq.gov/reports/statbriefs/sb277-Top-Reasons-Hospital-Stays-2018.pdf.

Ovbiagele, B. 2020. "HEADS-UP: Understanding and Problem-Solving: Seeking Hands-Down Solutions to Major Inequities in Stroke." *Stroke* 51 (11): 3375–3381.

Ovbiagele, B., L. B. Goldstein, R. T. Higashida, V. J. Howard, S. C. Johnston, O. A. Khavjou, D. T. Lackland, J. H. Lichtman, S. Mohl, et al. 2013. "Forecasting the Future of Stroke in the United States: A Policy Statement from the American Heart Association and American Stroke Association." *Stroke* 44 (8): 2361–2375. https://www.ahajournals.org/doi/full/10.1161/STR.0b013e31829734f2.

Sacco, R. L., H. Gardener, K. Wang, C. Dong, M. A. Ciliberti-Vargas, C. M. Gutierrez, N. Asdaghi, W. S. Burgin, O. Carrasquillo, et al. 2017. "Racial-Ethnic Disparities in Acute Stroke Care in the Florida-Puerto Rico Collaboration to Reduce Stroke Disparities Study." *Journal of the American Heart Association* 6 (2): e004073.

Schwamm, L. H., M. J. Reeves, W. Pan, E. E. Smith, M. R. Frankel, D. Olson, X. Zhao, E. Peterson, and G. C. Fonarow. 2010. "Race/Ethnicity, Quality of Care, and Outcomes in Ischemic Stroke." *Circulation* 121 (13): 1492–1501.

Schultz, Amy, and Mary E. Northridge. 2004. "Social Determinants of Health: Implications for Environmental Health Promotion." *Health, Education, & Behavior* 31 (4): 455–471.

Sedrak, A., and N. P. Kondamudi. 2021. "Sickle Cell Disease." Last modified February 26, 2021. National Library of Medicine. https://www.ncbi.nlm.nih.gov/books/NBK482384.

Skolarus, L. E., A. Sharrief, H. Gardener, C. Jenkins, and B. Boden-Albala. 2020. "Considerations in Addressing Social Determinants of Health to Reduce Racial/Ethnic Disparities in Stroke Outcomes in the United States." *Stroke* 51 (11): 3433–3439.

US Department of Health and Human Services, Office of Minority Heath. 2021. "Stroke and African Americans." Last modified February 11, 20201. Accessed July 28, 2021. https://minorityhealth.hhs.gov/omh/browse.aspx?lvl=4&lvlid=28.

Virani, S. S., A. Alonso, E. J. Benjamin, M. S. Bittencourt, C. W. Callaway, A. P. Carson, et al. 2020. "Heart Disease and Stroke Statistics—2020 Update: A Report From the American Heart Association." *Circulation* 141 (9): e139–e596. https://www.ahajournals.org/doi/10.1161/CIR.0000000000000757.

12

Disparities in Interpersonal Violence

CAMILLE BURNETT, PhD, MPA, APHN-BC, RN, BScN, DSW, CGNC, FAAN

Intimate partner violence (IPV) is a health issue of epidemic proportions in the United States and around the world. It is a form of violence against women that affects an estimated 1 in 4 women and 1 in 10 men in the United States (CDC 2020b; Smith et al. 2018). Intimate partner violence involves an array of abuses such as physical, sexual, and psychological aggression and stalking that occur within the context of an intimate partner relationship and vary in frequency and severity (CDC 2020b). Specifically, physical abuses involve the use of physical force against another person such as hitting, kicking, and punching. Sexual violence entails forced sex and sexual acts and touching without consent. Incidents involving verbal, mental, or emotional abuse fall under the category of psychological aggression, as do coercive acts. This spectrum includes reproductive coercion, or explicit acts to control reproduction and pregnancy outcomes, interference with contraception, and unprotected sex occur against the will of the partner (Basile et al. 2019). Stalking includes acts of unwanted contact and attention. These forms of violence constitute the many aspects of IPV that have serious and far-reaching consequences for individuals, families, and societies. Al'Uqdah, Maxwell, and Hill (2016) found higher rates of IPV victimization among African American men and women and referenced findings where African American men were more likely than other races to become victims of IPV. For Black women, the prevalence of certain forms of IPV has been found to be even higher (Smith et al. 2018; Black et al. 2011). In a recent study of Black women in Baltimore (N = 188) by Alexander et al. (2019), participants reported a lifetime exposure of 48.9% for IPV, 37.8% for reproductive coercion. Thirty-eight percent of the study participants had experienced both. Kapaya et. al. (2019) confirm also report a greater incidence of physical IPV for non-Hispanic Blacks (22.9%) than other racial/ethnic groups (13.1%). While IPV impacts both men and women, decades of research have clearly shown that African American women in particular experience "higher rates of overall severe, mutual, and recurrent past-year and lifetime IPV victimization and perpetration when compared with their White and Hispanic counterparts" (Lacey et al. 2016). Given such high rates of exposure to IPV, it is not surprising that negative health consequences are exacerbated within this group.

Negative health effects and the broader impacts of IPV are widespread and far reaching. IPV is associated with poor mental health and poor pregnancy outcomes such as low birth weight and adversely affects the economic status of its victims. Known health effects of IPV include posttraumatic stress disorder (PTSD), anxiety, depression, chronic pain, headaches, and fatigue (Lutwak 2018). If a victim of IPV suffers even a mild traumatic brain injury, they are at risk for adverse central nervous system symptoms. Campbell et. al (2018) found that 50% of their sample of women exposed to IPV had suffered a probable traumatic brain injury and reported at least one of the following central nervous system symptoms: memory loss, headaches, blacking out, ringing of the ears, dizzy spells, seizures, vision problems, hearing problems, and difficulty concentrating. Additionally, of those women who reported IPV (N = 270) slightly more than 70% had also experienced strangulation. Given the overabundance of negative health sequalae that IPV has on the lives of its victims and the higher prevalence of some forms of IPV in the Black population, it is expected that we would also find higher incidences of poor health outcomes, impairments to well-being, and a lower quality of life in this population. One critical precursor to IPV in adult relationships is exposure to previous abuse and adverse childhood experiences. Limited studies have explored the unique differences in the experiences of violence in the lives of African Americans and the salient factors that serve to mediate and/or protect Black women (Howell et al. 2018).

Contextualizing Our Understanding of Intimate Partner Violence

Understanding IPV in the lives of African American and Black people must be situated in our understanding of the root causes of violence globally and the experiences of violence for this specific group.

For decades, the Duluth Model has been recognized as the dominant paradigm for understanding IPV and its various forms (Domestic Abuse Intervention Programs 2017). Developed in 1981, this intervention model heavily focuses on power and control as the drivers of abuse tactics. However, its perspective that perpetrators of IPV (which this model understands to be male) have all the power and control in a relationship does not acknowledge the variation of experiences or identities. People have unique identities that play a significant role in shaping their experiences. Identities related to race, ethnicity, class, and sexual orientation merge into histories and exposures that cannot be unilaterally understood as rooted and shaped solely by the power and control of one individual. This is most evident and pronounced in the lives of Black and brown people in the United States, where history, oppression, and racist structures have affected their ability to live violence-free lives. Bohall, Bautista, and Musson's (2016) examination of the Duluth Model found that although some aspects of it are useful, it is limited in considering the full complexity of IPV, which cannot be explained away by patriarchal power and control. Any model that seeks to help Black men and women must factor in ethnicity; types of relationships; societal values, norms, and beliefs; and multiple forms of oppression such as racism that Black populations experience.

Discussions of race and racism in the United States are fraught with division, white fragility, and alternative dominant narratives that either portray an altered reality of the present-day impacts of racism or fail to even acknowledge its persistent existence. Racism is undeniably a root cause of the disparities that manifest today across and within groups, especially those experienced by Black and brown people. It is a key source of trauma that further perpetuates health disparities. The African American family experience has unfolded against the backdrop of the traumatizing effects of slavery and its structural and systemic derivatives that continue to present themselves in family dynamics (Al'Uqdah, Maxwell, and Hill 2016). The consequences of the disparities and historical oppression Black people face permeates both their experiences of IPV and their ability to escape it. Therefore, understanding IPV among Blacks has to account for the uniqueness of their experiences and their exposure to persistent inequities. Cheng and Lo (2016) used the multiple disadvantage model in an attempt to examine racial disparities in IPV and its connectedness to "social structural factors, social relationships, substance use, and health / mental health and access to related services." Although their study only partially supported these associative relationships, it illuminated distinct patterns associated with physical assault across ethnic groups. At a minimum, this indicates that addressing IPV must reconcile exposure to IPV with the lived reality of racialized populations by taking into account the multiple factors that negatively affect a family's ability to flourish.

Cumulative Trauma: A Catalyst for Increasing Vulnerability

Exposure to trauma is a critical determinant of a person's ability to create and sustain healthy relationships and achieve well-being. According to the Substance Abuse and Mental Health Services Administration of the United States Department of Health and Human Service, "trauma results from an event, series of events, or set of circumstances that is experienced by an individual as physically or emotionally harmful or threatening and that has lasting adverse effects on the individual's functioning and physical, social, emotional, or spiritual well-being" (Substance Abuse and Mental Health Services Administration 2014a, 7). Exposure to trauma elevates a person's risk of developing a variety of disorders such as mental health issues, substance use, disruptive behaviors, and sleep disturbances (Substance Abuse and Mental Health Services Administration 2014b). IPV is one source of trauma; others include but are not limited to adverse childhood experiences and racial trauma. Many such traumas are experienced concurrently (and cumulatively), and in the case of African Americans, racial trauma is experienced directly or vicariously in all aspects of life, further exacerbating the effects of trauma and impeding healing. Mental Health America (2022) recognizes that race-based trauma is experienced individually and systemically, often creating stressors that can be generationally transferred and can cause symptoms of PTSD. Roberts et al.'s (2010) study examined the ethnic and racial difference in exposure to trauma events, risk of PTSD, and access to treatment. They found that the lifetime prevalence of PTSD was highest in Blacks (8.7%), the risk for childhood trauma through witnessing IPV was greater in Blacks and Hispanics, and that seeking treatment PTSD was less across all minority groups. Seeking help is vital for overcoming trauma experiences and exposure to IPV. Furthermore, the accumulation of trauma can lead to accrued psychopathology and an increased vulnerability to violence and abuse (Anderson et al. 2018). How this cycle of trauma, vulnerability to IPV, and limited engagement with help-seeking behaviors serve to widen existing disparities among African American populations warrants far more exploration, as do solutions that redress and disrupt the virulence of the cycle. A deeper understanding is critical, given that historical and recurring trauma perpetrated by those who create and sustain inequitable structures and oppressive systems is pervasive. Communities of color and other minoritized groups bear the enormous burden of structural and systemic violence and injustice through the practices, policies, and institutions that have engaged in and reified inequitable practices such as mass incarceration, genocide, slavery, family separation, forced relocation, and redlining (Cockhren 2020).

Adverse childhood experiences (ACEs) include toxic events that create stress for children. They range from witnessing IPV to the divorce of parents, the alcoholism of parents or caregivers, and bullying. These stressors impact brain development, mental health, and stress response behaviors and are linked to epigenetic consequences, chronic health problems, mental illness, and substance misuse in adulthood (CDC 2019). In the United States, 61% of adults have experienced at least one ACE. Disturbingly, women and racial/ethnic minorities are "at greater risk for experiencing 4 or more ACEs" (CDC 2019). Given such prevalence, it is reasonable to assume that those exposed to violence have been exposed to adverse childhood experiences. This layered exposure means that IPV cannot be dealt with in a vacuum and without considering how these exposures to trauma intersect to increase a person's risk of IPV. In addition, overcoming abuse can be increasingly difficult for people who are more likely to have incurred cumulative trauma such as African Americans. Overcoming abuse requires various supports, resources, and opportunities that need to be tailored to African Americans and other communities of color because of the complexity and context of their lived experiences.

Intersectionality: An Informed Approach and Framework

Intersectionality is a concept that gained prominence in the early 1990s through the work of Black feminist activist and academic Kimberlé Crenshaw (1991). Crenshaw's work illuminates considerations that are important for contextualizing the experiences of violence against women because it emphasizes the importance of the multiple identities of Black women. This was deemed to be a necessary response to the identity politics movement that Crenshaw felt ignored intragroup differences, specifically as they relate to violence against women. Identity politics focuses on the narrative of the collective as a basis for political action and has struggled to be address personal identity (Brunila and Rossi 2017; Diamond 2012). Intersectionality, in contrast, does not ignore within-group differences, instead taking into account the totality of a person's multiple identities (i.e., race, gender, sexual orientation, class). These identities are respected and viewed as critical to understanding how worlds and experiences are constructed so people can transform them in ways that are meaningful for that them. However, an intersectional approach should be included within the mainstream IPV discourse. Otherwise, that discourse amounts to an inherent dismissal of contextual factors that contribute and shape IPV and its outcomes in communities of color.

African Americans have disproportionate experiences of cumulative trauma, oppression and subordination that frame their experience of IPV. Crenshaw (1991), who wrote about intersectionality as it pertains to Black women, noted the multiple layers and patterns of "routinized forms of domination that often converge on these women's lives," further impeding their ability to create alternatives to the abuse. Health inequities refers to differences in health that vary across populations and are unjust because they are preventable and unnecessary. They are systemic and could be avoided by reasonable means. They are inequitable distributions of health resources and risk that are allowed to persist (Arcaya, Arcaya, and Subramanian 2015). Yet they are multidimensional in their between-group impacts, which is why we must consider the experience of IPV through an intersectional lens.

Black women experience IPV within multiple identities of race, class, gender, age, and sexual orientation. These identities intersect with the inequitable distribution of the social determinants of health such as limited social mobility, affordable housing scarcity, discrimination, lower socioeconomic status, and lack of economic opportunity. Rates of violence are known to be higher in disadvantaged communities. Sabri and colleagues (2014) found that among Blacks, low levels of education, unemployment, low income, unemployment, and cohabitation without marriage contribute to a significant risk of violence.

The COVID-19 pandemic has influenced the prevalence of IPV and its associated risk factors. It has been well documented that people of color have borne the brunt of COVID-19 and its effects. In the United States, a nation with the highest COVID-19 infection rates and death rates per capita worldwide, this population suffers disproportionately (World Health Organization 2021). According to the Centers for Disease Control and Prevention

(CDC), African Americans account for 12.2% of COVID cases and 15.6% of COVID deaths (CDC 2020a), although they account for 13.4% of the US population (United States Census Bureau 2019). COVID-19 has magnified the inequities that existed before the pandemic. African Americans experience severe ramifications from a constellation of social and structural factors that include economic instability, unsafe housing, neighborhood violence, and lack of safe and stable child care and social support (Evans, Lindauer, and Farrell 2020). During the pandemic, stressors such as job loss, unemployment, and underemployment have ravaged families that were already struggling to make ends meet. Pending evictions and ongoing food insecurity loom heavily. Education has been upended, and many who already had insufficient resources have struggled to juggle access to technology, home schooling, and work while the economy plunged deeper into recession and the incidence of mental health issues increased. Black workers are overrepresented among lower-wage income earners relative to their total share of the workforce and along with Latinx community are among the most vulnerable to economic hardship (Ross and Bateman 2019). Many service sectors deemed to be essential are lower-wage jobs, so having a job deemed essential during a pandemic has increased these workers' exposure to the virus. Amid this intersecting turmoil are the brutal and horrific killings of Black people almost daily. George Floyd, Breonna Taylor, Ahmad Aubrey . . . #SayTheirNames. Personal stories shared on various media platforms have become the way to record the enormity of the impact that all of this has on the African American community. Many took to that forum to convey their frustration, sorrow, despondence, rage, and pain. Others used it as a call to action and worked to organize for change or publicize examples of resilience and humanity.

Meanwhile, social isolation mandates, although they were well intended and were necessary for slowing the spread of COVID-19, have created unintended consequences that are particularly harmful for those in abusive situations. Early on, government-sanctioned quarantine policies assumed that being home and isolated was the safest option for everyone. Van Gelder et al. (2020) noted that social isolating behaviors imposed by federal and local COVID-19 recommendations mimicked abusive tactics and that when paired with the various stressors resulting from the pandemic could also increase negative coping mechanisms. They warned of "an unprecedented wave of IPV." Sadly, what staying home means for those who are being abused has not been discussed in COVID-19 policies, guidelines, or practices. Victims of IPV seek opportunities when the abuser is not around to get help, which has become increasing difficult with modified working arrangements that can cause the abuser to be home more frequently. Moreover, the ever-ominous threat of exposure to a highly infectious and potentially deadly virus weighs heavily should the victim consider leaving (Kaufman and Garfin 2020). This has created an environment for increased IPV frequency and has decreased the privacy of victims and their ability to seek help. Further, COVID-19 disease control mechanisms have reduced access to services that victims have routinely turned to for support, interventions, and alternatives to being abused. Seeing health care providers is not as easy as it used to be, given their limited hours and options for contact. Telehealth works only if you have access to broadband internet. Even if you do, discussing the abuse situation from within the abusive home is unsafe. Shelters that have traditionally served as a respite and sanctuary from abuse have had to modify their entry requirements. Courts are not operating at full capacity, making it challenging to obtain an emergency protection order, another safety mechanism. Although data are limited and are still emerging, it should not be surprising that there is evidence of an alarming rise in domestic violence during COVID-19 (Boserup, McKenney, and Elkbuli 2020; Graham-Harrison et al. 2020). Bradbury-Jones and Isham (2020) reference emerging and disturbing reports of an increase in domestic homicides during the pandemic. An increase in the number of domestic violence hotline calls have been reported in some cases while decreasing call volume have been noted in others, which could be a result of the inability to access much-needed supports and resources during COVID restrictions (Evans, Lindauer, and Farrell 2020). Although the scale of the impact of IPV during COVID is still unfolding, evidence of its specific effects on IPV in the Black community and the associated risk factors must also be investigated.

Poverty and Housing

Research has established an association between economic abuse and psychological well-being. As experiences of economic abuse increase, so too do the accompanying hardships of unstable housing, lack of food, housing instability, food insufficiency, an inability to pay bills, and credit struggles (Adams et al. 2008; Adams and Beeble 2018). These stressful situations affect one's feeling of self-worth and self-esteem and often lead to depression and anxiety. It is known that individuals from financially disadvantaged backgrounds incur numerous strains and impacts, and poverty is a known risk factor for IPV (Cheng and Lo 2016). Gillium (2019) noted that poverty disproportionately affects Black communities within and outside the United States, which makes this a contextualizing factor for the disparities faced by those exposed to IPV in the Black community. Historic and perpetual economic subordination have diminished opportunities for African Americans at every turn. This has limited their education and housing options, social mobility, and access to healthy neighborhood environments. These are all critical factors in determining health outcomes. Wilson and Laughon's (2015) qualitative study of Black women's experiences in seeking housing in Baltimore showed that limited financial resources created barriers to obtaining housing and increased the risk for housing instability and IPV revictimization. The interconnectedness between IPV, poverty, and housing can create an inescapable cycle, rendering the attainment of an abuse-free life extremely difficult. It also repeatedly evokes high levels of stress that are detrimental to mental health. Because of the enormity and intersectionality of the disparities African Americans face, IPV interventions for this population should integrate solutions that redress inequities and are responsive to the impacts of structural violence and systemic racism.

How victims of IPV transition through IPV services and systems is deeply influenced by structures and actors who reflect the values of the service and the broader society (Burnett et al. 2016; Burnett et al. 2018). Options for living an abuse-free life are curtailed by a lack of access to equitable and affordable housing, economic opportunities, and sufficient resources. African Americans are disproportionately plagued and abused not only within IPV relationships but also within a society that has historically devalued their existence.

IPV Interventions and Help-Seeking Behaviors in the African American Community

Many interventions and sources of support exist to help victims of IPV. Domestic violence shelters, domestic violence helplines and advocacy centers, the police, and the medical community are among some the more commonly known and used formal supports. Interventions can take the form of IPV screening and brief counseling, which the United States Preventative Services Taskforce recommends as routine preventative measures that health care providers, family therapists, counselors, and crisis workers who can serve as a resource to support healthy family dynamics should use (De Boinville 2013). Other options include protective and no-contact court orders. Informally, those exposed to IPV can seek help from family and friends and within their own community networks. Yet help-seeking behaviors and patterns vary based on other factors that include the severity of abuse, socioeconomic status, immigration status, gender, culture, and race and ethnicity. A recent study by Cho et al. (2020) found that certain demographic characteristics such as gender and race were associated with patterns of help seeking. They found that women tend to seek help more than males and that Black and foreign-born survivors of IPV tended to use more informal sources of help than whites. Relatedly, African American women exposed to IPV are less likely to seek help from mental health care professionals (Cheng and Lo 2016) and African Americans are more likely to use informal sources of support (clergy, family, and friends) (Hays and Lincoln 2017).

IPV in the Black community is complex and intersectional and is further complicated by historical mistrust, structural/racial inequities, deep-rooted disparities and trauma, and cultural nuances. Interrupting patterns of abuse must account for and accommodate these contextual elements while integrating both nontraditional and culturally competent approaches that respond to the specific needs and challenges the African American community faces. Culturally tailored counseling is specific to racial groups and works to "address cultural issues that may reinforce violence or present barriers to stopping violence" (Al'Uqdah, Maxwell, and Hill 2016). One example is the use of intimate abuse circles led by domestic violence experts who use restorative justice principles to examine the social, historical, and political risk factors affecting the African American community in order to dismantle racial stereotypes (Al'Uqdah, Maxwell, and Hill 2016). St. Vil et al. (2017) found that low-income Black women who experienced IPV used (1) internal (using religion and becoming self-reliant), (2) interpersonal (leaving the abuser or fighting back), and (3) external (relying on informal, formal, or both kinds of sources of support) strategies. Such approaches showcase a resilience that Howell et. al. (2018, 2) defines as "the capacity of individuals facing adverse circumstances to navigate their way to the psychological, social, cultural, and physical resources that sustain their well-being." Howell et. al. found that Black women tended to use spirituality and informal networks of support (friends, family) as protective factors that bolstered their resilience. In the

Cheng & Lo study (2016), African American women were more inclined not to return to the abuser once the abuse was recognized. While it is understood that many factors contribute to the way IPV victims seek help, similarities and differences between the ways that African American men and women victims of IPV seek help needs further exploration. Moreover, appreciation for the resilience of black families and integration of resilience and cultural strategies that communities of color use are fundamental for programs and approaches that support and sustain human flourishing.

Conclusion

It is increasingly clear that while much is known about IPV, there are obvious limitations in the interventions and gaps in solutions for African Americans who experience IPV. Most resources fail to fully address the totality of the African American experience. Separating the issue of IPV from the context of the Black experience does not best serve the community or African American victims of IPV. Knowing that witnessing IPV is an identified adverse childhood experience requires us to find meaningful ways to intervene to eliminate IPV in the African American community and its impact on future generations.

Because the Black experience of IPV is not monolithic, it is critical that our work in this field be informed by a clear identification of and definition of the population of focus. This will help differentiate the unique and intersectional experiences of different populations of Blacks and African Americans (i.e., between experiences of those born in the United States and those naturalized as American citizens) so interventions can offer the most appropriate solutions. A tailored approach to addressing and eliminating IPV in the African American community is long overdue, as is research that examines what best-practice approaches could look like and how best to implement them. Integrating traditional resilience strategies and cultural practices that foster strengths and building on assets the Black community has identified are instrumental to such an approach.

Health care and social service providers are crucial in these efforts. It is critically important to educate and train providers in community and tertiary settings with programs that emphasize cultural humility and a racial equity lens when identifying and responding to IPV. These providers must be given the proper skills, knowledge, and training in culturally tailored best practices for the African American community. All providers must learn to engage in trauma-informed care practices and to recognize and respond appropriately to the presenting trauma while understanding its rootedness in the cumulative and historical traumas of the Black community.

The systems in place for addressing IPV are laden with structural impediments that are revictimizing and perpetuate structural violence for African Americans seeking to live violence-free lives. It is crucial that providers examine the unintended consequences of existing policies, activate policies that address the conditions that increase the risk for IPV in African Americans, and elucidate and rectify the structural inequities that create the most challenging obstacles for this community. Radical reform is needed to build policies and practices that work for the African American community into the system. The experience of IPV in the African American community is disparate and inequitable. It is essential to use frameworks that attend to and redress root causes if we are to move forward in addressing IPV in the African American community. This will require centering the voices and experiences of African Americans and using their expertise and traditions to co-create solutions that best meet their needs within the contexts of their lives.

REFERENCES

Adams, A., and M. Beeble. 2018. "Intimate Partner Violence and Psychological Well-Being: Examining the Effect of Economic Abuse on Women's Quality of Life." *Psychology of Violence* 9 (5): 517–525. https://dx.doi.org/10.1037/vi00000174.

Adams, A. E., C. M. Sullivan, D. Bybee, and M. R. Greeson. 2008. "Development of the Scale of Economic Abuse." *Violence Against Women* 14 (5): 563–588. https://journals.sagepub.com/doi/abs/10.1177/1077801208315529.

Al'Uqdah, S., C. Maxwell, and N. Hill. 2016. "Intimate Partner Violence in the African American Community: Risk, Theory, and Interventions." *Journal of Family Violence* 31 (7): 877–884. https://doi.org/10.1007/s10896-016-9819-x.

Alexander, K., T. Willie, R. McDonald-Mosley, J. Campbell, E. Miller, and M. Decker. 2019. "Associations between Reproductive Coercion, Partner Violence, and Mental Health Symptoms among Young Black Women in Baltimore, Maryland." *Journal of Interpersonal Violence* 36 (17–18): 1–25. https://doi.org/10.1177/0886260519860900.

Anderson, R., L. Edwards, K. Silver, and J. Johnson. 2018. "Intergenerational Transmission of Child Abuse: Predictors of Child Abuse Potential among Racially Diverse Women Residing in Domestic Violence Shelters." *Child Abuse & Neglect* 85 (November): 80–90. https://doi.org/10.1016/j.chiabu.2018.08.004.

Arcaya, M., A. Arcaya, and S. Subramanian. 2015. "Inequalities in Health: Definitions, Concepts and Theories." *Global Heath Action* 8 (1): article 27106. https://doi.org/10.3402/gha.v8.27106.

Basile, K., S. Smith, L. Yang, E. Miller, and M. Kresnow. 2019. "Prevalence of Intimate Partner Reproductive Coercion in the United States: Racial and Ethnic Differences." *Journal
of Interpersonal Violence* 36 (21–22): 1–17. https://doi.org/10.1177/0886260519888205.

Black, M., K. Basile, M. Breiding, S. Smith, M. Walters, M. Merrick, J. Chen, and M. Stevens.
2011. *National Intimate Partner and Sexual Violence Survey: 2010 Summary Report*. Atlanta, GA: National Center for Injury Prevention and Control, Centers for Disease Control and Prevention. Accessed January 27, 2021. https://www.cdc.gov/violenceprevention
/pdf/nisvs_report2010-a.pdf.

Bohall, G., M. Bautista, and S. Musson. 2016. "Intimate Partner Violence and the Duluth
Model: An Examination of the Model and Recommendations for Future Research and
Practice." *Journal of Family Violence* 31: 1029–1033. https://doi.org/10.1007/s10896-016
-9888.

Boserup, B., M. McKenney, and A. Elkbuli. 2020. "Alarming Trends in US domestic Violence
during the COVID-19 Pandemic." *American Journal of Emergency Medicine* 38 (12): 2753–
2755.

Bradbury-Jones, C., and L. Isham. 2020. "The Pandemic Paradox: The Consequences of
COVID-19 on Domestic Violence." *Journal of Clinical Nursing* 20 (13–14): 2047–2049.
https://doi.org/10.1111/jocn.15296.

Brunila, K., and L. Rossi. 2017. "Identity Politics, the Ethos of Vulnerability, and Education."
Educational Philosophy and Theory 50 (3): 287–298. https://doi.org/10.1080/00131857
.2017.1343115.

Burnett, C., M. Ford-Gilboe, H. Berman, N. Wathen, and C. Ward-Griffin. 2016. "The Day-
to-Day Reality of Shelter Service Delivery to Abused Women in the Context of System
and Policy Demands." *Journal of Social Service Research* 42 (4): 516–532. https://doi.org
/10.1080/01488376.2016.1153562.

Burnett, C., M. Swanberg, A. Hudson, and D. Schminkey. 2018. "Structural Justice: A Critical Feminist Framework Exploring the Intersection between Justice, Equity and Structural Reconciliation." *Journal of Health Disparities Research and Practice* 11 (4): 52–68.

Campbell, J., J. Anderson, A. McFadgion, J. Gill, E. Zink, M. Patch, G. Callwood, and D. Campbell. 2018. "The Effects of Intimate Partner Violence and Probable Traumatic Brain Injury on Central Nervous System Symptoms." *Journal of Women's Health* 27(6): 761–767.
https://doi.org/10.1089/jwh.2016.6311.

CDC. 2019. "Adverse Childhood Experiences (ACEs): Preventing Early Trauma to Improve
Adult Health." *Vital Signs* (November). Accessed December 29, 2020. https://www.cdc
.gov/vitalsigns/aces/index.html.

———. 2020a. "CDC COVID Data Tracker." Accessed December 29, 2020. https://covid.cdc
.gov/covid-data-tracker/#demographics.

———. 2020b. "Fast Facts: Preventing Intimate Partner Violence." Last reviewed November 2, 2021. Accessed November 9, 2020. https://www.cdc.gov/violenceprevention/inti
matepartnerviolence/fastfact.html.

Cheng, T., and C. Lo. 2016. "Racial Disparities in Intimate Partner Violence Examined
through the Multiple Disadvantage Model." *Journal of Interpersonal Violence* 31 (11):
2026–2051. https://doi.org/10.1177/0886260515572475.

Cho, H., D. Shamrova, J. Han, and P. Levchenko. 2020. "Patterns of Intimate Partner Violence Victimization and Survivors' Help-Seeking." *Journal of Interpersonal Violence* 35 (21–22): 4558–4582. https://doi.org/10.1177/0886260517715027.

Cockhren, I. 2020. "ACEs & African Americans Community on ACEs Connection." PACEs Connection, February 25. Accessed December 30, 2020. https://www.acesconnection .com/blog/aces-and-african-americans-online-community.

Crenshaw, K. 1991. "Mapping the Margins: Intersectionality, Identity Politics, and Violence against Women of Color." *Stanford Law Review* 43 (6): 1241–1299. https://doi.org/10 .2307/1229039.

De Boinville, M. 2013. "Screening for Domestic Violence in Health Care Settings." Office of the Assistant Secretary for Planning and Evaluation, U.S. Department of Health and Human Services. Accessed December 29, 2020. http://aspe.hhs.gov/hsp/13/dv/pb _screeningdomestic.cfm.

Diamond, E. 2012. "Identity Politics Then and Now." *Theatre Research International* 37 (1): 64–67. https://doi.org/10.1017/S0307883311000770.

Domestic Abuse Intervention Programs. 2017. "The Duluth Model." Accessed December 20, 2020. https://www.theduluthmodel.org/.

Evans, M., M. Lindauer, and M. Farrell. 2020. "A Pandemic within a Pandemic—Intimate Partner Violence during Covid-19." *New England Journal of Medicine* 383 (24): 2302–2303. https://doi.org/10.1056/NEJMp2024046.

Gillium, T. 2019. "The Intersection of Intimate Partner Violence and Poverty in Black Communities." *Aggression and Violence Behavior* 46 (May-June): 37–44. https://doi.org/10 .1016/j.avb.2019.01.008.

Graham-Harrison, E., A. Giuffrida, H. Smith, and L. Ford. 2020. "Lockdowns around the World Bring Rise in Domestic Violence." *The Guardian*, March 28. https://www.the guardian.com/society/2020/mar/28/lockdowns-world-rise-domestic-violence?CMP =Share_iOSApp_Other.

Hays, K., and K. Lincoln. 2017. "Mental Health Help-Seeking Profiles among African Americans: Exploring the Influence of Religion." *Race and Social Problems* 9 (2): 127–138. https://doi.org/10.1007/s12552-017-9193-1.

Howell, K., I. Thurston, L. Schwartz, L. Jamison, and A. Hasselle. 2018. "Protective Factors Associated with Resilience in Women Exposed to Intimate Partner Violence." *Psychology of Violence* 8 (4): 438–447. https://doi.org/10.1037/vio0000147.

Kapaya, M., S. Boulet, L. Warner, L. Harrison, and D. Fowler. 2019. "Intimate Partner Violence before and during Pregnancy, and Prenatal Counseling among Women with a Recent Live Birth, United States, 2009–2015." *Journal of Women's Health*, 28 (11): 1476–1486. https://doi.org/10.1089/jwh.2018.7545.

Kaufman, Y., and D. Garfin. 2020. "Home Is Not Always a Haven: The Domestic Violence Crisis Amid the COVID-19 Pandemic." *Psychological Trauma: Theory, Research, Practice, and Policy* 12 (S1): S199–S201. https://dx.doi.org/10.1037/tra0000866.

Lacey, K., C. West, N. Matusko, and J. Jackson. 2016. "Prevalence and Factors Associated with Severe Physical Intimate Partner Violence among U.S. Black Women: A Comparison of African American and Caribbean Blacks." *Violence Against Women* 22 (6): 651–670. https://doi.org/10.1177/1077801215610014.

Lutwak, N. 2018. "The Psychology of Health and Illness: The Mental Health and Physiological Effects of Intimate Partner Violence on Women." *Journal of Psychology* 152 (6): 373–387. https://doi.org/10.1080/00223980.2018.1447435.

Mental Health America. 2022. "Racial Trauma." Accessed December 24, 2020. https://www.mhanational.org/racial-trauma.

Roberts, A., S. Gilman, J. Breslau, N. Breslau, and K. Koenen. 2010. "Race/Ethnic Differences in Exposure to Traumatic Events, Development of Post-Traumatic Stress Disorder, and Treatment-Seeking for Post-Traumatic Stress Disorder in the United States." *Psychological Medicine* 41 (1): 71–83. https://doi.org/10.1017/S0033291710000401.

Ross, M., and N. Bateman. 2019. "Meet the Low-Wage Workforce." Metropolitan Policy Program at Brookings. Accessed January 27, 2021. https://www.brookings.edu/wp-content/uploads/2019/11/201911_Brookings-Metro_low-wage-workforce_Ross-Bateman.pdf.

Sabri, B., J. Stockman, J. Campbell, S. O'Brien, D. Campbell, G. Callwood, D. Bertrand, L. Sutton, and G. Hart-Hyndman. 2014. "Factors Associated with Increased Risk for Lethal Violence in Intimate Partner Relationships among Ethnically Diverse Black Women." *Violence Victims* 29 (5): 719–741. https://doi.org/10.1891/0886-6708.VV-D-13-00018.

Smith, S., S. Zhang, K. Basile, M. Merrick, J. Wang, M. Kresnow, and J. Chen. 2018. "National Intimate Partner and Sexual Violence Survey: 2015 Data Brief." Last reviewed July 9, 2021. Accessed January 21, 2021. https://www.cdc.gov/violenceprevention/datasources/nisvs/2015NISVSdatabrief.html.

St. Vil, N., V. Nwokolo, K. Alexander, and J. Campbell. 2017. "A Qualitative Study of Survival Strategies Used by Low-Income Black Women Who Experience Intimate Partner Violence." *Social Work* 62 (1): 63–71. https://doi.org/10.1093/sw/sww080.

Substance Abuse and Mental Health Services Administration. 2014a. *SAMHSA's Concept of Trauma and Guidance for a Trauma-Informed Approach*. Rockville, MD: Substance Abuse and Mental Health Services Administration, 2014. Accessed December 24, 2020. https://ncsacw.samhsa.gov/userfiles/files/SAMHSA_Trauma.pdf.

———. 2014b. *Trauma-Informed Care in Behavioral Health Services*. Treatment Improvement Protocol (TIP) Series 57. Rockville, MD: Substance Abuse and Mental Health Services Administration.

United States Census Bureau. 2019. "Quick Facts: United States," Accessed December 20, 2020. https://www.census.gov/quickfacts/fact/table/US/PST045219.

Van Gelder, N., A. Peterman, A. Potts, M. O'Donnell, K. Thompson, N. Shah, and S. Oertelt-Prigione. 2020. "COVID-19: Reducing the Risk of Infection Might Increase the Risk of Intimate Partner Violence." *eClinical Medicine* 21 (1–2). https://doi.org/10.1016/j.eclinm.2020.100348.

Wilson, P., and K. Laughon. 2015. "House to House, Shelter to Shelter: Experiences of Black Women Seeking Housing after Leaving Abusive Relationships." *Journal of Forensic Nursing* 11 (2): 77–83. https://doi.org/10.1097/JFN.0000000000000067.

World Health Organization. 2021. WHO Coronavirus Disease (COVID-19) Dashboard. Accessed January 27, 2021. https://covid19.who.int/.

13

Mental Health Disparities

DANIELLE L. McDUFFIE, MA,
and MARTHA R. CROWTHER, PhD, MPH

Overview

African Americans have a deeply entrenched history of being mistreated in America, starting with the transatlantic slave trade in the 1800s and continuing into modern times (Williams 1987). This mistreatment and the subsequent culture of fear Black individuals in the United States, particularly in the South, were subjected to could feasibly be identified as precursors to disparities in the mental health of African Americans living in the southern United States (Alexander 2010; Blackmon 2009; United Nations Office of the Commissioner of Human Rights 2016).

Historical Underpinnings of African American Mental Health

African Americans have a long history of justified mistrust of mental health institutions that dates back to some of the atrocities that occurred during and as a result of the transatlantic slave trade (Hunter and Schmidt 2010, 213). Western medicine has historically been exclusionary and discriminatory toward African Americans, as evidenced by foundational ideals such as phrenology, eugenics, social Darwinism, and polygenism (Byrd and Clayton 2003). Some in the African American community believe that psychological treatment systems are inherently racist (Williams, Beckmann-Mendez, and Turkheimer 2013, 35).

Particularly for African Americans living in the South, one of the most notable atrocities committed by health institutions was that of the Tuskegee Syphilis Study. Officially titled the U.S. Public Health Service Syphilis Study at Tuskegee, the study, which was conducted from 1932 to 1972, involved 399 Black male sharecroppers living in Macon County, Alabama. These men were all diagnosed with syphilis, but researchers withheld available medical treatment because they wanted to investigate the end-stage effects of the disease (Katz et al. 2009, 469). Many of these men infected others and subsequently died as a result of a lack of medical intervention. While the US government later issued a formal apology, it is hard to erase the legacy of the Tuskegee Syphilis Study and the impacts it has had on the trust of African Americans in health institutions of any modality, including mental health. American society has shown a disregard for the well-being of African Americans in the past, and it is feasible that African American mental health could be influenced by these events, particularly in the South, where the majority of these events took place. These events and the resulting justifiable mistrust on the part of African Americans also form the context for the fact that African American mental health is underaddressed and undertreated in the South.

African American Mental Health across the Lifespan

The first issue to address in a discussion of African American mental health disparities is the overall prevalence and diagnostic rate of mental illness among African Americans. Among African American children, there are notable disparities in the diagnosis of mental illness beginning at a young age. In early school settings, behaviors that are consistent with impulsivity, inattention, and difficulty with focus are often seen among male students. This behavior often brings two mental health diagnoses to mind: conduct disorder and attention deficit hyperactivity disorder (ADHD) (Spencer and Oatts 1999, 514–518). While the disorders share similar traits, conduct disorder often carries a heavier stigma and is associated with social maladjustment, whereas ADHD is often thought of as a neurodevelopmental disorder. Despite often shared presentations of impulsivity and difficulty with staying on task, African American adolescent males are diagnosed with conduct disorder at a much higher rate than their peers in other racial/ethnic groups (Spencer and Oatts 1999, 515–518). Additionally, African American adolescent girls are disproportionately mislabeled as "acting out" or being aggressive in school settings and are disciplined more frequently than their peers of different races/ethnicities, including non-Black male students (Crenshaw, Ocen, and Nanda 2015, 5–11; Hines-Datiri and Andrews 2017, 5–10). These findings suggest that there might be an issue of misdiagnosis regarding this group.

The literature is conflicting regarding the prevalence of mental illness among African American adults. Among young African American adults, evidence has been found that suggests an association between racial identity and psychological wellness (Sellers et al. 2003, 302–317). More specifically, it was found that young African American adults who consider race to be a more central part of their identity were likely to report lower levels of mental distress than African American peers who did not report race as a main component of their identity. Sellers and colleagues posited that strong identification with the Black race might be advantageous as a protective factor for young African American adults. Evidence largely suggests that African Americans have lower rates of depression than their non-Hispanic white counterparts. Although the prevalence is found to be lower, Budhwani, Hearld, and Chavez-Yenter (2015, 37–38) have suggested that when depression is seen among African Americans, is it more likely to be persistent. However, African American adults also report lower levels of any mental illness than non-Hispanic whites (Substance Abuse and Mental Health Services Administration 2015b). Among the psychotic disorders, there is a long history of higher diagnosis among African Americans (Schwartz and Feisthamel 2009). African Americans have historically been diagnosed with psychotic disorders (i.e., schizophrenia) at rates that have been noted as "unusually high" compared to other racial/ethnic groups (Chow, Jaffee, and Snowden 2003, 794; U.S. Department of Health and Human Services 2001). This diagnostic pattern among African Americans has had far-reaching consequences that will be detailed later in this section.

Additionally, even when considering more nuanced conditions such as clinical levels of grief, African Americans are diagnosed at higher rates. One such example is that of the diagnosis of prolonged grief between African American and non-Hispanic white bereaved adults. Prolonged grief is a condition characterized as being debilitating; it is exemplified by an overwhelming sense of longing for the deceased, a persistent inability to accept the loss, and dysfunction in normal life following the loss of a loved one (Boelen and van den Bout 2005, 2175–2177; Prigerson et al. 1995, 66). Investigations of this trend suggest that African Americans have significantly higher rates of this exacerbated level of grief than non-Hispanic whites (Goldsmith et al. 2008, 359–361). Finally, among African American adults, perceptions of stress across the lifespan might be impacted by depressive symptoms (Byrd, Thorpe, and Whitfield, 2020). African American adults who experience greater depressive symptoms are more likely to perceive higher amounts of stress as they age, such as when transitioning between middle and older adulthood.

Cognitive impairment is one of the most studied psychological conditions among older adults. Often when health care professionals attempt to diagnose cognitive impairment, they use screening tools that ask individuals a variety of questions in attempts to garner findings pertaining to their cognitive status. In the assessment of cognitive status, African American older adults show lower performance on screening tasks and are judged as being cognitively impaired more frequently than older non-Hispanic white adults (Manly, Jacobs, Sano et al. 1998; Manly Jacobs, Touradji et al. 2002; Unverzagt et al. 1996). This is particularly apparent in the diagnosis of various types of dementias (Carlson et al. 1998; Manly, Jacobs, Sano et al. 1998; Marcopulos, McLain, and Giuliano, 1997; Ripich, Carpenter, and Ziol 1997; Unverzagt et al. 1996, 180-190). Results of this nature pose the question of whether African American older adults are truly exhibiting signs of disparities in cognitive status as they age or whether there are structural issues with the tools being used to address cognitive impairment.

The fact that the literature that has uncovered a disproportionate prevalence of diagnoses of mental health difficulties among African Americans across the lifespan is potentially suggestive of a need for increased attention to mental health trends among African Americans, particularly in the South. However, this analysis of mental health trends and disparities among African Americans would be inadequate without consideration of the diagnostic issues and treatment disparities regarding Black Americans and the consequences of misdiagnosis for this population.

Diagnostic Issues in the Measurement of African American Mental Health

Evidence across the field of mental health suggests that there might be a fundamental lack of cultural sensitivity in the tools being used to address mental illness across racial/ethnic groups. The majority of the pioneer psychological tests were standardized, validated, and tested for reliability only in non-Hispanic, white, middle-class, English-speaking populations (Olmedo 1981; Reynolds 1982). Additionally, the scores of racial/ethnic minorities on psychological measures were often compared to the scores of samples of non-Hispanic white participants and decisions were made about "normality" or impairment based on such comparisons (Sue, Arredondo, and McDavis 1992, 479–480). While movements have attempted to foster greater norming and validation of measures using populations of racial/ethnic minorities, many tools still being used in the field suffer from these biases. This, in turn, creates larger disparities for African Americans (Council of National Psychological Associations for the Advancement of Ethnic Minority Interests 2016).

Education has been found to have a key role in explaining differences in cognition between groups (Schaie 1985). African Americans have been found to receive less education than non-Hispanic whites, regardless of cohort differences in educational attainment (Adams-Price 1993; Harper and Alexander 1990). Moreover, African Americans who attended school in the United States before the end of school segregation often attended schools that had fewer financial resources for education, shorter school years, and higher student-to-teacher ratios (Loewenstein et al. 1994; Whitfield and Wiggins, 2003, 277–278). The culmination of these factors could have manifested in lower reading-level attainment. Reading level in particular is something that has been associated with higher performance on neuropsychological tests (Manly, Jacobs, Sano et al. 1999).

Furthermore, evidence suggests that psychodiagnostic tools of mood disorders might not be reflective of the African American experience of depression. Within the African American community, there is often a large stigma attached to mental health, particularly among older cohorts (Conner, Copeland, Grote, Koeske et al. 2010, 974–975; Conner, Copeland, Grote, Rosen, et al. 2010, 536–539; Conner, Lee et al., 2010, 272–273). This stigma often manifests in feelings of depression among African Americans. Traditional measures of depression assess for many of the emotional and social factors of depression, for example, the Patient Health Questionnaire-9 (Kroenke, Spitzer, and Williams 2001) or the Center for Epidemiologic Studies Depression Scale (Radloff 1977). However, there is evidence to suggest that mood disorders in African Americans do not always have a "typical" presentation (Brown, Schulberg, and Madonia 1996, 185–187; Carrington 2006, 782–784; Pickering 2000, 345–346). African American expressions of depression have been linked to issues with somatization (Carrington 2006, 782–784), physical distress (Brown, Schulberg, and Madonia 1996, 185-187), and hypertension (Pickering 2000, 345–346). There is also evidence to suggest that conditions such as pathological grief are misdiagnosed due to a lack of cultural sensitivity in the measures (Granek and Peleg-Sagy 2017, 392–293). Improper measurement of mental illness among African Americans can lead to wide disparities in the expression and treatment of African American mental health.

Negative Implications Resulting from Misdiagnosis

One of the most notable places where disparities in the diagnosis of conditions among African Americans manifests is in rates of institutionalization among African Americans. Studies have shown exceptionally high rates of the diagnosis of psychotic disorders among African Americans (Chow, Jaffee, and Snowden 2003, 794; Neighbors et al. 2003, 242–246; U.S. Department of Health and Human Services 1999). Specifically, Cohen and Marino (2013, 1105) found a 15% lifetime prevalence of psychotic symptoms among African Americans, which is higher than any other racial/ethnic group. This rate is higher than epidemiological estimates would suggest, a fact that highlights the possibility of misdiagnosis. This high rate of diagnosis has often been attributed to misdiagnosis based on the prejudice of clinicians or a misinterpretation of African American personal and cultural factors (Chien and Bell 2008; Schwartz and Blankenship 2014, 139). Literature suggests that upon hospitalization (whether it is voluntary or involuntary), African American patients have a five times higher likelihood of being diagnosed with a psychotic condition or schizophrenia than non-Hispanic white patients (Barnes 2004, 250; Strakowski et al. 2003). Along with increased hospitalization, the misdiagnosis of psychotic symptoms among African Americans can also lead to overmedication and the associated adverse effects of medications (Barnes 2004, 243). Moreover, having a diagnosis of a psychotic disorder has been found to be associated with increased discrimination and potential stigmatization, which are both associated with poorer mental health outcomes (Thornicroft et al. 2009, 411–413).

Mental Health Treatment of African Americans

There are distinct barriers to seeking mental health treatment among African Americans. Research shows that Black Americans receive less mental health treatment than other racial/ethnic groups (Agency for Healthcare Research and Quality 2016; Diala et al. 2000). Only 1 in 3 African Americans who need mental health treatment receive any form of care (Dalencour et al. 2017, 370). Several notable factors have been cited as potential barriers to effective mental health treatment for racial/ethnic minorities, including lack of insurance, heightened stigma attached to mental illness, a lack of diversity among behavioral health providers, a lack of cultural competency among providers, language barriers, distrust on the part of racial/ethnic minorities in health care systems, and an overall lack of support for mental health services (American Psychiatric Association 2017). African Americans who do seek mental health care are less likely to receive care that is consistent with proven mental health guidelines, are less often included in mental health research, and are more likely to use emergency departments or primary care for mental health treatment (US Department of Health and Human Services 2001). African Americans seeking mental health care are also less likely to be offered evidence-based medications or psychotherapy to help treat their conditions (Wang, Berglund, and Kessler 2000, 287–288).

A particularly relevant disparity to consider in the treatment of mental health among African Americans is the criminalization of African American mental illness. From a young age, racial/ethnic minority youth with behavioral health problems are more readily referred to law enforcement and juvenile justice systems than to mental health treatment than their non-Hispanic white peers are (Substance Abuse and Mental Health Services Administration 2015a). Racially Black individuals with mental health conditions, particularly schizophrenia, bipolar disorders, or psychosis, are overwhelmingly more likely to be incarcerated than individuals in other racial/ethnic groups (Carson and Anderson 2016; Hawthorne et al. 2012, 28–29). An additional factor contributing to the criminalization of African American mental health is substance use. Not only has substance use has been found to be highly comorbid with existing mental health conditions, it also has grounds for being a standalone mental health diagnosis (American Psychiatric Association 2013). African Americans represent a substantial percentage of drug offenders in federal prisons (Taxy, Samuels, and Adams 2015). Not only has this criminalization of substance use among African Americans disproportionately affected the lives of millions of African Americans, it also acts as a barrier to African Americans seeking treatment for substance use disorders.

Evidence of African American mental health diagnosis and misdiagnosis, historical trends in African American mental health, and negative implications of disparities in African American mental health treatment demonstrate an urgent need to address the mental health of African Americans dwelling in the South. However, if mental health professionals are to properly treat and work with African Americans, they must understand some of the more nuanced cultural considerations.

Cultural Considerations

Impacts of Discrimination

Experiences of discrimination and feelings of marginalization across the lifespan have been found to have enduring effects on adults with minority identities (Meyer 2003). This is particularly true for African Americans, who have been the targets of consistent discrimination in American society. African Americans report perceived discrimination at significantly higher rates than other minority groups. African American youth who identify more closely with their racial identity might perceive more racial discrimination in their daily lives (Sellers et al. 2003, 312). Discrimination can have detrimental mental health effects on its recipients (Williams, Neighbors, and Jackson 2003, 200). For instance, feelings of racial discrimination have been associated with higher levels of depression among African American women (Gibbons et al. 2014, 11). Additionally, perceptions of discrimination can factor into an unwillingness to seek care from health institutions. African Americans who perceive higher levels of discrimination display higher levels of mistrust toward medical researchers and health care professionals (Corbie-Smith et al. 1999, 543–544; Goodin et al. 2013, 1121). African American youth have been cited as being particularly sensitive to the effects of racial discrimination. For example, Walker et al. (2017, 95) found that perceived racism directly affects the risk of suicide and death-related thinking among African American youth. African American youth who have experienced racism also have an increased chance of having thoughts of death later in life. This finding is particularly important, as most studies of stress in the lives of African American youth do not treat discrimination and its effects as a standalone cause of emotional distress. Given its extensive history of strained race relations, the South is an area where African Americans are likely to experience high levels of discrimination. Given the effects that discrimination can have on mental health, there is an urgent need to consider how social discrimination and perceived discrimination in the medical and mental health fields could impact African Americans in the South.

Adverse Childhood Experiences

Adverse childhood experiences (ACEs) include all types of abuse or other neglect a child under the age of 18 receives at the hands of a parent, guardian, caregiver, or any other person acting in a custodial capacity (Fortson et al. 2016). Evidence suggests that African American children have higher specific ACEs and a higher cumulative number of ACEs than non-Hispanic white children (Maguire-Jack, Lanier, and Lombardi 2020, 109). In an experimental study of ACEs, people who were found to have encountered four or more categories of ACEs had significantly higher levels of alcoholism, drug abuse, depression, suicide attempts, and smoking; poorer self-reported health; and more sexual partners and sexually transmitted diseases than those who reported no ACEs (Felitti et al. 1998, 249–250).

Among African American adults, individuals who were historically exposed to trauma during childhood have a higher likelihood of being diagnosed with posttraumatic stress disorder, panic disorder (with and without agoraphobia), major depressive disorder, schizophrenia, schizoaffective disorder, bipolar disorder, anxiety disorders, psychosis, mood disorders, personality disorders, and substance abuse or dependence disorders (Bell, Jackson, and Bell 2015, 39). Many of these disorders also manifest in African American children at the time of or soon after the trauma (Bell 1997, 336–339). A great deal of this trauma might be associated with disruptions in childhood caregiving and distrust of close relationships (Van der Kolk 2005, 401–404). This could have pertinent effects for African American children, adolescents, and adults, not only in daily social settings but also in treatment-based interactions (Bell, Jackson, and Bell 2015, 40). The ever-shifting nature of social settings and treatment settings (i.e., rotating therapists, client transferring) could exacerbate some of these trauma-related reactions and have further negative impacts on African American mental health.

The South is a unique environment where generational racial trauma might be present among African American children, adolescents, and adults. From the late 1800s through the early 1900s, African Americans were forced on an almost daily basis to see Black bodies brutalized. Unfortunately, these atrocities failed to spare children (e.g., Emmett Till). African Americans of all ages in the South were often made to bear witness to the most grotesque expressions of racism and prejudice. Lynchings were public spectacles in the

South. African American parents conveyed folklore and warnings to even the youngest children about the dangers of being Black in the South. Contemporarily, the brutalization of Black bodies continues to be openly on display. With the advent of social media, young African American children are often in positions where they see the deaths of Black men and women consistently (Chama 2019, 206; Cohen and Lewis 2016). While this topic is not thoroughly studied in the literature, it is important to consider what effects seeing the repeated assaults on Black bodies has on the mental health of African American children and adolescents today and the effects it might have on adults and older adults who encountered similar traumatic racial images during their childhood.

Rurality and Other Geographic Factors

Many racial/ethnic minorities have been found to live in geographic areas that limit their access to essential health care (Green et al. 2005, 693–695; Morrison et al. 2000, 1024–1025). Particularly for residents of the South, this trend is seen in areas categorized as rural. Rurality is associated with higher rates of mental illness, specifically substance use and suicidality (CDC 2020). Rural communities have higher rates of disability and limited access to health care services. Over the past decade, rural areas have been severely underresourced. More than 100 hospitals have closed in rural areas of the United States, and 60% of those closures happened in the South (Democratic Policy and Communications Committee 2020, 7). Minority patients who are able to access essential health care often receive worse treatment, less preventative care, and a lower availability of primary care (McCarthy et al. 2011). People living in the South often have less access to health care and live in communities that spend less money annually on public health (Koma et al. 2020). Health disparities are often associated with significant differences between racial/ethnic minorities and non-Hispanic whites in poverty levels and policies (Kaiser Family Foundation 2018).

About 27% of African Americans live below the poverty level, compared to 10.8 percent of non-Hispanic whites (United States Census Bureau 2016a). Evidence suggests that mental illness is overrepresented in low-income neighborhoods (Chow, Jaffee, and Snowden 2003, 792; Schwartz and Feisthamel 2009, 295–296). African Americans are often forced to live in low-income neighborhoods and because of that are vulnerable to overdiagnosis and misdiagnosis of mental health conditions. African Americans are the most highly concentrated in the Southeast (specifically Louisiana, Alabama, Georgia, South Carolina, and North Carolina) (United States Census Bureau 2016b). The combination of almost one-third of African Americans living below the poverty level and a vast majority of African Americans living in the Southeast has direct connections with the deleterious effects of rurality. This might have significant mental health consequences for impoverished African Americans in the rural South. It is also highly likely that this population has limited access to resources to aid them.

Stoicism

While similar attitudes might be present in other racial/ethnic groups, some African Americans believe that mental illness is not something Black Americans encounter (Alvidrez, Snowden, and Kaiser 2008, 874–875; Sibrava et al. 2013, 1053). Within the African American community, even mental illnesses that are considered to be "milder," such as anxiety disorders, can be equated with being "crazy" (Alvidrez, Snowden, and Kaiser 2008, 874-893). The stigma associated with mental illness among African Americans can lead to an underreporting of mental illness (Hunter and Schmidt 2010, 211–235). It is conceivable that African Americans might not present for treatment or that by the time they do, their symptomology could be severely exacerbated. It is important to consider and understand the historical reasons why African Americans might be hesitant to report their mental health struggles and to make attempts to provide maximally efficacious and culturally competent care. It is also important to understand that this stoicism is likely steeped in generations of having to steel one's self against discrimination and oppression, and for that reason it might also be protective.

Bereavement

Loss is something that affects everyone at some point in time. However, bereavement tends to trend higher among African Americans. African American young adults have been found to experience a higher rate of loss by homicide than any other cultural group (Laurie and Neimeyer 2008, 182). Traumatic and/or unexpected loss has been found to be strongly associated with negative grief outcomes (Goldsmith et al. 2008, 359). African Americans, who as a group are more likely to encounter unexpected loss, might face unique mental health challenges resulting from these losses. Young African American adults have been found to express deeper levels of grief for those outside the immediate family and to spend less time talking about their grief than non-Hispanic whites (Laurie and Neimeyer 2008, 183–184). This reflects the importance of kinship among African Americans, including during times of grief. Evidence suggests that African Americans might face the double burden of processing the lingering effects of racism in their lives and the lives of the deceased in the midst of grieving (Rosenblatt and Wallace 2005, 232–233). While bereavement is associated with negative mental health outcomes for all ethnic/racial groups, it should be particularly attended to among African Americans, who might be susceptible to repeated, unexpected losses over the lifespan.

Substance Use

The rate of illicit substance use among African Americans is slightly higher than the national average (12.4% versus 10.2%). However, rates of alcohol use, heavy drinking, and binge drinking among African Americans were all lower than national averages (CDC 2016). As of 2018, 7.3% (2.2 million) of African Americans aged 18 or older had a diagnosable substance use disorder. Marijuana was the most widely used illicit substance among African Americans aged 12 or older (17.8% versus 15.9% of the nation) (US Department of Health and Human Services 2020). African Americans have a lower rate of opioid overdose than non-Hispanic whites (6.6% versus 13.9%) but higher rates of synthetic opioid misuse (Kaiser Family Foundation 2017). In 2017, African Americans had the highest rates of opioid-related (~70%) and total drug (43%) overdose deaths by synthetic opioids (Substance Abuse and Mental Health Services Administration 2020). Startlingly, drug overdose deaths involving synthetic opioids increased by 818% from 2014 to 2017 among African Americans. Factors that substance use among African Americans include increased age and negative life circumstances (i.e., low socioeconomic status) (Assari et al. 2019, 1831; Cobb et al. 2019, 170).

It is likely that a greater stigma is associated with seeking treatment for mental illness and/or substance use based on the criminalization of substance use among African Americans both historically and currently (Taxy, Samuels, and Adams 2015). It could follow that African Americans in the South who are struggling with mental illness might be more likely to turn to substance use than to mental health treatment. That would be consistent with a historical mistrust of practitioners in the health fields. However, with this turn to substances to cope with mental illness, African Americans might also be in a doubly detrimental position in that they might need substance use and mental health care but also be apprehensive about seeking care because of fear of imprisonment or extensive punishment.

Racial Stereotypes

One of the most prevalent racial stereotypes relating to the mental health of African Americans is that of the strong Black woman. Dating back to the transatlantic slave trade, Black women have been placed in positions that called for excessive strength (Beauboeuf-Lafontant 2008, 395). In contrast to women in other racial/ethnic groups, African American women's strength was defined as their ability to overcome hardships while not reacting to mistreatment (Harris-Lacewell 2001, 24). The "strong Black woman" race-sex schema encompasses the beliefs that Black women must display unwavering strength and self-reliance and a resistance to negative mental health outcomes regardless of circumstances (Watson and Hunter 2015, 609–610). West, Donovan, and Daniel (2016, 402) note that African American cite projecting the image of the strong Black woman as protection against the stress of a white-dominated society.

However, the unwavering strength that is expected of Black women could lead to a minimization of mental illness or an inadvertent failure on the part of Black women to identify symptoms of mental illness (West, Donovan, and Daniel 2016, 406). Embracing the strong Black woman schema might help African American women steel themselves against the repeated hardships of life and maintain a sense of mental well-being. However, endorsement of this schema could also place African American women in a position where they fail to attend to their mental health, burn out, and/or present for treatment at a time when their symptomology is dangerously exacerbated. Mental health professionals who work with African American women need to know and understand the implications of racial stereotypes such as this one and the ways these stereotypes can affect the lives of African American women in particular.

The Mental Health of Black Men

Black male mental health is a topic of particular interest when considering the mental health of African Americans in the South. Black men often face the double burden of battling cultural expectations for both men and African Americans (Watkins 2012, 195). Black men were also brutally and directly affected by injustices in America historically (i.e., slavery, Jim Crow), as they still do today (i.e., police brutality). One mental health condition that is worthy of further investigation among Black men is depression. It has been found that Black men's presentations of depression might vary from what is described in current diagnostic manuals. Specifically, evidence suggests that irritability and anger might be important elements to consider in the expression of depression among Black men (Watkins, Walker, and Griffith 2010, 321). Depression in this group might also manifest through increased rates of alcohol, tobacco, and illegal substance use. Presentations of depression among Black men are further associated with a heightened engagement in violence and a higher rate of suicide. Factors such as racial injustice, socioeconomic status, lack of access to education, and stoicism and/or Black men's need to engage in responses to stress that are more "culturally appropriate" (i.e., instead of engaging in strategies for coping with stress such as openly emoting) are all directly linked to violence among Black men. Exposure to violence among Black men can lead to depression, anxiety, and suicidal thoughts (Watkins 2012, 200). Additionally, unresolved health and social well-being outcomes from earlier years have the potential to directly influence psychological challenges Black men face during adulthood (Watkins 2012, 199).

Low socioeconomic status is one of the most pervasive challenges Black men face. Having a lower socioeconomic status and/or feeling economically marginalized has been posited to have long-term negative mental health consequences for Black males. Accompanying cultural perceptions that a man should be a provider, there is an increased likelihood that African American men will neglect self-care and personal wellness to prioritize financial outcomes. Evidence shows that experiencing socioeconomic struggles during their youth and early adult years increases their likelihood for depression over the life course. Moreover, stress among Black men (examined through "allostatic load") has been significantly linked with higher levels of depression regardless of age, level of education, current income, and health-related behaviors (Thorpe et al. 2020, 5–6). Mental health among Black men can be fraught with cultural, social, and personal challenges that make it exceptionally important that mental health care professionals find culturally appropriate ways to intervene to better their overall psychological health.

Protective Factors for African American Mental Health
Faith

Religious and spiritual beliefs constitute one of the most notable strengths of the African American community. African Americans have been identified as more spiritual and religious than other racial/ethnic groups (Taylor and Chatters 2010, 284). Since the South is often cited as being the most religious area of the United States (Norman 2018) and the majority of African Americans live in the South, it follows that African Americans have a deep investment in their religious faith. It has been posited that the Black church can serve as a means of healing for African Americans, particularly those suffering from trauma. The Black church often provides African Americans with hope, the sense that they can reconstruct meaning in their lives, and empowerment. It rests strongly on the notion that individuals can be "reborn" through their belief in God (Bell, Jackson, and Bell 2015, 40). In some spheres, religious faith can provide African Americans with a sense of comfort, which is particularly relevant to mental health.

Social Support

Social support often holds the distinction of being a maximally important resource for African Americans. Family and kinship networks are highly valued in African American communities (Billingsley 1992). Particularly during times of distress, African Americans seek out kinship networks (i.e., family, friends, and fictive kin) rather than the services of professionals (Stack 1974, 90–107; Sudarkasa, 1997). Even in response to one of the most insidious forms of distress among African Americans (i.e., race-based stress), social support was found to partially buffer the relationship between such stress and feelings of hopelessness (Odafe, Salami, and Walker 2017, 566). Further illustrating the importance of social support within the African American community, Miller et al. (2004) found that the absence of perceived social support among African Americans is the most important risk factor for depression. It is clear that social support and collectivism play important roles for African Americans. In conceptualizing the mental health of African Americans in the South, it is important to consider the high concentration of African Americans living in the region and how protective that might be for their mental health generally. It is also important to consider the role of community when investigating the mental health outcomes of

African Americans who might be in circumstances where they either have no community or have been distanced from their primary community.

Resilience

African Americans have historically demonstrated an astounding level of resilience through their ability to turn inward within the community (Boyd-Franklin 2003, 52–72; Hines and Boyd-Franklin 1996). Clay (2019, 6) has conceptualized this resilience as "black resilience neoliberalism." This concept posits that African Americans are constantly in positions where the available human capital for combating structural racism and other social disadvantages is depleted. This further extends to the notion that African Americans have a normalized expectation of overcoming deeply entrenched systems that were built against them (Clay 2019, 82). Clay highlights the reality that despite centuries of being disadvantaged and facing systems that were built to exclude and harm them, African Americans have managed to preserve a sense of hope and have continued to persist. This resilience is tied to the concept of stoicism, the idea that African Americans often steel themselves from negativity in order to continue on in their lives, even in the face of mental health challenges.

Clinical Implications

What follows are a few suggestions for working with African Americans in the South regarding mental health issues:

1. Attempt to meet African Americans where they are. Given that the majority of African Americans in America live in the Southeast, possibly in rural areas, and that a third live below the poverty level, it is important for those seeking to engage in work with African Americans to attempt to go out into communities of color to reach clients who might not have access to transportation or treatment nearby. Meeting the client where they are also extends to matching clients in terms of cognitive and emotional functioning. It should be understood that African Americans are at a significant disadvantage in society and oftentimes might be prevented from engaging in services by other factors. This consideration calls for grace from mental health workers in the treatment of African American clients.

2. Understand and do not attempt to invalidate the lived experiences of

African American clients. African Americans generally but particularly those living in the South may have deeply entrenched, justifiable biases relative to American society and some of the systems in place. In working with African Americans, do not try to dissuade them from their opinions or attempt to instill in them the perception that conditions in America are better for African Americans now than they were in the past. Listen, affirm, and validate their feelings. Particularly in the South, manifestations of social inequity such as unfair policing and overcriminalization of African Americans are rampant. Be considerate of the fact that African American men and women in the South might have a particular stigma about major institutions or be guarded in the interactions with members of the dominant society in the South.

3. Be mindful of the treatment screeners, measures, protocols, and/or techniques being used with African American clients. Many of the leading theories and techniques in the field of mental health were created, normed, and validated using non-Hispanic white clients of middle to high socioeconomic status. This is not sensitive to the African American experience, and in using these measures, you might be inadvertently conceptualizing African American clients as "abnormal" when in fact it might be that the wrong parameters of normality are in place.

4. Enlist the institutions African Americans find value in. The Black church has been studied in multiple bodies of literature as a location that is helpful in disseminating information to African Americans about health and well-being. The same is true for African American community organizations and/or leaders. When trying to reach African Americans, consider meeting first with representatives of some of these institutions to ascertain the best ways to engage with African Americans and to potentially help with treatment adherence.

5. Train primary care physicians to better address African American mental health. Many African Americans do not engage with mental health institutions, instead receiving much of their behavioral health care from their primary care physicians. Because of this, it might be important to provide additional training and support to these physicians, many of whom will be the only line of defense for accurately addressing, assessing, and treating African American mental health. This is particularly relevant for southern African Americans who might be

living in more rural areas where only limited specific mental health treatment is available.

Conclusion

African Americans living in the South are a unique group in terms of balancing generations of institutionalized racism, trauma, and mistreatment. This group might be at a particular risk for negative mental health outcomes consistent with rurality, poverty, unequal educational quality and attainment levels, and other factors that are the result of generations of struggle. However, African Americans are also resilient as a group. Despite centuries of second-class treatment and its associated disadvantages, African Americans have proven through their reliance on social support, faith, and internal strength that they will continue to endure. Our job as those seeking to aid African Americans in the area of mental health should be to provide them as much unconditional support, compassion, and validation as possible.

REFERENCES

Adams-Price, C. E. 1993. "Age, Education, and Literacy Skills of Adult Mississippians." *Gerontologist* 33 (6): 741–46. https://doi.org/10.1093/geront/33.6.741.

Agency for Healthcare Research and Quality. 2016. *2015 National Healthcare Quality and Disparities Report and 5th Anniversary Update on the National Quality Strategy.* AHRQ Pub. No. 16-0015. Rockville, MD: AHRQ.

Alexander, Michelle. 2010. *The New Jim Crow: Mass Incarceration in the Age of Color Blindness.* New York: New Press.

Alvidrez, Jennifer, Lonnie R. Snowden, and Dawn M. Kaiser. 2008. "The Experience of Stigma among Black Mental Health Consumers." *Journal of Health Care for the Poor and Underserved* 19 (3): 874–93. https://doi.org/10.1353/hpu.0.0058.

American Psychiatric Association. 2013. *Diagnostic and Statistical Manual of Mental Disorders.* 5th ed. Washington, DC: American Psychiatric Association.

———. 2017. "Mental Health Disparities: African Americans." Washington, DC: American Psychiatric Association. Accessed November 15, 2020 https://www.psychiatry.org/File%20Library/Psychiatrists/Cultural-Competency/Mental-Health-Disparities/Mental-Health-Facts-for-African-Americans.pdf.

Assari, Shervin, James Smith, Ritesh Mistry, Mehdi Farokhnia, and Mohsen Bazargan. 2019. "Substance Use among Economically Disadvantaged African American Older Adults: Objective and Subjective Socioeconomic Status." *International Journal of Environmental Research and Public Health* 16 (10): 1826. https://doi.org/10.3390/ijerph16101826.

Barnes, Arnold. 2004. "Race, Schizophrenia, and Admission to State Psychiatric Hospitals." *Administration and Policy in Mental Health* 31 (3): 241–52. https://doi.org/10.1023/b:apih.0000018832.73673.54.

Beauboeuf-Lafontant, Tamara. 2008. "Listening Past the Lies That Make Us Sick: A Voice-Centered Analysis of Strength and Depression among Black Women." *Qualitative Sociology* 31: 391–406. https://doi.org/http://dx.doi.org/10.1007/s11133-008-9113-1.

Bell, Carl C. 1997. "Stress-Related Disorders in African-American Children." *Journal of the National Medical Association* 89 (5): 335–340.

Bell, Carl C., Willie Mae Jackson, and Briatta H. Bell. 2015. "Misdiagnosis of African-Americans with Psychiatric Issues—Part II." *Journal of the National Medical Association* 107 (3): 35–41. https://doi.org/10.1016/s0027-9684(15)30049-3.

Billingsley, Andrew. 1992. *Climbing Jacob's Ladder: Enduring Legacy of African-American Families*. New York: Simon & Schuster.

Blackmon, Douglas A. 2009. *Slavery by Another Name: The Re-Enslavement of Black Americans from the Civil War to World War II*. New York: Anchor Books.

Boelen, Paul A, and Jan van den Bout. 2005. "Complicated Grief, Depression, and Anxiety as Distinct Postloss Syndromes: A Confirmatory Factor Analysis Study." *American Journal of Psychiatry* 162: 2175–2177. https://doi.org/10.1176/appi.ajp.162.11.2175.

Boyd-Franklin, Nancy. 2003. *Black Families in Therapy: Understanding the African American Experience*. New York: Guilford Press.

Brown, Charlotte, Herbert C. Schulberg, and Michael J. Madonia. 1996. "Clinical Presentations of Major Depression by African Americans and Whites in Primary Medical Care Practice." *Journal of Affective Disorders* 41 (3): 181–191. https://doi.org/10.1016/s0165-0327(96)00085-7.

Budhwani, Henna, Kristine Ria Hearld, and Daniel Chavez-Yenter. 2015. "Depression in Racial and Ethnic Minorities: The Impact of Nativity and Discrimination." *Journal of Racial and Ethnic Health Disparities* 2 (1): 34–42. https://doi.org/10.1007/s40615-014-0045-z.

Byrd, DeAnnah R., Roland J. Thorpe Jr., and Keith E. Whitfield. 2020. "Do Depressive Symptoms Shape Blacks' Perceptions of Stress Over Time?" *Innovation in Aging* 4 (5): 1–10. https://doi.org/10.1093/geroni/igaa022.

Byrd, W. Michael, and Linda A Clayton. 2003. "Racial and Ethnic Disparities in Healthcare: A Background and History." In *Unequal Treatment: Confronting Racial and Ethnic Disparities in Health Care*, ed. Brian D. Smedley, Adrienne Y. Stith, and Alan R. Nelson, 455–527. Washington, DC: National Academies Press.

Carlson, Michelle C., Jason Brandt, Kathryn A. Carson, and Claudia H. Kawas. 1998. "Lack of Relation between Race and Cognitive Test Performance in Alzheimer's Disease." *Neurology* 50 (5): 1499–1501. https://doi.org/10.1212/wnl.50.5.1499.

Carrington, Christine H. 2006. "Clinical Depression in African American Women: Diagnoses, Treatment, and Research." *Journal of Clinical Psychology* 62 (7): 779–791. https://doi.org/10.1002/jclp.20289.

Carson, E. Ann, and Elizabeth Anderson. 2016. *Prisoners in 2015*. NCJ 250229. Washington, DC: US Department of Justice.

CDC (Centers for Disease Control and Prevention). 2016. Table 50. Use of Selected Substances in the Past Month among Persons Aged 12 and Over, by Age, Sex, Race, and Hispanic Origin: United States, Selected Years 2002–2014. In *Health, United States 2015*. accessed November 12, 2020. https://www.cdc.gov/nchs/data/hus/hus15.pdf.

———. 2020. "Rural Communities." Last updated July 7, 2021. Accessed November 12, 2020. https://www.cdc.gov/coronavirus/2019-ncov/need-extra-precautions/other-at-risk-populations/rural-communities.html.

Chama, Brian. 2019. "The Black Lives Matter Movement, Crime and Police Brutality: Comparative Study of New York Post and New York Daily News." *European Journal of American Culture* 38 (3): 201–216. https://doi.org/10.1386/ejac_00002_1.

Chien, Peter L, and Carl C Bell. 2008. "Racial Differences in Schizophrenia." *Directions in Psychiatry* 28 (4): 297–304.

Chow, Julian Chun-Chung, Kim Jaffee, and Lonnie Snowden. 2003. "Racial/Ethnic Disparities in the Use of Mental Health Services in Poverty Areas." *American Journal of Public Health* 93 5 (2003): 792–797. https://doi.org/10.2105/ajph.93.5.792.

Clay, Kevin L. 2019. "'Despite the Odds': Unpacking the Politics of Black Resilience Neoliberalism." *American Educational Research Journal* 56 (1): 75–110. https://doi.org/10.3102/0002831218790214.

Cobb, Sharon, Mohsen Bazargan, James Smith, Homero E. Del Pino, Kimberly Dorrah, and Shervin Assari. 2019. "Marijuana Use among African American Older Adults in Economically Challenged Areas of South Los Angeles." *Brain Sciences* 9 (7): 166. https://doi.org/10.3390/brainsci9070166.

Cohen, Carl I., and Leslie Marino. 2013. "Racial and Ethnic Differences in the Prevalence of Psychotic Symptoms in the General Population." *Psychiatric Services* 64 (11): 1103–1109. https://doi.org/10.1176/appi.ps.201200348.

Conner, Kyaien O., Valire Carr Copeland, Nancy K. Grote, Gary Koeske, Daniel Rosen, Charles F. Reynolds, and Charlotte Brown. 2010. "Mental Health Treatment Seeking among Older Adults with Depression: The Impact of Stigma and Race." *The American Journal of Geriatric Psychiatry* 18 (6): 531–543. https://doi.org/10.1097/jgp.0b013e3181cc0366.

Conner, Kyaien O., Valire Carr Copeland, Nancy K. Grote, Daniel Rosen, Steve Albert, Michelle L. McMurray, Charles F. Reynolds, Charlotte Brown, and Gary Koeske. 2010. "Barriers to Treatment and Culturally Endorsed Coping Strategies among Depressed African-American Older Adults." *Aging & Mental Health* 14 (8): 971–983. https://doi.org/10.1080/13607863.2010.501061.

Conner, Kyaien O., Brenda Lee, Vanessa Mayers, Deborah Robinson, Charles F. Reynolds, Steve Albert, and Charlotte Brown. 2010. "Attitudes and Beliefs about Mental Health among African American Older Adults Suffering from Depression." *Journal of Aging Studies* 24 (4): 266–277. https://doi.org/10.1016/j.jaging.2010.05.007.

Corbie-Smith, Giselle, Stephen B. Thomas, Mark V. Williams, and Sandra Moody-Ayers. 1999. "Attitudes and Beliefs of African Americans toward Participation in Medical Research." *Journal of General Internal Medicine* 14 (9): 537–546. https://doi.org/10.1046/j.1525-1497.1999.07048.x.

Council of National Psychological Associations for the Advancement of Ethnic Minority Interests. 2016. *Testing and Assessment with Persons & Communities of Color.* Washington, DC: American Psychological Association. Accessed November 1, 2020. https://www.apa.org/pi/oema/resources/testing-assessment-monograph.pdf.

Cohen, Deborah, and Nemoy Lewis. 2016. "Anti-Blackness and Urban Geopolitical Economy: Reflections on Ferguson and the Suburbanization of the 'Internal Colony.'" Society & Space, August 2. Accessed October 30, 2020. https://www.societyandspace.org/articles/anti-blackness-and-urban-geopolitical-economy.

Crenshaw, Kimberlé W., Priscilla Ocen, and Jyoti Nanda. 2015. *Black Girls Matter: Pushed Out, Overpoliced, and Underprotected*. New York: Center for Intersectionality and Social Policy Studies.

Dalencour, Michelle, Eunice C. Wong, Lingqi Tang, Elizabeth Dixon, Aziza Lucas-Wright, Kenneth Wells, and Jeanne Miranda. 2017. "The Role of Faith-Based Organizations in the Depression Care of African Americans and Hispanics in Los Angeles." *Psychiatric Services* 68 (4): 368–374. https://doi.org/10.1176/appi.ps.201500318.

Democratic Policy and Communications Committee. 2020. *Rural America and COVID–19: Small Towns and Rural Communities Are at High Risk*. Washington, DC: Democratic Policy and Communications Committee.

Diala, Chamberlain, Carles Muntaner, Christine Walrath, Kim J. Nickerson, Thomas A. LaVeist, and Philip J. Leaf. 2000. "Racial Differences in Attitudes toward Professional Mental Health Care and in the Use of Services." *American Journal of Orthopsychiatry* 70 (4): 455–464. https://doi.org/10.1037/h0087736.

Felitti, Vincent J., Robert F. Anda, Dale Nordenberg, David F. Williamson, Alison M. Spitz, Valerie Edwards, Mary P. Koss, and James S. Marks. 1998. "Relationship of Childhood Abuse and Household Dysfunction to Many of the Leading Causes of Death in Adults: The Adverse Childhood Experiences (ACE) Study." *American Journal of Preventive Medicine* 14: 245–258.

Fortson, Beverly L., Joanne Klevens, Melissa T. Merrick, Leah K. Gilbert, and Sandra P. Alexander. 2016. *Preventing Child Abuse and Neglect: A Technical Package for Policy, Norm, and Programmatic Activities*. Atlanta, GA: National Center for Injury Prevention and Control.

Gibbons, Frederick X., John H. Kingsbury, Chih-Yuan Weng, Meg Gerrard, Carolyn Cutrona, Thomas A. Wills, and Michelle Stock. 2014. "Effects of Perceived Racial Discrimination on Health Status and Health Behavior: A Differential Mediation Hypothesis." *Health Psychology* 33 (1): 11–19. https://doi.org/10.1037/a0033857.

Goldsmith, B., R. Sean Morrison, L. C. Vanderwerker, and Holly G. Prigerson. 2008. "Elevated Rates of Prolonged Grief Disorder in African Americans." *Death Studies* 32 (4): 352–365. https://doi.org/10.1080/07481180801929012.

Goodin, Burel R., Quyen T. Pham, Toni L. Glover, Adriana Sotolongo, Christopher D. King, Kimberly T. Sibille, Matthew S. Herbert, S. H. Sanden, R. Staud, et al. 2013. "Perceived Racial Discrimination, but Not Mistrust of Medical Researchers, Predicts the Heat Pain Tolerance of African Americans with Symptomatic Knee Osteoarthritis." *Health Psychology* 32 (11): 1117–1126. https://doi.org/10.1037/a0031592.

Granek, Leeat, and Tal Peleg-Sagy. 2017. "The Use of Pathological Grief Outcomes in Bereavement Studies on African Americans." *Transcultural Psychiatry* 54 (3): 384–399. https://doi.org/10.1177/1363461517708121.

Green, Carmen R., S. Khady Ndao-Brumblay, Brady West, and Tamika Washington. 2005.

"Differences in Prescription Opioid Analgesic Availability: Comparing Minority and White Pharmacies Across Michigan." *Journal of Pain* 6 (10): 689–699. https://doi.org/10 .1016/j.jpain.2005.06.002.

Harper, Mary S., and Camille D. Alexander. 1990. "Profile of the Black Elderly." In *Minority Aging: Essential Curricula Content for Selected Health and Allied Health Professions,* ed. Mary S. Harper, 193–222. DHHS Publication No. HRS-R-DV 90-4. Washington, DC: United States Department of Health and Human Services.

Harris-Lacewell, Melissa. 2001. "No Place to Rest: African American Political Attitudes and the Myth of Black Women's Strength." *Women & Politics* 23 (3): 1–33. https://doi.org /10.1300/J014v23n03_01.

Hawthorne, William B., David P. Folsom, David H. Sommerfeld, Nicole M. Lanouette, Marshall Lewis, Gregory A. Aarons, Richard M. Conklin, Ellen Solorzano, Laurie A. Lindamer, and Dilip V. Jeste. 2012. "Incarceration among Adults Who Are in the Public Mental Health System: Rates, Risk Factors, and Short-Term Outcomes." *Psychiatric Services* 63 (1): 26–32. https://doi.org/10.1176/appi.ps.201000505.

Hines, Paulette, and Nancy Boyd-Franklin. 1996. "African American Families." In *Ethnicity and Family Therapy,* 2nd ed., ed. Monica McGoldrick, Joe Giordano, and John K. Pearce, 66–84. New York: Guilford Press.

Hines-Datiri, Dorothy E., and Dorinda Carter Andrews. 2017. "The Effects of Zero Tolerance Policies on Black Girls: Using Critical Race Feminism and Figured Worlds to Examine School Discipline." *Urban Education* 55 (10): 1419–1440. https://doi.org/10.1177 /0042085917690204.

Hunter, Lora Rose, and Norman B. Schmidt. 2010. "Anxiety Psychopathology in African American Adults: Literature Review and Development of an Empirically Informed Sociocultural Model." *Psychological Bulletin* 136 (2): 211–235. https://doi.org/10.1037/ a0018133.

Kaiser Family Foundation. 2017. "Opioid Overdose Deaths by Race/Ethnicity (2012–2015)." Accessed October 30, 2020. https://www.kff.org/other/state-indicator/opioid-overdose -deaths-by-raceethnicity/?currentTimeframe=0&sortModel=%7B%22colId%22:%22 Location%22,%22sort%22:%22asc%22%7D.

———. 2018. "Total Population in U.S. Correctional Systems by Correctional Status." kff .org/other/state-indicator/total-population-in-u-s-adult-correctional-systems-by -correctional-status/?dataView=1&currentTimeframe=0&sortModel=%7B"colId" :"Incarcerated,""sort":"desc"%7D (accessed October 30, 2020).

Katz, Ralph V., Germain Jean-Charles, B. Lee Green, Nancy R. Kressin, Cristina Claudio, Minqi Wang, Stefanie L. Russell, and Jason Outlaw. 2009. "Identifying the Tuskegee Syphilis Study: Implications of Results from Recall and Recognition Questions." *BMC Public Health* 9 (1): 468–476. https://doi.org/10.1186/1471-2458-9-468.

Koma, Wyatt, Tricia Neuman, Gary Claxton, Matthew Rae, Jennifer Kates, and Josh Michaud. 2020. "How Many Adults Are at Risk of Serious Illness if Infected with Coronavirus? Updated Data." Last modified April 23, 2020. https://www.kff.org/global-health -policy/issue-brief/how-many-adults-are-at-risk-of-serious-illness-if-infected-with -coronavirus/.

Kroenke, Kurt, Robert L. Spitzer, and Janet B. Williams. "The PHQ–9: Validity of a Brief

Depression Severity Measure." *Journal of General Internal Medicine* 16 (9): 606–613. https://doi.org/10.1046/j.1525-1497.2001.016009606.x.

Laurie, Anna, and Robert A. Neimeyer. 2008. "African Americans in Bereavement: Grief as a Function of Ethnicity." *OMEGA—Journal of Death and Dying* 57 (2): 173–193. https://doi.org/10.2190/om.57.2.d.

Loewenstein, David A., Trinidad Argüelles, Soledad Argüelles, and Patricia Linn-Fuentes. 1994. "Potential Cultural Bias in the Neuropsychological Assessment of the Older Adult." *Journal of Clinical and Experimental Neuropsychology* 16 (4): 623–629. https://doi.org/10.1080/01688639408402673.

Maguire-Jack, Kathryn, Paul Lanier, and Brianna Lombardi. 2020. "Investigating Racial Differences in Clusters of Adverse Childhood Experiences." *American Journal of Orthopsychiatry* 90 (1): 106–114. https://doi.org/10.1037/ort0000405.

Manly, Jennifer J., Diane M. Jacobs, Mary Sano, Karen Bell, Carol A. Merchant, Scott A. Small, and Yaakov Stern. 1998. "Cognitive Test Performance among Nondemented Elderly African Americans and Whites." *Neurology* 50 (5): 1238–1245. https://doi.org/10.1212/wnl.50.5.1238.

———. 1999. "Effect of Literacy on Neuropsychological Test Performance in Nondemented, Education-Matched Elders." *Journal of the International Neuropsychological Society* 5 (3): 191–202. https://doi.org/10.1017/s135561779953302x.

Manly, Jennifer J., Diane M. Jacobs, Pegah Touradji, Scott A. Small, and Yaakov Stern. 2002. "Reading Level Attenuates Differences in Neuropsychological Test Performance between African American and White Elders." *Journal of the International Neuropsychological Society* 8 (3): 341–348. https://doi.org/10.1017/s1355617702813157.

Marcopulos, Bernice A., Carol A. Mclain, and Anthony J. Giuliano. 1997. "Cognitive Impairment or Inadequate Norms? A Study of Healthy, Rural, Older Adults with Limited Education." *Clinical Neuropsychologist* 11 (2): 111–131. https://doi.org/10.1080/13854049708407040.

McCarthy, Douglas, Sabrina K. H. How, Ashley-Kay Fryer, David C. Radley, and Cathy Schoen. 2011. "Why Not The Best? Results from the National Scorecard on U.S. Health System Performance, 2011." Last modified October 18, 2011. https://www.commonwealthfund.org/publications/fund-reports/2011/oct/why-not-best-results-national-scorecard-us-health-system.

Meyer, Ilan H. 2003. "Prejudice, Social Stress, and Mental Health in Lesbian, Gay, and Bisexual Populations: Conceptual Issues and Research Evidence." *Psychological Bulletin* 129 (5): 674–697. https://doi.org/10.1037/0033-2909.129.5.674.

Miller, Douglas K., Theodore K. Malmstrom, Seema Joshi, Elena M. Andresen, John E. Morley, and Fredric D. Wolinsky. 2004. "Clinically Relevant Levels of Depressive Symptoms in Community-Dwelling Middle-Aged African Americans." *Journal of the American Geriatrics Society* 52 (5): 741–748. https://doi.org/10.1111/j.1532-5415.2004.52211.x.

Morrison, R. Sean, Sylvan Wallenstein, Dana K. Natale, Richard S. Senzel, and Lo-Li Huang. 2000. "'We Don't Carry That'—Failure of Pharmacies in Predominantly Nonwhite Neighborhoods to Stock Opioid Analgesics." *New England Journal of Medicine* 342 (14): 1023–1026. https://doi.org/10.1056/NEJM200004063421406.

Neighbors, Harold W., Steven J. Trierweiler, Briggett C. Ford, and Jordana R. Muroff. 2003.

"Racial Differences in DSM Diagnosis Using a Semi-Structured Instrument: The Importance of Clinical Judgment in the Diagnosis of African Americans." *Journal of Health and Social Behavior* 44 (3): 237–256. https://doi.org/10.2307/1519777.

Norman, Jim. 2018. "The Religious Regions of the U.S." Last modified April 6, 2018. https://news.gallup.com/poll/232223/religious-regions.aspx.

Odafe, Mary O., Temilola K. Salami, and Rheeda L. Walker. 2017. "Race-Related Stress and Hopelessness in Community-Based African American Adults: Moderating Role of Social Support." *Cultural Diversity and Ethnic Minority Psychology* 23 (4): 561–569. http://dx.doi.org/10.1037/cdp0000167.

Olmedo, Esteban L. 1981. "Testing Linguistic Minorities." *American Psychologist* 36 (10): 1078–1085. https://doi.org/10.1037/0003-066x.36.10.1078.

Pickering, Thomas G. 2000. "Effects of Stress and Behavioral Intervention in Hypertension, Headache and Hypertension: Something Old, Something New." *Journal of Clinical Hypertension* 2 (5): 345–346.

Prigerson, Holly G., Paul K. Maciejewski, Charles F. Reynolds, Andrew J. Bierhals, Jason T. Newsom, Amy Fasiczka, Ellen Frank, Jack Doman, and Mark Miller. 1995. "Inventory of Complicated Grief: A Scale to Measure Maladaptive Symptoms of Loss." *Psychiatry Research* 59 (1–2): 65–79. https://doi.org/10.1016/0165-1781(95)02757-2.

Radloff, Lenore Sawyer. 1977. "The CES-D Scale: A Self-Report Depression Scale for Research in the General Population." *Applied Psychological Measurement* 1 (3): 385–401. https://doi.org/10.1177/014662167700100306.

Reynolds, Cecil R. 1982. "Methods for Detecting Construct and Predictive Bias." In *Handbook of Methods for Detecting Test Bias*, ed. Ronald A. Berk, 192–227. Baltimore, MD: Johns Hopkins University Press.

Ripich, Danielle N., Brian Carpenter, and Elaine Ziol. 1997. "Comparison of African-American and White Persons with Alzheimer's Disease on Language Measures." *Neurology* 48 (3): 781–783. https://doi.org/10.1212/wnl.48.3.781.

Rosenblatt, Paul C., and Beverly R. Wallace. 2005. "Narratives of Grieving African-Americans about Racism in the Lives of Deceased Family Members." *Death Studies* 29 (3): 217–235. https://doi.org/10.1080/07481180590916353.

Schaie, K. Warner. 1985. *Schaie-Thurstone Adult Mental Abilities Test Manual*. Palo Alto, CA: Consulting Psychologists Press.

Schwartz, Robert C., and David M. Blankenship. 2014. "Racial Disparities in Psychotic Disorder Diagnosis: A Review of Empirical Literature." *World Journal of Psychiatry* 4 (4): 133–140. https://doi.org/10.5498/wjp.v4.i4.133.

Schwartz, Robert C., and Kevin P. Feisthamel. 2009. "Disproportionate Diagnosis of Mental Disorders Among African American Versus European American Clients: Implications for Counseling Theory, Research, and Practice." *Journal of Counseling & Development* 87 (3): 295–301. https://doi.org/10.1002/j.1556-6678.2009.tb00110.x.

Sellers, Robert M., Cleopatra H. Caldwell, Karen H. Schmeelk-Cone, and Marc A. Zimmerman. 2003. "Racial Identity, Racial Discrimination, Perceived Stress, and Psychological Distress among African American Young Adults." *Journal of Health and Social Behavior* 44 (3): 302–317. https://www.jstor.org/stable/1519781.

Sibrava, Nicholas J., Courtney Beard, Andri S. Bjornsson, Ethan Moitra, Risa B. Weisberg, and Martin B. Keller. 2013. "Two-Year Course of Generalized Anxiety Disorder, Social Anxiety Disorder, and Panic Disorder in a Longitudinal Sample of African American Adults." *Journal of Consulting and Clinical Psychology* 81 (6): 1052–1062. https://doi.org/10.1037/a0034382.

Spencer, Leon E., and Terry Oatts. 1999. "Conduct Disorder vs. Attention-Deficit Hyperactivity Disorder: Diagnostic Implications for African-American Adolescent Males." *Education* 119 (3): 514–518.

Stack, Carol B. 1974. *All Our Kin*. New York: Basic Books.

Strakowski, Stephen M., Paul E. Keck, Lesley M. Arnold, Jacqueline Collins, Rodgers M. Wilson, David E. Fleck, Kimberly B. Corey, Jennifer Amicone, and Victor R. Adebimpe. 2003. "Ethnicity and Diagnosis in Patients with Affective Disorders." *Journal of Clinical Psychiatry* 64 (7): 747–754. https://doi.org/10.4088/jcp.v64n0702.

Substance Abuse and Mental Health Service Administration. 2015a. "Emerging Issues in Behavioral Health and the Criminal Justice System." Accessed November 1, 2020. www.samhsa.gov/criminal-juvenile-justice/behavioral-health-criminal-justice.

———. 2015b. "Racial/Ethnic Differences in Mental Health Service Use among Adults." Accessed November 1, 2020. https://www.samhsa.gov/data/sites/default/files/MHServicesUseAmongAdults/MHServicesUseAmongAdults.pdf.

———. 2020. *The Opioid Crisis and the Black/African American Population: An Urgent Issue*. Publication No. PEP20-05-02-001. Rockville, MD: Office of Behavioral Health Equity.

Sudarkasa, Niara. "African American Families and Family Values." In *Black Families,* edited by Harriette Pipes McAdoo, 9–40. Thousand Oaks, CA: Sage, 1997.

Sue, Derald Wing, Patricia Arredondo, and Roderick J. Mcdavis. 1992. "Multicultural Counseling Competencies and Standards: A Call to the Profession." *Journal of Counseling & Development* 70 (4): 477–486. https://doi.org/10.1002/j.1556-6676.1992.tb01642.x.

Taxy, Sam, Julie Samuels, and William Adams. 2015. *Drug Offenders in Federal Prison: Estimates of Characteristics Based on Linked Data*. Washington, DC: Office of Justice Programs,

Taylor, Robert Joseph, and Linda M. Chatters. 2010. "Importance of Religion and Spirituality in the Lives of African Americans, Caribbean Blacks and Non-Hispanic Whites." *Journal of Negro Education* 79 (3): 280–294.

Thornicroft, Graham, Elaine Brohan, Diana Rose, Norman Sartorius, and Morven Leese. 2009. "Global Pattern of Experienced and Anticipated Discrimination against People with Schizophrenia: a Cross-Sectional Survey." *The Lancet* 373 (9661): 408–415. https://doi.org/10.1016/s0140-6736(08)61817-6.

Thorpe, Roland J., Jr., Ryon Cobb, Keyonna King, Marino A. Bruce, Paul Archibald, Harlan P. Jones, Keith C. Norris, Keith E. Whitfield, and Darrell Hudson. 2020. "The Association Between Depressive Symptoms and Accumulation of Stress Among Black Men in the Health and Retirement Study." *Innovation in Aging* 4 (5): 1–9. https://doi.org/10.1093/geroni/igaa047.

United Nations. Officer of the Commission of Human Rights. 2016. Working Group of Experts on People of African Descent on Its Mission to the United States of America. Last modified August 18, 2016. https://www.ohchr.org/en/issues/racism/wgafricandescent/pages/wgepadindex.aspx.

United States Census Bureau. 2016a. *Income and Poverty in the United States: 2015*. Accessed November 1, 2020. https://www.census.gov/library/publications/2016/demo/p60-256.html.

———. 2016b. "[Population of] Black or African American Alone, Percent, [by State, United States, 2016]." Quick Facts. Accessed November 12, 2020. https://www.census.gov/quickfacts/fact/map/US/RHI225220.

US Department of Health and Human Services. 1999. *Mental Health: A Report of the Surgeon General*. Rockville, MD: DHHS.

———. 2001. *Mental Health: Culture, Races, and Ethnicity–A Supplement to Mental Health: A Report of the Surgeon General*. Accessed November 10, 2020. https://www.ncbi.nlm.nih.gov/books/NBK44243/.

———. 2020. *2018 National Survey on Drug Use and Health: African Americans*. Center for Behavioral Health Statistics and Quality. Accessed November 10, 2020. https://www.samhsa.gov/data/sites/default/files/reports/rpt23247/2_AfricanAmerican_2020_01_14_508.pdf.

Unverzagt, Frederick W., Kathleen S. Hall, Alexia M. Torke, Jeff D. Rediger, Nenette Mercado, Oye Gureje, Benjamin O. Osuntokun, and Hugh C. Hendrie. 1996. "Effects of Age, Education, and Gender on CERAD Neuropsychological Test Performance in an African American Sample." *Clinical Neuropsychologist* 10 (2): 180–190. https://doi.org/10.1080/13854049608406679.

Van Der Kolk, Bessel. 2005. "Developmental Trauma Disorder: Toward a Rational Diagnosis for Children with Complex Trauma Histories." *Psychiatric Annals* 35 (5): 401–408. https://doi.org/10.3928/00485713-20050501-06.

Walker, Rheeda, David Francis, Gene Brody, Ronald Simons, Carolyn Cutrona, and Frederick Gibbons. 2017. "A Longitudinal Study of Racial Discrimination and Risk for Death Ideation in African American Youth." *Suicide and Life-Threatening Behavior* 471: 86–102. https://doi.org/ 10.1111/sltb.12251.

Wang, Philip S., Patricia Berglund, and Ronald C. Kessler. 2000. "Recent Care of Common Mental Disorders in the United States: Prevalence and Conformance with Evidence-Based Recommendations." *Journal of General Internal Medicine* 15 (5): 284–292. https://doi.org/10.1046/j.1525-1497.2000.9908044.x.

Watkins, Daphne C. 2012. "Depression over the Adult Life Course for African American Men: Toward a Framework for Research and Practice." *American Journal of Men's Health* 6 (3): 194–210. https://doi.org/10.1177/1557988311424072.

Watkins, Daphne C., Rheeda L. Walker, and Derek M. Griffith. 2010. "A Meta-Study of Black Male Mental Health and Well-Being." *Journal of Black Psychology* 36 (3): 303–330. https://doi.org/10.1177/0095798409353756.

Watson, Natalie N., and Carla D. Hunter. 2015. "Anxiety and Depression among African American Women: The Costs of Strength and Negative Attitudes toward Psychological Help-Seeking." *Cultural Diversity and Ethnic Minority Psychology* 21 (4): 604–612. https://doi.org/10.1037/cdp0000015.

West, Lindsey M., Roxanne A. Donovan, and Amanda R. Daniel. 2016. "The Price of Strength: Black College Women's Perspectives on the Strong Black Woman Stereotype." *Women & Therapy* 39 (3–4): 390–412. https://doi.org/10.1080/02703149.2016.1116871.

Whitfield, Keith E., and Sebrina A. Wiggins. 2003. "The Impact of Desegregation on Cognition among Older African Americans." *Journal of African American Psychology* 29 (3): 275–91. https://doi.org/10.1177/0095798403254209.

Williams, Chancellor. 1987. *The Destruction of Black Civilization: Great Issues of a Race from 4500 BC to 2000 AD*. Chicago: Third World Press.

Williams, David R., Harold W. Neighbors, and James S. Jackson. 2003. "Racial/Ethnic Discrimination and Health: Findings From Community Studies." *American Journal of Public Health* 93 (2): 200–208. https://doi.org/10.2105/ajph.93.2.200.

Williams, Monnica T., Diana A. Beckmann-Mendez, and Eric Turkheimer. 2013. "Cultural Barriers to African American Participation in Anxiety Disorders Research." *Journal of the National Medical Association* 105 (1): 33–41. https://doi.org/10.1016/s0027-9684(15) 30083-3.

14

Prostate Cancer

FOLAKEMI ODEDINA, PhD,

CLAYTON YATES, PhD,

and ERNEST KANINJING, DrPH

Roots of Prostate Cancer Disparities in Black Men

Prostate cancer is the second most common cancer among men in the United States (American Cancer Society 2019). It is the result of mutations in the genes of the prostate cells that occur when normal prostate cells divide too quickly or die too slowly. Prostate cancer is more prevalent among men with a positive family history and men of African ancestry (American Cancer Society 2019). Increased prostate cancer incidence in the United States peaked in the period 1989 to 1992 with the introduction of the prostate specific antigen (PSA) test. However, there has been a decline in the trend of new cases since the early 2000s. It is estimated that in 2021, about 248,530 new cases of prostate cancer will be diagnosed in the United States representing 13.1% of all new cancer cases (Surveillance, Epidemiology, and End Results Program 2021). While it is common among all ethnic and racial groups, Black men are disproportionately affected by prostate cancer.

We begin by describing some key aspects of the US South and its Black population. The southern region includes Delaware, the District of Columbia, Maryland, Virginia, West Virginia, North Carolina, South Carolina, Kentucky, Arkansas, Oklahoma, Texas, Alabama, Mississippi, Louisiana, Tennessee, Georgia, and Florida (United States Bureau of the Census 1994). In 2019, the estimated Black population in the United States was 46.8 million and the highest concentration (56%) lived in southern states (Tamir 2021). This population is diverse and dynamic and its members have varied histories and identities. It includes both individuals whose ancestors were brought to the United States during the transatlantic slave trade, which was active from the fifteenth century and into the nineteenth century (Eltis 2001), and more recent immigrants and their descendants (Tamir 2021).

America's Black Population: The Racial Context for Prostate Cancer Disparities

The forefathers of African Americans were originally taken from Africa as slaves. The greatest concentration of enslavers was in the southern United States. In total, about 4.4% of the slaves who were removed from Africa during the transatlantic slave trade ended up in British North America and United States (Curtin 1969). The African regions that most enslaved people came from were Senegambia, Upper Guinea, the Windward Coast, the Gold Coast, the Bight of Benin, the Bight of Biafra, west-central Africa, and southeast Africa (Boddy-Evans 2019). Over 10 million slaves were removed from Africa to various parts of the world in the period 1650 to 1900. In addition to the African-origin population from the slave era (native-born Blacks), immigration has led to significant increase in the US Black population. US foreign-born Blacks include Black immigrants from Africa, the Caribbean, South America, and Europe. The number of foreign-born Blacks in the United States more than tripled in the period 1980–2005, from 0.8 million to about 3 million (Tamir 2022). By 2019, the Black immigrant population was estimated to be 4.6 million; it is expected to be 9.5 million by 2050. Immigration contributed to more than 20% of the growth in the US Black population in the period 2001–2006. The growth of sub-Saharan African immigrants in the United States, which increased by 53% in the period 2010–2018, is notable. This growth outpaced the 12% growth rate for the overall foreign-born population in the United States during that same period (Echeverria-Estrada and Batalova 2019). Foreign-born Blacks continue to transform the ethnic composition of the Black population in the United States. Unfortunately, native-born and foreign-born Blacks are grouped together in health disparities research. Disaggregated data based on nativity or country of birth are important for effectively addressing prostate cancer disparities. With this context in mind, we use the term "African American" to refer to the native-born Black population and the term "Black" to refer to all Black populations, including Black immigrants to the United States.

The Black population within and outside the United States bears the greatest prostate cancer burden of all racial/ethnic groups. In the United

States, Black men have a 1 in 7 lifetime probability of developing prostate cancer and 1 in 25 lifetime probability of dying from it (American Cancer Society 2019). In comparison, non-Hispanic white men have 1 in 9 lifetime probability of developing prostate cancer and 1 in 45 lifetime probability of dying from it. On average, about 30,000 Black men will hear the words "You have prostate cancer" each year. The prostate cancer disparities Black men experience in the United States is a microcosm of the global burden of prostate cancer in Blacks (Odedina et al. 2006; Odedina et. al. 2009). For example, the World Health Organization has estimated that the top ten countries leading prostate cancer mortality in the world are nations countries with predominantly Black populations (Ferlay et al. 2020). Additionally, prostate cancer is the leading cancer among men within the World Health Organization African region for estimated age-standardized incidence rates, age-standardized mortality rates, and estimated cases of five years' prevalence of the disease (GLOBOCAN 2018).

Geographical Pattern and Trend of Prostate Cancer Incidence and Mortality

Since most Black men in the United States live in the southern states, the burden of prostate cancer is more pronounced in the South than it is in other regions. Data for prostate cancer among Blacks in the United States from 2014–2018 shows that the southern states were impacted more than other regions (Surveillance, Epidemiology, and End Results Program 2021). Each of the southern states had age-adjusted rates higher than the national average (which is 111.3/100,000) among men of all racial and ethnic groups. A cluster of six states (Georgia, Tennessee, Arkansas, Alabama, Mississippi, and Louisiana) had elevated rates of new cases between the range of 181/100,000 and 200/100,000 men. North and South Carolina were also severely impacted, with incidence rates of 180/100,000 and 167/100,000 men, respectively. The rate for Texas, which is home to the largest Black population in the South, was 158/100,000, for Kentucky it was 159/100,000, for Virginia it was 161/100,000, and for Oklahoma it was 164/100,000. Florida had slightly lower rates at 143/100,000 (see fig. 14.1). The most current data (2018) indicates a prostate cancer incidence rate of 164/100,000 in Black men. Thirteen of the sixteen southern states had age-adjusted incidence rates higher than the national average (United States Cancer Statistics Working Group 2021) Virginia, South Carolina, and Florida were the only three

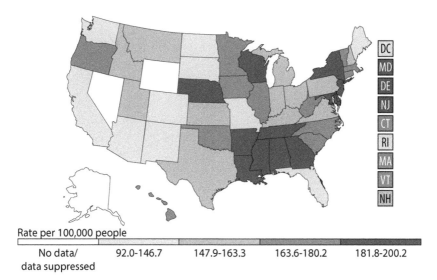

Rate per 100,000 people

| No data/ data suppressed | 92.0-146.7 | 147.9-163.3 | 163.6-180.2 | 181.8-200.2 |

Figure 14.1. Incidence of prostate cancer among US Black men, 2014–2018. CDC, "Number of New Cancers in the United States, 2014–2018, Prostate, All Ages, Black, Male," Cancer at a Glance, https://gis.cdc.gov/Cancer/USCS/#/AtAGlance. Accessed August 5, 2021.

southern states in 2018 with incidence rates below the national average. No-tably, Arkansas (206/100,000) and Louisiana (200/100,000) had the highest prostate cancer incidence rates in the South.

Data on long-term mortality trend for prostate cancer in the United States shows a decline among all racial and ethnic groups, from a peak rate of 70/100,000 in 1999 to 38/100,000 in 2017 (CDC 2019). However, this decline has not been equal across all racial/ethnic groups. As figure 14.2 shows, Black men continue to experience mortality disparities. Moreover, age-adjusted data for the United States in the period 2012–2016 shows that the death rate for non-Hispanic white men was 18.1/100,000 but was more than double for Black men at 39.8/100,000 (American Cancer Society 2019). The mortality rate for Black men in the South follows the pattern of prostate cancer incidence. A cluster of five states (South Carolina, Georgia, Tennes-see, Alabama, Mississippi, and Oklahoma) had rates ranging from 41 to 49 per 100,000, which is double the national average for men of all races. West Virginia, Virginia, and North Carolina represent a cluster of states with mor-tality rates ranging from 36/100,000 to 41/100,000. Texas had the lowest mortality rates in the South at 33/100,000 (fig. 14.3). The 2018 data indicated

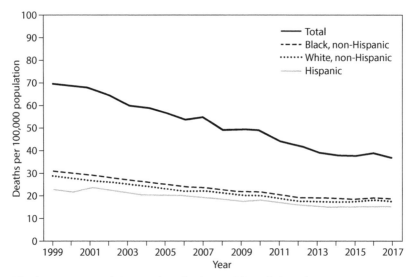

* Deaths per100,000 population, age-adjusted to the 2000 U.S. standard population.

Figure 14.2. Prostate cancer mortality among US males by race/ethnicity, 1999–2017. CDC, "QuickStats: Age-Adjusted Death Rates from Prostate Cancer, by Race/ Ethnicity—National Vital Statistics System, United States, 1999–2017," *Mortality and Morbidity Weekly Report* 68, no. 23 (2019), https://www.cdc.gov /mmwr/volumes/68/wr/mm6823a4.htm?s_cid=mm6823a4_w.

that a cluster of seven southern states (Virginia, North Carolina, Georgia, Alabama, Mississippi, Arkansas and Oklahoma) had age-adjusted mortality rates above the national average for Black men (37/100,000) (United States Cancer Statistics Working Group 2021). Oklahoma had the highest death rate in the South at 50/100,000. Although Virginia had a lower incidence rate in 2018 (143/100,000) than the national average, it was among the seven states with mortality rates above the national average at 41/100,000. Overall, the mortality burden in 2018 was not concentrated in the South; three midwestern states (Illinois, Missouri, and Nebraska) and two western states (Colorado and Nevada) had death rates above the national average. It is worth noting that the two leading southern states for incidence rates in 2018 (Arkansas and Louisiana) did not report the highest death rates. The highest prostate cancer deaths rates for Black men were in Oklahoma and Mississippi.

Increased used of diagnostic and screening tests has contributed to early detection and treatment of prostate cancer in the United States. As a result,

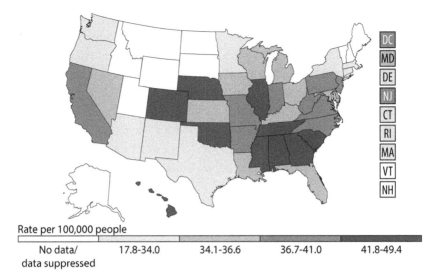

Rate per 100,000 people

| No data/
data suppressed | 17.8–34.0 | 34.1–36.6 | 36.7–41.0 | 41.8–49.4 |

Figure 14.3. Rate of prostate cancer death among US Black men, 2014–2018. CDC, "Rate of Cancer Deaths in the United States, 2014-2018," Cancer at a Glance, https://gis.cdc.gov/Cancer/USCS/#/AtAGlance/. Accessed August 5, 2021.

data for 2010–2016 shows that the 97.5% of men survive five years or more after being diagnosed with prostate cancer in the United States (the five-year relative survival rate) (Surveillance, Epidemiology, and End Results Program 2021). About 86% of all prostate cancer diagnosed among Black men in the period 2014–2018 were at a local or regional stage and the five-year relative survival rate approached 100% (American Cancer Society 2019).

Factors Associated with the Burden of Prostate Cancer

Several factors have been implicated in prostate cancer disparities in US Black men. Social determinants of health are notable. Health insurance coverage is the main avenue for accessing care in the United States. In 2019, about 11% of Blacks in the United States were uninsured, compared to 8% of non-Hispanic whites (Artiga et al. 2021). This unequitable access to care, particularly for preventive services such as prostate cancer screening, contributes to late-stage diagnosis in Black men (American Cancer Society 2015; Klassen and Platz 2006). Geographic variations in the prostate cancer death rate have been found to be positively associated with the incidence of late-stage disease (Fletcher et al. 2020). In addition, limited access to standard prostate cancer treatment and care persists for Black men. Research studies have found that Black and Hispanic men are significantly less likely to receive definitive treatment (prostatectomy or radiation treatment) than white men (Fletcher et al. 2020; Moses et al. 2017; Underwood et al. 2004). A recent review by Coughlin (2020) documented the social determinants of health associated with the risk level, stage at diagnosis, and survival rate associated with prostate cancer. In a review of 833 publications, Coughlin found that 17 converged on the evidence that poverty, lack of education, immigration status, lack of social support, and social isolation impact prostate cancer survival.

Another important factor is that Black prostate cancer patients are more likely to have comorbidities than their white counterparts. This affects both their care and their participation in clinical trials that may be beneficial to them. Health conditions such as hypertension, diabetes mellitus, and insulin resistance are common comorbid conditions in cancer patients (Roy et al. 2018). Williams et al. (2018) found a higher comorbidity index among Blacks in the South than their white counterparts, putting them at increased risk for poorer outcomes. In an earlier study, Fleming and colleagues (2006) reported a higher likelihood of late-stage prostate cancer for Black men with coronary artery disease, dyslipidemia, and severe renal disease. The authors reported that Black prostate cancer patients with two or more comorbidities had a 40% higher probability of a late-stage prostate cancer diagnosis than Black patients with no comorbidities.

Studies have also suggested an elevated incidence of prostate cancer among farmers (Blair et al. 1992; Meyer, Coker, and Sanderson 2007; Welton et al. 2015), which is relevant in the South, where agriculture is the economic base in several southern states and the history of Blacks working in agriculture reaches back to the slavery era. In a study based in Georgia, researchers found an association between prostate cancer incidence rates, expenditure on agricultural chemicals, and expenditures on commercial fertilizers. Notably, these findings were statistically significant in counties with higher than median percentages of Black residents (Welton et al. 2015).

Factors Implicated in Prostate Cancer Disparities
Prostate Cancer Risk Factors

The primary risk factors for prostate cancer are increasing age, family history, and genetic factors. In a Florida cancer registry study of Black men diagnosed with prostate cancer in the period 2006–2010, Dagne et al. (2017) found that most African American men were diagnosed with prostate cancer aged 60 to 69 years (38.4% of 2,614 men diagnosed). Similarly, Caribbean-born Black men and African-born Black men were mostly diagnosed within this age bracket. It was interesting to note that African-born Black men were more likely to be diagnosed at a younger age. About 11% were diagnosed with prostate cancer before age 50, compared to about 5% for African American men and 4% for Caribbean-born Black men in that age group. Fletcher et al. (2020) found a similar pattern for Black men in a study of 18 cancer registries within the Surveillance, Epidemiology, and End Results database. Most (41.4%) of the 35,000 men included in the study were diagnosed at 60 to 69 years of age; only 6.5% were diagnosed before the age of 50.

Prostate cancer is known to be heritable. The relationship between a family history of prostate cancer and a prostate cancer diagnosis has been well established in the literature, especially for men who have a brother or a father who was diagnosed with this cancer (Cerhan et al. 1999; Chen et al. 2008; Kalish, McDougal, and McKinlay 2000; Whittemore et al. 1995). A family history of breast cancer has also been linked to prostate cancer diagnosis (Chen et al. 2008; Rodriguez et al. 1998), although the association is stronger for men with a prostate cancer family history. In the Health Professionals Follow-Up Study, Barber et al. (2018) found that men with a family history of prostate cancer had a 68% increased risk for prostate cancer compared to the 21% increased risk for men with a family history of breast cancer. As expected, there is a higher chance of developing prostate cancer if a man has a family history that includes both breast cancer and prostate cancer.

Behavioral Risk Factors Associated with Prostate Cancer

About 42% of cancer cases and 45% of cancer deaths can be linked to lifestyle factors (Islami, Sauer et al. 2018), the most significant of which are cigarette smoking, excess body weight, and alcohol use. However, the evidence about the association between prostate cancer and modifiable risk factors is mixed. The expert panel review conducted by the World Cancer Research Fund and the American Institute for Cancer Research (2018) reported that global evidence points to strong evidence that while advanced prostate cancer is positively linked to excess body weight and prostate cancer risk is positively linked to height, levels of beta-carotene are not associated with the risk of prostate cancer. Additionally, there is some evidence that an increased risk of prostate cancer is associated with higher consumption of dairy products, a diet high in calcium, a low concentration of vitamin E in plasma, and a low concentration of selenium in plasma. Currently, there is little or no consensus about several modifiable risk factors, including the consumption of fruits, meat, poultry, fish, or alcohol; the use of vitamin supplements; and levels of physical activity.

In a study of the cancer morbidity and mortality attributable to modifiable risk factors, Islami, Goding, and colleagues (2018) did not find that a substantial proportion of prostate cancer cases or deaths was caused by modifiable risk factors in men. The body of evidence strongly suggests that smoking is not linked to prostate cancer incidence. However, some studies have reported associations of prostate cancer mortality with smoking and excess body weight. Smoking has been linked to prostate cancer recurrence (Joshu et al. 2011; Moreira et al. 2014; Rieken et al. 2015; Kenfield et al. 2011) and to mortality from prostate cancer in multiple studies (Gansler et al. 2018; Giovannucci et al. 1999; Islami et al. 2014). This information is important because Black men have a higher smoking prevalence than Black women, white men, or white women (American Cancer Society 2021). Excess body weight has also been reported to increase fatal prostate cancer.

Prostate Cancer Screening Controversy

The common screening tests for prostate cancer are the digital rectal exam and the PSA test. The overall decline in prostate cancer mortality has been attributed to the discovery of the PSA test, although its use continues to be controversial. Currently, routine PSA screening is not recommended by most organizations because of concerns about overdiagnosis and side effects associated with prostate cancer treatment. The American Cancer Society recommends that all Black men aged 45 years and above (and who have at least ten years of life expectancy) should discuss prostate cancer with their physician so they can make informed decisions about prostate cancer screening. The recommendation for Black men with a family history of prostate cancer is that they start the discussion with their physicians beginning at 40 years of age. The United States Preventive Services Taskforce recommends that men aged 55 to 69 should make an individual decision about PSA screening after discussing the pros and cons with their physicians. There was no specific recommendation made for Black men, despite the significant disparities this group experiences. Multiple organizations and associations have made other recommendations. The lack of consensus on prostate cancer screening has significantly impacted the opportunity for early detection and put Black men at a greater health disadvantage compared to other racial groups (Chornokur et al. 2011; DeSantis et al. 2016; Kelly et al. 2017; Kinlock et al. 2016; Mahal et al. 2017; Siegel, Miller, and Jema 2017; Singh and Jemal 2017). For example, the percentage of Black men who report that they have had PSA screening is lower than that of white men (American Cancer Society 2019). Given the prostate cancer disparities experienced by Black men, it has been argued that tailored screening should be considered for Black men (Powell et al. 2014; Saltzman et al. 2015; Smith, Eggener, and Murphy 2017).

Biological Etiology of Prostate Cancer in Black Men

Molecular Features of Prostate Cancer in Black Men

A number of recent discoveries have focused on the distinct molecular features that drive tumor aggressiveness in Black men with prostate cancer. Epigenetic modulations of gene expression are at the forefront of these studies. DNA methylation is responsible for modulating gene expression in a number of critical mechanisms for prostate cancer progression such as metabolism, epithelial-to-mesenchymal transition, and immunosurveillance (Apprey et al. 2019; Devaney et al. 2015; Kwabi-Addo et al. 2010; Rubicz et al. 2019). While most of these studies have been limited by a small cohort size, Apprey and colleagues (2019) recently reported that genetic ancestry influences DNA methylation and that this modifying factor has been shown in epigenetic association studies in populations of admixed patients. Furthermore, in a comparison of methylation frequency in the normal and prostate cancer tissue samples by race, Black samples showed a significantly higher prevalence of methylation for androgen receptors *RARβ2, SPARC, TIMP3,* and *NKX2-5* than white samples. Interestingly, Black patients who are TMPRSS-ERG negative have lower levels of androgen receptor expression (Farrell et al. 2014; Powell et al. 2014; Yamoah et al. 2015). However, whether this loss of expression is associated with DNA methylation is yet to be determined. The increased methylation pattern in Black patients appears to extend to microRNAs. Theodore and colleagues (2014) reported differentially expressed microRNA in ancestry-verified African prostate cancer cell lines and tissue samples from Alabama. In 2017, Yates and colleagues followed up this study, demonstrating that Black prostate cancer patients with TMPRSS-ERG negative tumors have an enrichment of microRNAs associated with DNA methylation. While there are currently no published studies that compare DNA methylation in northern and southern states, Yates's lab identified that Kaiso, a bimodal BTB/POZ protein, is overexpressed in Black men with prostate cancer (Jones et al. 2012). Kaiso binds methylated DNA to epigenetically suppress gene expression. Interestingly, Kaiso expression was predominately located in the cytoplasm in low Gleason-grade tumors, while high Gleason-grade and metastatic tumors displayed increased nuclear Kaiso expression (Abisoye-Ogunniyan et al. 2018; Pierre et al. 2019; Wang et al. 2016). In a subsequent study, Abisoye-Ogunniyan et al. (2018) found that this cytoplasmic to nuclear shift is induced by epidermal growth factor receptor (EGFR) and mitogen-activated protein (MAP) kinase signaling, resulting in an epithelial to mesenchymal transition and increased migration and invasiveness.

In addition to these findings, several groups have identified metabolic differences in Black and white prostate cancer patients. Gohlke et al. (2019) demonstrated that methionine and homocysteine were both higher in plasma from Black prostate cancer patients than in case-control, positive, or negative biopsies or samples from men of self-reported race or West African ancestry (Gohlke et al. 2019). Elevated levels of homocysteine and the degeneration of bone matrix that is critical for metastasis is also consistent with the increased methylation found in Black prostate tumors (Gohlke et al. 2019). Since Kaiso regulates epigenetic silencing of methylated DNA, this further suggests an overall phenotype that drives aggressive in the patient population. Multiple reports have demonstrated that Black prostate tumors overexpress EGFR (Douglas et al. 2006; Nwaneri, McBeth, and Hinds 2016; Shuch et al. 2004). Thus, it is tempting to speculate that upstream EGFR signaling could play a role in these observations. Furthermore, given the robust literature on the available therapeutics that target EGFR and downstream signaling pathways for a number of tumor types to limit disease progression, this pathway could be a viable approach for Black men with prostate cancer.

A second major finding in Black men with prostate cancer is elevated levels of systemic inflammation. These findings were first published by Reams et al. (2009), who conducted a micro-array pilot study of Florida men with prostate tumors with a Gleason score of 6. A comparison of genes differentially expressed in Black and white patients revealed at least 97 statistically significant genes that were predominantly in the interleukins chemokine family (Devaraj et al. 2010). Since this initial report, multiple groups have now added to this finding and have identified that Black men with prostate cancer differentially express many immune-related genes, including interleukins, cytokines, and growth factors. While varying immune genes have been reported, a differential immune signature in the INF-γ-STAT1 signaling cascade is consistent among these reports (Wallace et al. 2008). Leveraging existing data from two independent prostate cancer Gene Expression Omnibus datasets (GSE6956 and GSE21032) that contain race annotations, Taylor et al. (2010) and Prueitt et al. (2016) found that STAT1 was overexpressed in tumors from Black patients compared to those of white patients ($p < 0.001$ and $p < 0.01$, respectively). Furthermore, in unpublished whole transcriptome sequencing data from both Black and white men with high-grade prostate cancer from Alabama, Yates lab (Levy and Darnell 2002) similarly found that Black men with prostate cancer exhibited elevated RNA levels of STAT1 while white patients express low levels. Collectively, these findings provide evidence that STAT1 is associated with tumors in Black men. Since STAT1 is a well characterized transcription factor to active multiple downstream genes, multiple reports have demonstrated that determining STAT1-inducible genes is a reliable predictor of STAT1 activity and inflammation (Levy and Darnell 2002). To determine its regulatory role in tumors of men with African ancestry, we examined STAT-inducible genes in both Black and white prostate cancer patients within the Alabama cohort. Using STAT1 chromatin immunoprecipitation with sequencing data from independent studies (Satoh and Tabunoki 2013) and the TRRUST database (Han et al. 2017; Satoh and Tabunoki 2013), the lab identified STAT1-related genes (N = 1,507). The expression of these genes was then overlapped in mRNA from whole transcriptome Black and white prostate cancer sequencing data. Using relatively stringent filtering criterion, we identified 18 genes associated with STAT1. Interestingly, within this list were common STAT1-inducible genes such as IRF9, PARP9, IFI35, UBE2L6, IFIT3, DTX3L, and TAP1 (Gongora and Mechti 1999; Katsoulidis et al. 2008; Legrier et al. 2016) for both races. However, we observed that 11 of the 18 genes found in Black men (TMEM140, DOCK3, GFM1, SLC38A11, NEDD9, GEN1, EFHD2, MREG, GINS3, SLCO2A1) were not correlated with STAT1 in white patients with prostate cancer tumors (figs. 14.4 and 14.5). These findings further highlight that evaluated STAT1 expression could have a differential impact in men of African ancestry.

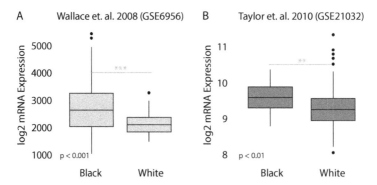

Figure 14.4. Box plot of GEO datasets GSE6956 and GSE21032 for STAT1 expression in Black and white patients with prostate cancer.

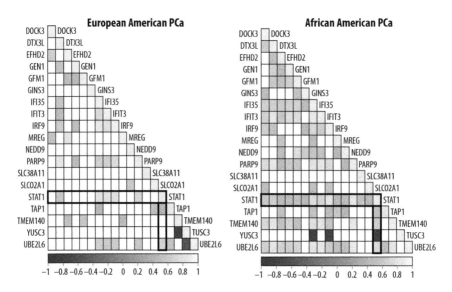

Figure 14.5. Significant STAT1 target interaction for Black and white US men with prostate cancer, 2013 and 2017. STAT1 ChIP-Seq data (from Satoh and Tabunoki 2013) and the TRRUST database (Han et. al 2017). STAT1 target genes (n =1,507) were extracted from differentially expressed genes within the Alabama cohort of men with prostate cancer.

Lifestyle Factors Influence the Molecular Features of Prostate
Tumors in African American Men

Recent studies have focused on the influence of dietary supplements
in Black prostate cancer patients (Pierre et al. 2019), including vitamin E
(α-tocopherol) and vitamin D. While the majority of such studies have not
been completed for Black patients, it is well known that a large population of Black men exhibit decreased serum 1,25 dihydroxy vitamin D levels
(Jerabek-Willemsen et al. 2011; Rosenberg et al. 2019). Although both vitamin D_3 and vitamin D_2 can be derived from the diet, sunlight, or UVB radiation, is by far the most important source. The synthesis of 1,25-dihydroxy
vitamin D begins with the production of vitamin D_3 cholecalciferol after
7-dehydrocholesterol in the skin is exposed to UVB radiation. The average
American receives different amounts of exposure based on geographical
location. For example, a study measured UV exposure in northern states (Se-
attle, Washington, and Burlington, Vermont) and southern states (Phoenix,
Arizona, and Miami, Florida) that have extreme differences in UV exposure.
Interestingly, during the winter, nearly 70% of Blacks living in southern
states were vitamin D deficient. Furthermore, Blacks living in Miami during
the summer only had a 20% increase in vitamin D and 25-hydroxy levels of
less than 50 nmol/L (Marvel 2006; Park and Johnson 2005). This data is
further supported by studies of Blacks in Nigeria, which have high UV exposure year round and similarly low vitamin D levels despite overwhelmingly
high UVB exposure (Sajo et al. 2020; Wang et al. 2018).

To determine if vitamin D supplementation could mitigate prostate
cancer, Hardiman and colleagues (2016) examined 27 men (10 Black and 17
white) who had low vitamin D_3 levels prior to prostatectomy (Hardiman et
al. 2016) to examine the biological effects of vitamin D supplementation.
Similar to previous reports, they observed that Black men with prostate cancer exhibit differential expression of immune-related genes, categorized into
lymphocyte activation, T-cell activation, and dendritic cell maturation and
crosstalk with natural killer cells (Hardiman et al. 2016; Kiely and Ambs 2021;
Wallace et al. 2008). Of these multiple pathways, the researchers demonstrated that growth differentiation factor 15, which belongs to the transforming growth factor beta superfamily, was lower in Black patients than
in white patients (–1.65-fold and highly significant at a false discovery rate
of 0.16). Of the 27 patients, 14 received 4,000 IU of vitamin D_3 daily and 13

subjects received a placebo for two months before surgery. Interestingly, growth differentiation factor 15 mRNA expression, which is a marker for overall inflammation, was significantly increased relative to those in the control group, further suggesting that Black men have a specific benefit from vitamin D_3 supplementation.

Given the high level of inflammation and immune deregulation observed with prostate cancer, the role of aspirin in mitigating prostate cancer has also been explored. The hypothesis is that the use of anti-inflammatory compounds would limit aggressive prostate cancer in Black men. The first study to explore this hypothesis was performed by the Ambs lab (Smith et al. 2017) using the National Cancer Institute—Maryland Prostate Cancer Case Control Study consisting of 823 men with incident prostate cancer (422 Black and 401 white) and 1,034 population-based men without the disease diagnosis (486 Black and 548 white). They reported that daily long-term use of aspirin for more than three years significantly decreased the risk of advanced disease and that tumors recurred only in Black men (Smith et al. 2017). In 2002–2009, this same group followed up their observation with 22,426 Black men from the Southern Community Cohort Study, which collected patients from a twelve-state area (Alabama, Arkansas, Florida, Georgia, Kentucky, Louisiana, Mississippi, North Carolina, South Carolina, Tennessee, Virginia, and West Virginia) (Tang et al. 2021). While only 5,486 men (25.1%) reported taking any aspirin (regular strength, low-dose or baby aspirin, or half tablets of aspirin) and 2,634 men (12.1%) reported regular strength aspirin at the time of enrollment, there was still a significant reduction in mortality attributable to prostate cancer in these men. Interestingly, in both studies there was no statistically significant association between aspirin usage and the incidence of prostate cancer.

Behavioral Models of Prostate Cancer Disparities in Black Men

Influence of Intrapersonal Factors in Prostate Cancer Disparities

Individual (intrapersonal) factors are among the most significant sources of disparities in health care (Smedley, Stith, and Nelson 2003). These factors, which include knowledge (Abbott, Taylor, and Barber 1998; Agho and Lewis 2001; Ashford et al. 2001; Baguet 1991; Barber et al. 1998; Coughlin et al. 2021; Forrester-Anderson 2005; Freedland and Isaacs 2005; Jones et al. 2005; Magnus 2004; Miller, Hamler, and Qin. 2020; McWhorter 1989; Ogunsanya et al. 2017; Pruthi et al. 2006; Richardson, Webster, and Fields 2004; Ross, Uhler, and Williams 2005; Steele et al. 2000; Smith, Dorsey et al. 1997; Smith, Eggener, and Murphy 1997; Woods et al. 2004), perceived barriers (Cobran, Hall, and Aiken 2018; Shelton, Weinrich, and Reynolds 1999), and cues to action from health care providers (Nievens et al. 2001; Weinrich et al. 1998), have been found to significantly determine whether a man receives prostate cancer screening. In a study of 1,373 Black men (Odedina et al. 2008), only 26% of respondents reported that they were screened annually. About 42% of respondents had never been screened. Some of the key issues that led respondents to get screened were prostate cancer signs and symptoms, a recommendation from a doctor, having appropriate information, having access to screening, less invasive screening procedures, knowledge of risk factors, encouragement from family members, the perception that they would benefit from screening, media campaigns, perceived seriousness of prostate cancer, prostate cancer screening awareness, and knowing someone who has prostate cancer. In turn, participants noted that they were deterred by fear of testing positive for prostate cancer, low perceived susceptibility to prostate cancer, limited access to screening, lack of information from a doctor, lack of trust in the doctor, no regular primary care provider, the discomfort of the screening procedure, and lack of information about the disease.

A limited area of prostate cancer disparities research is the role that varying personal cultural beliefs and values play in individual behavior among Black men (Odedina et al. 2011a). Leininger (1995) has noted that fundamental elements related to ethnicity and culture shape health perceptions, attitudes, and behaviors and that it is important to acknowledge cultural diversity and study the specific cultural beliefs of each ethnic group related to health and health behaviors. Researchers, including those at the United States Department of Health and Human Services, recognized the importance of culture in the Black community decades ago (Bailey 1987; Harrison and Harrison 1971; Heckler 1985; Hogle 1982). Unfortunately, there is still a dearth of literature in this area. Learning about the cultural world view of Black men will further improve our understanding of prostate cancer risk reduction and early detection behaviors (Hughes et al. 2003) and will ultimately improve the design of successful interventions.

Leininger (1970) defines culture as the beliefs, values, customs, behaviors, and artifacts a society uses to cope with other people and the world in general that are passed down from one generation to another through learning. The cultural world view of individuals is rooted in the values, beliefs, and behaviors of their ethnic population (Jackson and Sears 1992; Myers 1998). Cultural beliefs and values such as cancer fatalism, religion and spirituality, temporal orientation, and acculturation affect beliefs and assumptions about health and behavior related to health. Cancer fatalism, or an individual's belief that death is inevitable when they are diagnosed with cancer, is a major barrier to cancer detection and control (Powe and Finnie 2003). Although the number of reports on the impact of religion and spiritual beliefs on cancer prevention or detection is limited, it has been suggested that such beliefs may deter women from seeking treatment for breast cancer (Lannin et al. 1998). Temporal orientation, which refers to the role of the social psychology of time, or an individual's perception of time as being in the past, present, or future (Brown and Segal 1997; Holman and Silver 1998), has a significant influence on individual thoughts and actions (Graham 1981). In general, health promotion and disease prevention behavior such as prostate cancer risk reduction and detection requires a future time perspective. It is interesting to note that Black adults' time orientation has been reported to be in the present (Brown and Segal 1996; Jones 1988). This is likely to have a negative impact on Black men's prostate cancer risk reduction behavior. Acculturation is a cross-cultural psychology concept that "reflects the extent to which individuals (from a non-dominant culture) learn the values, behaviors, lifestyles, and language of the host (dominant) culture" (Zane and Mak 2003, 39). Since Black men belong to a nondominant group in the United States, over the years many will adopt values, behaviors, and lifestyles of the dominant white group. The level and process of acculturation differs for each individual and are likely to influence prostate cancer risk reduction and early detection behaviors.

The Personal Integrative Model of Prostate Cancer Disparity Model: Findings from Black Men in Florida

Odedina et al. (2000, 2004, 2008, 2011b) developed the Personal Integrative Model of Prostate Cancer Disparity (PIPCaD) in the first decade of the twenty-first century (see fig. 14.6). The model proposes that potential sources of prostate cancer disparity among Black men are personal factors such as lack of behaviors that would reduce the risk of prostate cancer or

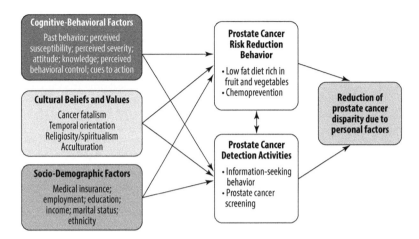

Figure 14.6. Proposed PIPCaD model for Black men prior to test of hypotheses.

lead to early detection and that these personal factors are further impacted by cognitive and behavioral factors, cultural beliefs and values, and socio-demographic factors. The model was tested among 3,410 Black men in Florida (Odedina et al. 2011b). Table 14.1 provides the operational definition of the PIPCaD constructs. (Reliability estimates of the scales ranged from 0.71 to 0.94.)

Most of the Black men who participated in the validation study of the PIPCaD model were African Americans aged 40 to 49 who had a high school diploma, were married, were employed full time, earned less than $20,000 per year, had health insurance, and had a regular doctor. In addition, most of the participants reported that they had an physical examination each year and preferred to see a physician for their medical care.

BLACK MEN'S RISK REDUCTION BEHAVIORS, SCREENING
BEHAVIORS, SOCIOCOGNITIVE CHARACTERISTICS, AND
PROSTATE CANCER HISTORY

The participants' score on the index of risk reduction behavior was very low; the median was 18 on a 0–71 index scale. This was because a majority of the men were not taking vitamins or supplements to prevent prostate cancer. Most of the participants reported that they ate fruits, vegetables, dairy products, and butter or oil 1–3 times a week. Most of the men, however, consumed meat products 4–6 times a week and indicated that meat

Table 14.1. Operational definitions of PIPCaD study variables

Study construct	Operational definitions
Prostate cancer risk reduction behavior	An index of prostate cancer risk reduction behavior was created by totaling the responses of participants about their consumption of fruits, vegetables, meat products (reversed scale), dairy products (reversed scale), and butter/oil (reversed scale) within the previous week and their use of the following supplements to prevent prostate cancer within the previous week: selenium, lycopene and other retinoids, vitamin D, or soy. The index score ranged from 0 to 71.
Prostate cancer early detection behavior	An index of prostate cancer detection behavior was created by totaling the responses of participants regarding prostate cancer screening by DRE in the previous year (5 if yes, and 0 if no); prostate cancer screening by PSA in the previous year (5 if yes, and 0 if no); behavior to seek information about prostate cancer (measured on a 5-point Likert scale); discussion of prostate cancer with a physician (measured on a 5-point Likert scale); and paying attention to prostate cancer information (measured on a 5-point Likert scale). The index score ranged from 0 to 25.
Past behavior	Past behavior was assessed with three items on a yes/no scale. Participants indicated if they had been screened for prostate cancer in the previous year via PSA or DRE and if they had participated in medical research on prostate cancer during the previous year.
Perceived susceptibility	Perceived susceptibility was measured of three statements about participants' perceptions of their chances of getting prostate cancer. Responses ranged from strongly agree (5) to strongly disagree (1). A higher score for this construct indicated a high perception of susceptibility to prostate cancer.
Perceived severity	Perceived severity was measured by three items about the seriousness and consequences of prostate cancer. The score ranged from 1 (strongly disagree) to 5 (strongly agree). A higher score indicated high perceived seriousness of prostate cancer.
Attitude	Five items measured participants' attitude about prostate cancer screening, prostate cancer risk reduction, and participating in prostate cancer medical research on a Likert scale that ranged from very favorable to very unfavorable scale. A higher score indicated a positive attitude about these three issues.
Knowledge	Ten questions assessed participants' knowledge about prostate cancer knowledge. The possible responses were true, false, or don't know. Each correct response was worth 1 point and each incorrect or I don't know response was worth 0 points. A higher score indicated high knowledge about prostate cancer.

(*continued*)

Table 14.1. *Continued*

Study construct	Operational definitions
Perceived behavioral control	Five items assessed how easy or difficult it is for respondents to participate in prostate cancer screening, prostate cancer risk reduction, and prostate cancer medical research. Possible responses ranged from 1 (very difficult) to 5 (very easy). A higher score indicated that a participant believed they had significant control over their behavior vis-à-vis these three issues.
Cues to action	Seven items measured participants' cues to action on a yes (1 point) or no (0 points) response scale. The items included a physician's recommendation that the participant be screened for prostate cancer, participation in an education forum, and prostate cancer signs/symptoms.
Cancer fatalism	The measure of cancer fatalism was adapted from the Powe Fatalism Inventory (Powe 1995a, 1995b; Powe and Finnie 2003). Participants responded to three items. One of the items was "I believe that if someone has prostate cancer, it is already too late to do something about it." A high score on this scale is an indication of strong belief that death is bound to happen when a person is diagnosed with cancer,
Temporal orientation	The three items used to assess temporal orientation were based on Brown and Segal's (1996) Hypertension Temporal Orientation scale. A response scale that ranged from strongly disagree (1) to strongly agree (5) captured participants' responses. A low score on this measure indicated a future time perspective.
Religiosity/ spirituality	Carver et al.'s (1989) scale provided the items for religious coping, which included the statement "I usually put my trust in God." Responses ranged from strongly disagree (1) to strongly agree (5). A higher score indicated high spirituality.
Acculturation	The measure of acculturation was based on Klonoff & Landrine's (2000) acculturation scale. It included items such as "When it comes to the music I listen to and the movies I watch, they are mostly by African American artists." Four items with responses ranging from strongly disagree (1) to (strongly agree (5) were employed for this study. A high score on the acculturation scale indicated a low level of acculturation, i.e., a low adoption of the values, behaviors, and lifestyles of others.

products made up the biggest portion of their meals. In addition, most of the men had not consumed chemoprevention products such as selenium, lycopene, vitamin A, vitamin D, or soy within the previous week.

The participants scored average on index of early detection behaviors (a median of 12 on a 0–25 index scale). About 31% of the men had been tested for prostate cancer with PSA screening and 26% had been tested with a digital rectal exam. Fifty-eight percent had actively sought information about prostate cancer, 60% had been attentive to health information about the disease, and 41% had discussed the disease with a physician. It is interesting to note that only 24% of the men had received a recommendation from a physician for a digital rectal exam and 29% had received a recommendation from a physician for PSA screening within the previous year. About 18% of the men had been asked to participate in prostate cancer medical research and 12% had participated in such research in the previous year.

The men's attitude towards prostate cancer screening was favorable and their perceived behavioral control was high. However, their perception of the severity of and their susceptibility to prostate cancer were low. Furthermore, the participants had a low level of acculturation, did not hold fatalistic beliefs about cancer, had religious coping skills, and had a future time perspective. The mean score on the knowledge scale was about 52%. Only 5.28% reported a personal history of prostate cancer, 8.26% reported that their father had been diagnosed with prostate cancer, 4.19% reported a prostate cancer diagnosis for their brother, and 2.60% reported a prostate cancer diagnosis for their son. Almost 18% of the men reported that they did not know if their father had been diagnosed with prostate cancer, about 16% did not know if their brother had been diagnosed, and 10% did not know if their son had been diagnosed. Thus, over 10% of the men did not know their family history with this disease.

Associated PIPCaD Variables. The confirmed associations among the PIPCaD study variables are summarized in figure 14.7. The results indicated a positive association between practices for detecting prostate cancer and perceived susceptibility ($\beta = 0.086$, $p < 0.001$); attitude about screening, risk reduction, and participating in prostate cancer research ($\beta = 0.164$, $p < 0.001$); perceived behavioral control ($\beta = 0.318$, $p < 0.001$); acculturation ($\beta = 0.069$, $p = 0.006$); and knowledge ($\beta = 0.195$, $p = 0.024$). These data suggest that a typical Black man with higher scores on perceived susceptibility, attitude, perceived behavioral control, acculturation, and knowledge level has better prostate cancer detection practices than a Black man with lower scores. The results showed negative associations between prostate cancer risk reduction behavior and perceived severity ($b = -0.017$, $p = 0.013$) and acculturation

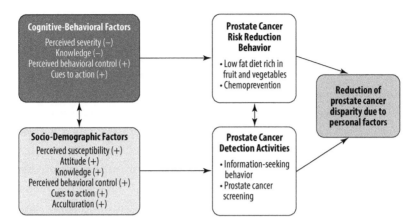

Figure 14.7. Confirmed PIPCaD model for Black men after test of hypotheses showing negative (−) and positive (+) relationships with dependent variables.

(b = −0.016, p = 0.048). This suggests that as scores on perceived severity and acculturation increase, the level of risk reduction behavior for Black men decreases. However, the level of risk reduction behavior of Black men increased when the level of perceived behavioral control (b = 0.034, p = 0.007) was higher.

The Prostate Cancer Care and Survivorship Model for Black Prostate Cancer Survivors

Currently, there is little published research on the prostate cancer care and survivorship (CaPCaS) experiences of Black men, especially the psychosocial effects and coping mechanisms Black men use. Some of the CaPCaS experiences that have been highlighted in the literature include shock when diagnosed with prostate cancer (Sinfield et al. 2009), perception of a "death sentence" (Maliski et al. 2010), receiving helpful information from physicians that helped with anxiety (Jones et al. 2010), receiving inadequate information to make informed decisions about treatment (Sinfield et al. 2008), and receiving limited treatment options that are usually tailored to the physician's expertise. Considering that patients going through the CaPCaS process will be experiencing different emotions and may not be prepared or have the knowledge to be fully involved in their treatment decisions, it is not surprising that some patients have regret about the decisions they made about treatment (Sinfield et al. 2009). The transition to prostate cancer survivorship can be mentally and physically trying, especially for those who lack emotional and financial support.

Odedina, Young, Pereira et al. (2017a, 2017b) developed the CaPCaS model to explain the experiences Black men go through during prostate cancer prevention, screening, diagnosis, treatment, and survivorship. The model is based on the principles of community-engaged research and used qualitative methodology. Odedina and interviewed Black prostate cancer survivors who were identified through the Florida Cancer Data System database. Black prostate cancer survivors, including US-born Black men, African-born Black men, and Caribbean-born Black men, were included in the study. Grounded theory methodology was employed to study the CaPCaS process among Black men, using audio and video recordings. The data analysis plan included preparing and verifying the narrative data, coding data, and developing an interpretive framework for Black men's experiences.

Constructivist grounded-theory methods (Charmaz 2014) were used to explore the experience of prostate cancer prevention, screening, diagnosis, treatment, survivorship, and advocacy from the perspective of Black men in depth, giving participants the opportunity to provide a rich narrative and to explore both the positive and negative aspects of their experience (see fig. 14.8). Forty-one participants (20 US-born Black men, 20 Caribbean-born Black men, and 1 African-born Black man) were recruited for the study. Data saturation was achieved with 17 US-born Black man and 14 Caribbean-born Black men, after which we ended data collection. Data saturation is the standard for deciding that we are not finding anything different from the interviews first coded and last coded. Only one African-born Black man agreed to participate in the interview phase. The majority of the participants were married US-born Black men aged 50 to 69 years who did not have a college degree. Over 80% of the participants did not have any support person with them at the point of prostate cancer diagnosis.

The contextual factors participants reflected on included the immigration patterns of Blacks, the African diaspora, the construct of Black men's masculinity, and sociodemographic factors such as age, marital status, educational status, employment, and income. Prostate cancer prevention and advocacy anchor each end of the process model, as these processes are in play but do not necessarily impact the experience of the disease directly.

Some of the unique themes that emerged for prostate cancer prevention were participants' perception of limited awareness about prostate cancer in

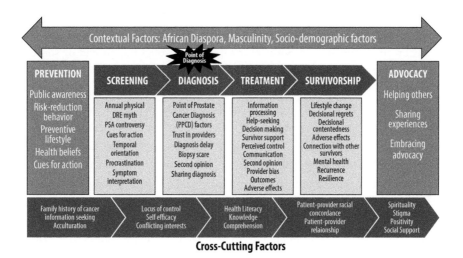

Figure 14.8. The prostate cancer care and survivorship (CaPCaS) model.

the Black community and the need for public awareness/education. Other themes were the need for behavior to reduce the risk of prostate cancer, a preventive lifestyle, health beliefs, and cues for action. Participant 1086 described the importance of lifestyle: *"It's very important for us to eat better and to leave a lot of that sodas, and drink more water, okay? It's very important for you to do that."* Participant 355 mentioned the importance of public awareness: *"Until recently, I don't think they are aware of it to be honest with you, but, um, recently more, um, of our daughters—sons and daughters—are more aware of it and it's more publicized now."* Participant P001 stated that *"Black men as a whole need to become, uh, more aware of things that affect them primarily other than, uh, other races, prostate cancer being one of them."* Some participants also felt that beliefs about health were important: *"I think we—we really have a negative view of it, and then, too, even though it's negative, it's not something that's really taken seriously. Uh, I think, uh, cancer is a serious thing, but I don't think we take prostate cancer serious. When—when—when—when the doctor says you have a elevated PSA count or somethin' like, and—and it's, like, 'Okay. So what?'"* (Participant 1881).

The factors that related to prostate cancer advocacy included helping others, sharing experiences, and embracing advocacy. A few of the men considered themselves to be prostate cancer advocates and expressed their willingness to share their prostate cancer journey with other Black men. Some discussed their prostate cancer diagnosis as a "calling to become a prostate cancer advocate" and have embraced advocacy, especially by sharing information about the disease. Some of the men also brought up providing social support for newly diagnosed Black men: "*I'm not ashamed of it. I'm ready to discuss it anytime, anywhere because if that way helped them—for that is another reason why I do this—if that way helped them, that's very good. So they don't have to go through what I went through*" (Participant 355).

Prostate cancer screening was discussed in terms of the digital rectal exam and PSA screening. The words and phrases that emerged as subthemes for the digital rectal exam were "unmanly," "rape," "overcoming the digital rectal exam myth," and "just something you have to do," while the words and phrases that emerged as subthemes for PSA screening were "limited access," "routine," and "not recommended." In general, participants emphasized the importance of screening for their prostate cancer journey.

> *In the beginning, I realized, you know, the screening portion, uh, it was scary. You know, all you hear is, when you hear the word prostate cancer you hear, uh, you didn't hear white guys dying. You were hearing the Black man disease, or the blacks dying at a higher rate because of stats saying they're not getting medical treatment, they're getting diagnosis late, or they're not adequate getting medical care. Those were the things I heard. Did I know anything about the disease? No. You just seen public service announcement: Black mens are dying from prostate cancer, you know, at a higher rate from their white counterparts.* (Participant 2039)

Participants also highlighted the role of physicians and wives in providing cues to take action to get screened. Additional themes were the importance of annual physicals to facilitate screening, procrastination that delays screening, interpretation of symptoms, and temporal orientation. On symptom interpretation, Participant 1086 stated, "*Also pay attention to, um, you-your-your go—your bathroom use, you know, how often you wakin' up at night. Does it feel like you completin' your urine, um, stuff like that? And, and if that PSA level is going up, then go get checked.*" Given that Blacks have been noted to exhibit present temporal orientation, the implication in terms of health is that prevention and screening activities are limited when there are no symptoms.

> *I basically ignored it for almost eight years. I basically just ignored it because my life was normal. Doctor told me that my prostate was enlarged, but that was not a prob-*

lem. I went on television and saw they had prostate pills so I ordered some of those thinking yeah take the pills and everything's gonna be fine. And everything was fine! I was not sick. Didn't feel any way ill. So my life was normal, there was nothing abnormal about my life except when I went to the restroom to urinate sometime and it was slow, but that was it I thought it was no big deal. So your PSA count is high? What does that really mean? It meant nothing to me because it was not affecting me in any way. (Participant 1881)

The men's discussion of their diagnosis centered on treatment decisions and outcomes. The need to be comfortable with the physician at the time of diagnosis, the need for emotional support, and the need for time to reflect on the diagnosis were key themes. The moment when they were diagnosed with prostate cancer was a crucial point for all the men who participated in the CaPCaS process (Odedina et al. 2017a, 2017b). We found that Black men who had been diagnosed had emotions and reactions that included shock, hope, fear, resilience, a need for immediate action, acceptance, leaning on religiosity/faith, and expressing the will to live. Additional factors identified at the moment of diagnosis were denial, cancer fatalism, disbelief, and thoughts about impact of disease on manhood. Faith and the will to live emerged as coping mechanisms during the diagnosis phase. Some of the comments by the men were:

I mean, um, it—put it in the hands of God, really, you know, and-and-and, um, let him lead you. (Participant 1086)

And I found it is good to take someone with you who's been through it, even if they sit there and don't say nothing. That's somebody who, when the doctor tell you, "You got cancer." . . . When they told me, I didn't hear him. I didn't hear him! My wife was in there when the man said cancer. Everything after that sentence I didn't hear. So my point is, you take someone who's going to hear what they say so they can repeat it to you when you get away and get your mind back and say "What did they say?" They can repeat it to you because you're gonna miss—I don't care who you are. Once that doctor says "it came back positive and we gotta do this," your mind goes everywhere except listening to what that cat say. And then when you finally listen, your mind is so screwed up on "am I gonna die? How bad is it? Are you gonna lose your friend?" (Participant 2039)

For the treatment phase, the importance of processing information, seeking help, shared-decision making with a physician, support, perceived control, good communication from health care providers, positive outcomes, and learning from the experience of other prostate cancer patients or survivors emerged from the interview data. In addition, provider bias and adverse effects were identified. Participant 1086 justified his choice of surgery as "*I just wanted it outta me. I wanted the cancer outta me*" and said that he was "*100 percent satisfied with my decision.*" Participant 355 spoke of the importance of having a physician he could trust: "*The advantage of having home boy or home girl as your doctor . . . is that you speak the same language. On [the] weekend, you can go to their house and ask free questions which you don't pay for.*"

Another theme that came across clearly was the need for second opinion. The decision-making process and outcomes were clear drivers of prostate cancer treatment:

> *You take anybody word that's in a white coat. Now, I don't take nobody word just from my experience—not to say that I know everything. I'm saying by my experience on misdiagnosis, different side effects—it's important when somebody tell me "now you got this," I want to know how is this going to affect me down the road. Am I going to be better or am I going to be worse? If I'm going to be worse, then why am I doing this? When I don't understand—what I want people to understand is, when you don't understand something, don't leave the office like I did. I left the office in the first couple of years—this is my fourth year—the first two years, I just do whatever Joe Blow or Mary Ann say, I thought it was God. Now, in these last two years, I'm not taking it anymore. I'm asking the questions because the quality of life is what you want to know. How is my quality of life going to be better with the decision they say you need?* (Participant 2039)

Participant P001 spoke about how helpful having a positive attitude was: "*I knew I had to have a positive attitude about this because it had been explain to me that the more positive I was, uh, the more successful our treatments would probably be, so I had to have a very positive attitude with what was going on with me.*" If there is one primary thing that is clear in the CaPCaS process, it is that there is no stupid question:

> *One of the things that I found out now is it ain't no stupid question. You ask and you ask and you ask till you get the answer. I found out they don't like it, but I make it clear to them I don't understand. Can you–I have a tendency to tell the doctor "Can you talk down to my level and say it in English?" And they'll laugh at it—you make a joke of because one we have a tendency—we don't want to upset the doctor, we don't want to*

offend the doctor, we don't want to get a second opinion. Here's the problem: it's your damn health. You can't worry about offending them. There's only two options: they say "I don't want to see you no more" or "I'm going to refer you to another doctor." At the end of the day, you must ask those questions. If you don't—I repeat it again—if you don't understand something they saying, you raise your hand. "Excuse me sir, I know you done said that." I say, "Help the old dog out. I don't understand. Can you bring it down a little?" They be like, "Mr. So-and-so, you crazy." I break it down to them. I understand—I want to know how this will affect me. When I talk to someone in the street, I tell them you don't want nobody to talk above you or act like they know everything. When I talk to my friends or church members, I tell them the same thing. When you go, I tell them what to ask, what I been through, don't be afraid to ask no question because it ain't no stupid question. The doctor may say, "I explained that two or three times." You getting offended? This is a decision that can have very bad, uh, very bad decision on you and your family if you don't make the right health decision. (Participant 2039)

Post-treatment survivorship generated a lot of discussion among the Black study participants. They talked about side effects and regrets about decisions. One of the key themes that emerged is the need for lifestyle changes. The men also discussed challenges they experienced during survivorship, including dealing with side effects of treatment (such as impotence), continuous monitoring (especially for recurrence), and dealing with depression. They expressed dissatisfaction when their physician gave them unrealistic expectations.

My physician told me, "Okay, 6 months to a year, you'll be back to normal." That's what he told me. "6 months to a year, you'll be back to normal." He kept preaching that, he didn't tell me anything different. He told me [emphasizes] 6 months to a year you'll be back to normal." So when I, when I went into surgery, I went into surgery with that in mind. "Hey doc, in 6 months to a year, you'll be back to normal, okay, and you won't have that problem." [It's] still ongoing. It's almost 5 years, and it's not back to normal. (Participant 1881)

As expected, the adverse outcomes arising from treatments presented some challenges for the men during survivorship:

The incontinence—yes, it does weigh on you because, again, we're men, and we don't wanna go around knowin' that we have to be wearin' Pamper and all of that. Now get this. When I came out, they—the doctor said that I had to be out of work for six weeks.

I had the bag on my leg and so forth or whatever, and after two weeks I went back to work with the Pamper. And the reason why is because, again, I ran a business and so forth, and I—I had to be there just to make sure that I had a business when I came back. (Participant 866)

Participants said that helpful information on prostate cancer survivorship and the ability to connect with other Black men who had undergone the same experience were helpful in the survivorship phase.

Also crucial to understanding the CaPCaS process are the crosscutting factors the participants identified, which are listed at the bottom of figure 14.8. These themes across the continuum of prostate cancer care include a family history of cancer, seeking information, acculturation, locus of control, self-efficacy, conflicting interests, health literacy, prostate cancer knowledge, comprehension of prostate cancer across the care continuum, access to care, racial concordance between patients and providers, the relationship of patients with their providers, spirituality, prostate cancer stigma, positivity, and social support. Participants reported that the communication style of their providers (paternalistic versus shared decision-making) impacted their relationships with them. Locus of control emerged multiple times as an issue; participants reported that they struggled with control over prostate cancer screening and prostate cancer risk reduction while going through the process. Also of primary concern was access to care, especially in terms of health insurance. Participant 1881 spoke about this issue: *"And I think—but I was guided—I think I was led that way by—by options that were not viable, that were not given to me with the—once again, it was the policy beginning to lapse, not bein' renewed, not knowin' whether or not I'm gonna be able to get insurance to—to follow through on that. And so there's an urgency situation here as well. "I gotta get up under this before that policy lapse and get this done."*

The CaPCaS model summarizes factors of significant importance to Black men across the prostate cancer care continuum. The lives of Black men who receive a diagnosis of prostate cancer change dramatically as they go through the CaPCaS process. The themes participants identified for each stage of the prostate cancer care continuum (prevention, screening, diagnosis, treatment, survivorship, and advocacy) and the themes that cut across stages provide critical information that providers can use to support Black men. For example, the experiences Black men reported at the time of diagnosis provide information that physicians can use to prepare for the consultation when they deliver a diagnosis and for developing a support system for Black men.

Conclusion

The body of literature on prostate cancer disparities shows a complex interplay of social, structural (health system), lifestyle, and biological factors are implicated in prostate cancer disparities among Black men in the South. To effectively address the prostate cancer disparities Black men experience, it is necessary to understand the social, biological, and behavioral factors related to prostate cancer across the cancer care continuum, including prevention, screening, detection, treatment, survivorship, and end of life. These are all components of the science of survivorship, which is important for Black men, given that about 30,000 Black men are diagnosed with prostate cancer each year in the United States. The moment of diagnosis is a crisis point for Black men and a critical point for intervention. The transition from the time of diagnosis to survivorship can be trying and is significantly affected by social determinants of health, biological, and personal factors. The uncertainties surrounding the diagnosis, management, and treatment of prostate cancer can cause psychological distress (Mehnert et al. 2010). Prostate cancer patients have noted significant unmet needs regarding social determinants of health and psychosocial and emotional support after diagnosis (Lintz et al. 2003; Perczek et al. 2002). Furthermore, the experience of uncertainty related to cancer diagnosis and treatment may be influenced by the cultural perspectives of patients and their families (Germino et al. 1998). Therefore, it is important to optimize the experience of receiving a prostate cancer diagnosis and the treatment and survivorship of Black men based on a comprehensive research framework that incorporates social, behavioral, and biological influences.

REFERENCES

Abbott, R., D. Taylor, and K. Barber. 1998. A Comparison of Prostate Knowledge of African-American and Caucasian Men: Changes from Prescreening Baseline to Post Intervention." *Cancer J Sci Am* 4 (3):175–177.

Abisoye-Ogunniyan, A., H. Lin, A. Ghebremedhin, A. B. Salam, B. Karanam, S. Theodore, J. Jones-Trich, M. Davis, W. Grizzle, et al. 2018. "Transcriptional Repressor Kaiso Promotes Epithelial to Mesenchymal Transition and Metastasis in Prostate Cancer through Direct Regulation of MiR–200c." *Cancer Lett* 431: 1–10. https://doi.org/10.1016/j.canlet.2018.04.044.

Agho, A. O., and M. A. Lewis. 2001. "Correlates of Actual and Perceived Knowledge of Prostate Cancer among African Americans." *Cancer Nursing* 24 (3):165–171.

American Cancer Society. 2015. *Global Cancer Facts & Figures*. 3rd ed. Atlanta, GA: American Cancer Society.

———. 2019. *Cancer Facts and Figures for African Americans, 2019–2021*. Atlanta: American Cancer Society. https://www.cancer.org/content/dam/cancer-org/research/cancer-facts -and-statistics/cancer-facts-and-figures-for-african-americans/cancer-facts-and-figures -for-african-americans-2019-2021.pdf.

———. 2021. "Cancer Facts & Figures 2021." Atlanta, GA: American Cancer Society. https:// www.cancer.org/research/cancer-facts-statistics/all-cancer-facts-figures/cancer-facts -figures-2021.html.

Apprey, V., S. Wang, W. Tang, R. A. Kittles, W. M. Southerland, M. Ittmann, and B. Kwabi-Addo. 2019. "Association of Genetic Ancestry with DNA Methylation Changes in Prostate Cancer Disparity." *Anticancer Res* 39 (11): 5861–5866. https://doi.org/10.21873/anti canres.13790.

Artiga Samantha, Latoya Hill, Kendal Orgera, and Anthony Damico. 2021. "Health Coverage by Race and Ethnicity, 2010–2019." Kaiser Family Foundation, July 16. https://www .kff.org/racial-equity-and-health-policy/issue-brief/health-coverage-by-race-and -ethnicity/.

Ashford, A. R., S. M. Albert, G. Hoke, L. F. Cushman, D. S. Miller, and M. Bassett. 2001. "Prostate Carcinoma Knowledge, Attitudes, and Screening Behavior among African-American Men in Central Harlem, New York City." *Cancer* 91 (1): 164–172.

Baguet, C. R., J. W. Horm, T. Gibbs, and P. Greenwald. 1991. "Socioeconomic Factors and Cancer Incidence among Blacks and Whites." *J Natl Cancer Inst* 83:551–557.

Bailey, E. J. 1987. "Sociocultural Factors and Health Care-Seeking Behavior among Black Americans." *J Natl Med Assoc* 79 (4): 389–392.

Barber, L., T. Gerke, S. C. Markt, S. F. Peisc, K. M. Wilson, T. Ahearn, E. Giovannucci, G. Parmigiani, and L. A. Mucci. 2018. Family History of Breast or Prostate Cancer and Prostate Cancer Risk. *Clin Cancer Res* 24 (23): 5910–5917. doi:10.1158/1078-0432.CCR-18-0370.

Barber, K. R., R. Shaw, M. Folts, D. K. Taylor, A. Ryan, M. Hughes, V. Scott, and R. R. Abbott. 1998. "Differences between African American and Caucasian Men Participating in a Community-Based Prostate Cancer Screening Program." *J Community Health* 23 (6): 441–451.

Blair, A., S. H. Zahm, N. E. Pearce, E. F. Heineman, and J. F. Fraumeni. 1992. "Clues to Cancer Etiology from Studies of Farmers." *Scandinavian Journal of Work, Environment & Health* 18 (4): 209–215. https://doi.org/10.5271/SJWEH.1578.

Boddy-Evans, A. 2019. "How Many Enslaved People Were Taken from Africa?" Thought.co. Last updated October 24, 2019. Accessed January 18, 2005. http://afrcanhistory.about .com/cs/slavery/a/slavenumbers.htm.

Brown, C. M., and R. Segal. 1996. "Ethnic Differences in Temporal Orientation and Its Implications for Hypertension Management." *J Health Soc Behav* 37: 350–361.

———. 1997. "The Development and Evaluation of the Hypertension Temporal Orientation (HTO) Scale." *Ethn Dis* 7: 41–54.

Carver, C. S., M. F. Scheier and J. K. Weintraub. 1989. "Assessing Coping Strategies: A Theoretically Based Approach." *J Pers Soc Psychol* 56: 267–283.

CDC (Centers for Disease Control and Prevention). 2019. "QuickStats: Age-Adjusted Death Rates from Prostate Cancer, by Race/Ethnicity—National Vital Statistics System, US 1999–2017." https://www.cdc.gov/mmwr/volumes/68/wr/mm6823a4.htm?s_cid=mm 6823a4_w.

Cerhan, J. R., A. S. Parker, S. D. Putnam, B. C. Chiu, C. F. Lynch, M. B. Cohen, J. C. Torner, and K. P. Cantor. 1999. "Family History and Prostate Cancer Risk in a Population-Based Cohort of Iowa Men." *Cancer Epidemiol Biomarkers Prev* 8 (1): 53–60.

Charmaz, K. 2014. *Constructing Grounded Theory*. Los Angeles: SAGE Publications.

Chen, Y., J. H. Page, R. Chen, and E. Giovannucci. 2008. "Family History of Prostate and Breast Cancer and the Risk of Prostate Cancer in the PSA Era." *Prostate* 68 (14): 1582–1591. doi: 10.1002/pros.20825.

Chornokur, G., K. Dalton, M. E. Borysova, and N. B. Kumar. 2011. "Disparities at Presentation, Diagnosis, Treatment, and Survival in African American Men, Affected by Prostate Cancer." *Prostate* 71 (9): 985–997.

Cobran, E. W., J. N. Hall, and W. D. Aiken. 2018. "African-American and Caribbean-Born Men's Perceptions of Prostate Cancer Fear and Facilitators for Screening Behavior: A Pilot Study." *J Cancer Educ* 33 (3): 640–648. doi: 10.1007/s13187-017-1167-x.

Coughlin, S. S. 2020. "A Review of Social Determinants of Prostate Cancer Risk, Stage, and Survival." *Prostate Int* 8 (2): 49–54.

Coughlin, S. S., M. Vernon, Z. Klaassen, M. S. Tingen, and J. E. Cortes. 2021. "Knowledge of Prostate Cancer among African American Men: A Systematic Review." *Prostate* 81 (3): 202–213. doi: 10.1002/pros.24097.

Curtin, P. D. 1969. *Atlantic Slave Trade: A Census*. Madison: University of Wisconsin Press.

Dagne, G., F. Odedina, N. Aime, and M. Young. 2017. "Area-Level Factors Associated with Spatial Variation of Prostate Cancer Incidence for Black Men." *International Journal of Cancer Therapy and Oncology* 5(1):5123.

DeSantis C. E., R. L. Siegel, A. G, Sauer, K. D. Miller, S. A, Fedewa, K. I. Alcaraz, and A. Jemal. 2016. "Cancer Statistics for African Americans, 2016: Progress and Opportunities in Reducing Racial Disparities." *CA Cancer J Clin* 66 (4): 290–308.

Devaney, J. M., S. Wang, P. Furbert-Harris, V. Apprey, M. Ittmann, B. D. Wang, J. Olender, N. H. Lee, and B. Kwabi-Addo. 2015. "Genome-Wide Differentially Methylated Genes in Prostate Cancer Tissues from African-American and Caucasian Men." *Epigenetics* 10 (4): 319–328. https://doi.org/10.1080/15592294.2015.1022019.

Devaraj, B., A. Lee, B. L. Cabrera, K. Miyai, L. Luo, S. Ramamoorthy, T. Keku, R. S. Sandler, K. L. McGuire, and J. M. Carethers. 2010. "Relationship of EMAST and Microsatellite Instability among Patients with Rectal Cancer." *J Gastrointest Surg* 14 (10): 1521–1528. https://doi.org/10.1007/s11605-010-1340-6.

Douglas, D. A., H. Zhong, J. Y. Ro, C. Oddoux, A. D. Berger, M. R. Pincus, J. M. Satagopan, W. L. Gerald, H. I. Scher, et al. 2006. "Novel Mutations of Epidermal Growth Factor Receptor in Localized Prostate Cancer." *Front Biosci* 11: 2518–2525. https://doi.org/10.2741/1986.

Echeverria-Estrada, Carlos, and Jeanne Batalova. 2019. "Sub-Saharan African Immigrants in the United States." Migration Policy Institute. November 6. https://www.migration policy.org/article/sub-saharan-african-immigrants-united-states-2018.

Eltis, David. 2001. "The Volume and Structure of the Transatlantic Slave Trade: A Reassessment." *William and Mary Quarterly* 58 (1): 17–46. https://doi.org/10.2307/2674417.

Farrell, J., D. Young, Y. Chen, J. Cullen, I. L. Rosner, J. Kagan, S. Srivastava, D. G. McLeod, I. A. Sesterhenn, et al. 2014. "Predominance of ERG-Negative High-Grade Prostate Cancers in African American Men." *Mol Clin Oncol* 2 (6): 982–986. https://doi.org/10 .3892/mco.2014.378.

Ferlay, J., M. Ervik, F. Lam, M. Colombet, L. Mery, M. Piñeros, A. Znaor, I. Soerjomataram, and F. Bray. 2020. "Cancer Today: Data Visualization Tools for Exploring the Global Cancer Burden in 2020." International Agency for Research on Cancer. Accessed May 21, 2021. https://gco.iarc.fr/today.

Fleming, Steven T., Kathleen McDavid, Kevin Pearce, and Dmitri Pavlov. 2006. "Comorbidities and the Risk of Late-Stage Prostate Cancer." *TheScientificWorldJOURNAL* 6: 2460– 2470. https://doi.org/10.1100/tsw.2006.383.

Fletcher, Sean A., Maya Marchese, Alexander P. Cole, Brandon A. Mahal, David F. Friedlander, Marieke Krimphove, Kerry L. Kilbridge, S. R. Lipsitz, P. L. Ngyuen, et al. 2020. "Geographic Distribution of Racial Differences in Prostate Cancer Mortality." *JAMA Network Open*. https://doi.org/10.1001/jamanetworkopen.2020.1839.

Forrester-Anderson, I. T. 2005. "Prostate Cancer Screening Perceptions, Knowledge, and Behaviors among African American Men: Focus Group Findings." *J Health Care Poor U* 16 (4 Suppl. A): 22–30.

Freedland, S. J., and W. B. Isaacs. 2005. "Explaining Racial Differences in Prostate Cancer in the United States: Sociology or Biology?" *The Prostate* 62: 243–252.

Gansler, T., R. Shah, Y. Wang, V. L. Stevens, B. Yang, C. C. Newton, S. M. Gapstur, and E. J. Jacobs. 2018. "Smoking and Prostate Cancer-Specific Mortality after Diagnosis in a Large Prospective Cohort." *Cancer Epidemiol Biomarkers Prev* 27(6): 665–672. doi: 10.1158 /1055-9965.EPI–17-0890.

Germino, B. B., M. H. Mishel, M. Belyea, L. Harris, A. Ware, and J. Mohler. 1998. "Uncertainty in Prostate Cancer: Ethnic and Family Patterns. *Cancer Pract* 6 (2): 107–113. https://doi.org/10.1046/j.1523-5394.1998.1998006107.x.

Giovannucci, E., E. B. Rimm, A. Ascherio, G. A. Colditz, D. Spiegelman, M. J. Stampfer, and W. C. Willett. 1999. "Smoking and Risk of Total and Fatal Prostate Cancer in United States Health Professionals." *Cancer Epidemiol Biomarkers Prev* 8 (4 Pt. 1): 277–282.

GLOBOCAN. 2018. Global Cancer Observatory. International Agency for Research on Cancer. Accessed May 21, 2021. https://gco.iarc.fr/.

Gohlke, J. H., S. M. Lloyd, S. Basu, V. Putluri, S. K. Vareed, U. Rasaily, D. W. B. Piyarathna, H. Fuentes, T. Rajendiran, et al. 2019. "Methionine-Homocysteine Pathway in African-American Prostate Cancer." *JNCI Cancer Spectr* 3 (2): pkz019. https://doi.org/10.1093 /jncics/pkz019.

Gongora, C., and N. Mechti. 1999. "[Interferon Signaling Pathways]." *Bull Cancer* 86 (11): 911–919. https://www.ncbi.nlm.nih.gov/pubmed/10586107.

Graham, R. J. 1981. "The Role of Perception of Time in Consumer Research." *J Consum Res* 7: 335–342.

Han, H., J. W. Cho, S. Lee, A. Yun, H. Kim, D. Bae, S. Yang, C. Y. Kim, M. Lee, et al. 2017. "TRRUST v2: An Expanded Reference Database of Human and Mouse Transcriptional Regulatory Interactions." *Nucleic Acids Res*. 46 (D1): D380–386. https://doi.org/10.1093/nar/gkx1013.

Hardiman, G., S. J. Savage, E. S. Hazard, R. C. Wilson, S. M. Courtney, M. T. Smith, B. W. Hollis, C. H. Halbert, and S. Gattoni-Celli. 2016. "Systems Analysis of the Prostate Transcriptome in African-American Men Compared with European-American Men." *Pharmacogenomics* 17 (10): 1129–1143. https://doi.org/10.2217/pgs-2016-0025.

Harrison, I., and D. Harrison. 1971. "The Black Family Experience and Health Behavior." In *Health and the Family: A Medical-Sociological Analysis*, ed. C. Crawford, 171–199. New York: Macmillan.

Heckler, Margaret. 1985. *Report of the Secretary's Task Force: Black and Minority Health*. Vol. 1, *Executive Summary*. Washington, DC: U.S. Department of Health and Human Services.

Hogle, J. 1982. "Ethnicity and Utilization of Health Services: An Urban Response to a Community Health Center." PhD diss., University of Connecticut.

Holman, E. A., and R. C. Silver. 1998. "Getting Stuck in the Past: Temporal Orientation and Coping with Trauma." *J Pers Soc Psychol* 74: 1146–1163.

Hughes, C., G. A. Fasaye, V. H. LaSalle, and C. Finch. 2003. "Sociocultural Influences on Participation in Genetic Risk Assessment and Testing among African American Women." *Patient Educ Couns* 51: 107–114.

Islami, F., S. A. Goding, K. D. Miller, R. L. Siegel, S. A. Fedewa, E. J. Jacobs, M. L. McCullough, A. V. Patel, J. Ma, I. Soerjomataram, W. D. Flanders, O. W. Brawley, S. M. Gapstur, and A. Jemal, 2018. "Proportion and Number of Cancer Cases and Deaths Attributable to Potentially Modifiable Risk Factors in the United States." *CA Cancer J Clin* 68 (1): 31–54. doi: 10.3322/caac.21440.

Islami F., D. M. Moreira, P. Boffetta, and S. Freedland. 2014. "A Systematic Review and Meta-Analysis of Tobacco Use and Prostate Cancer Mortality and Incidence in Prospective Cohort Studies." *J Eur Urol* 66 (6): 1054–1064. doi: 10.1016/j.eururo.2014.08.059.

Islami, F. A. G. Sauer, K. D. Miller, R. L. Siegel, S. A. Fedewa, E. J. Jacobs, M. L. McCullough, A. V. Patel, J. Ma, et al. 2018. "Proportion and Number of Cancer Cases and Deaths Attributable to Potentially Modifiable Risk Factors in the United States." *CA Cancer J Clin* 68 (1): 31–54. doi: 10.3322/caac.21440.

Jackson, A. P., and S. J. Sears. 1992. "Implications of an Afrocentric Worldview in Reducing Stress for African American Women. *J Couns Dev* 71:184–190.

Jerabek-Willemsen, M., C. J. Wienken, D. Braun, P. Baaske, and S. Duhr. 2011. "Molecular Interaction Studies Using Microscale Thermophoresis." *Assay Drug Dev Technol* 9 (4): 342–353. https://doi.org/10.1089/adt.2011.0380.

Jones, A. R., M. Shipp, C. J. Thompson, and M. K. Davis. 2005. "Prostate Cancer Knowledge and Beliefs among Black and White Older Men in Rural and Urban Counties." *J Cancer Educ* 20: 96–102.

Jones, J. M. 1988. "Cultural Differences in Temporal Perspectives: Instrumental and Expressive Behaviors in Time." In *The Social Psychology of Time*, ed. J. E. McGrath, 21–38. Newbury Park, CA: Sage Publications.

Jones, J., H. Wang, J. Zhou, S. Hardy, T. Turner, D. Austin, Q. He, A. Wells, W. E. Grizzle, and C. Yates. 2012. "Nuclear Kaiso Indicates Aggressive Prostate Cancers and Promotes Migration and Invasiveness of Prostate Cancer Cells." *Am J Pathol* 181 (5): 1836–1846. https://doi.org/10.1016/j.ajpath.2012.08.008.

Jones, R. A., J. Wenzel, I. Hinton, M. Cary M, N. R. Jones, S. Krumm, and J. G. Ford. 2011. "Exploring Cancer Support Needs for Older African-American Men with Prostate Cancer." *Support Care Cancer* 19 (9):1411–1419. doi: 10.1007/s00520-010-0967-x.

Joshu, C. E., A. M. Mondul, C. L. Meinhold, E. B. Humphreys, M. Han, P. C. Walsh, and E. A. Platz. 2011. "Cigarette Smoking and Prostate Cancer Recurrence after Prostatectomy." *J Natl Cancer Inst* 103 (10): 835–838. doi: 10.1093/jnci/djr124.

Kalish, L. A, W. S. McDougal, and J. B. McKinlay. 2000. "Family History and the Risk of Prostate Cancer." *Urology* 56 (5): 803–806. doi: 10.1016/s0090-4295(00)00780-9.

Katsoulidis, E., A. Sassano, B. Majchrzak-Kita, N. Carayol, P. Yoon, A. Jordan, B. J. Druker, E. N. Fish, and L. C. Platanias. 2008. "Suppression of Interferon (IFN)-Inducible Genes and IFN-Mediated Functional Responses in BCR-ABL-Expressing Cells." *J Biol Chem* 283 (16): 10793–10803. https://doi.org/10.1074/jbc.M706816200.

Kelly, S. P., P. S. Rosenberg, W. F. Anderson, G. Andreotti, N. Younes, S. D. Cleary, and M. B. Cook. 2017. "Trends in the Incidence of Fatal Prostate Cancer in the United States by Race." *Eur Urol* 71 (2): 195–201.

Kenfield, S. A., M. J. Stampfer, J. M. Chan, E. Giovannucci. 2011. "Smoking and Prostate Cancer Survival and Recurrence." *JAMA* 305 (24): 2548–2555. doi: 10.1001/jama.2011.879.

Kiely, M., and S. Ambs. 2021. "Immune Inflammation Pathways as Therapeutic Targets to Reduce Lethal Prostate Cancer in African American Men." *Cancers (Basel)* 13 (12): 2874. https://doi.org/10.3390/cancers13122874.

Kinlock, B. L., R. J. Thorpe Jr., D. L. Howard, J. V. Bowie, L. E. Ross, D. O. Fakunle, and T. A. LaVeist. 2016. "Racial Disparity in Time between First Diagnosis and Initial Treatment of Prostate Cancer." *Cancer Control* 23 (1): 47–51.

Klassen, Ann C., and Elizabeth A. Platz. 2006. "What Can Geography Tell Us about Prostate Cancer?" *Am J Prev Med* 30 (2 suppl.): 7–9. https://doi.org/10.1016/j.amepre.2005.09.004.

Klonoff, E. A., and H. Landrine. 2000. "Revising and Improving the African American Acculturation Scale." *J Black Psychol* 26 (2): 235–261.

Kwabi-Addo, B., S. Wang, W. Chung, J. Jelinek, S. R. Patierno, B. D. Wang, R. Andrawis, N. H. Lee, V. Apprey, et al. 2010. "Identification of Differentially Methylated Genes in Normal Prostate Tissues from African American and Caucasian Men." *Clin Cancer Res* 16 (14): 3539–3547. https://doi.org/10.1158/1078-0432.CCR-09-3342.

Lannin, D. R., H. F. Mathews, J. Mitchell, M. S. Swanson, F. H. Swanson, and M. S. Edwards. 1998. "Influence of Socioeconomic and Cultural Factors on Racial Differences in Late-Stage Presentation of Breast Cancer." *JAMA* 279: 1801–1807.

Legrier, M. E., I. Bieche, J. Gaston, A. Beurdeley, V. Yvonnet, O. Deas, A. Thuleau, S. Château-Joubert, J.-L. Servely, et al. 2016. "Activation of IFN/STAT1 Signalling Predicts Response to Chemotherapy in Oestrogen Receptor-Negative Breast Cancer." *Br J Cancer* 114 (2): 177–187. https://doi.org/10.1038/bjc.2015.398.

Leininger, M. 1970. *Nursing and Anthropology: Two Worlds to Blend*. New York: John Wiley & Sons.

Leininger, M. 1995. "Nursing Theories and Culture: Fit or Misfit? *J Transcult Nurs* 7 (1): 41–42.

Levy, D. E., and J. E. Darnell Jr. 2002. "Stats: Transcriptional Control and Biological Impact." *Nat Rev Mol Cell Biol* 3 (9): 651662. https://doi.org/10.1038/nrm909.

Lintz, K., C. Moynihan, S. Stegina, A. Norman, R. Eeles, R. Huddart, D. Dearnaley, and M. Watson. 2003. "Prostate Cancer Patients' Support and Psychological Care Needs: Survey from a Non-Surgical Oncology Clinic." *Psycho-Oncology* 12: 769–783. doi:10.1002/pon.702.

Magnus, M. 2004. "Prostate Cancer Knowledge among Multiethnic Black Men." *J Natl Med Assoc* 96: 650–656.

Mahal, B. A., W. Chen, V. Muralidhar, A. R. Mahal, T. K. Choueiri, K. E. Hoffman, J. C. Hu, C. J. Sweeney, J. B. Yu, et al. 2017. "Racial Disparities in Prostate Cancer Outcome among Prostate-Specific Antigen Screening Eligible Populations in the United States." *Ann Oncol* 28 (5): 1098–1104.

Maliski, S. L., S. E. Connor, L. Williams, and M. S. Litwin. 2010. "Faith among Low-Income, African American / Black Men Treated for Prostate Cancer." *Cancer Nurs* 33 (6): 470–478. doi: 10.1097/NCC.0b013e3181e1f7ff.

Marvel, Kathryn. 2006. "Difference in Prostate Cancer Rates between the United States and Spain: Effect of Vitamin D." Honors thesis, Oregon State University. https://ir.library.oregonstate.edu/concern/honors_college_theses/wd375z10w.

McWhorter, W. B., A. G. Schatzkin, J. W. Horm and C. C. Brown. 1989. "Contribution of Socioeconomic Status to Black/White Differences in Cancer Incidence." *Cancer* 63: 982–987.

Mehnert, A., C. Lehmann, M. Graefen, H. Huland, and U. Koch. 2010. "Depression, Anxiety, Post-Traumatic Stress Disorder and Health-Related Quality of Life and Its Association with Social Support in Ambulatory Prostate Cancer Patients." *Eur J Cancer Care* 19: 736–745. doi:10.1111/j.1365-2354.2009.01117.x.

Meyer, Tamra E., Ann L. Coker, and Maureen Sanderson. 2007. "A Case-Control Study of Farming and Prostate Cancer in African-American and Caucasian Men." *Texas Health Science Center Occup Environ Med* 64: 155–160. https://doi.org/10.1136/oem.2006.027383.

Miller, D. B., T. C. Hamler, and Q. Weidi. 2020. "Prostate Cancer Screening in Black Men: Screening Intention, Knowledge, Attitudes, and Reasons for Participation." *Soc Work Health Care* 59 (8): 543–556.

Moreira, D. M., W. J. Aronson, M. K. Terris, C. J. Kane, C. L. Amling, M. R. Cooperberg, P. Boffetta, and S. J. Freedland. 2014. "Cigarette smoking Is Associated with an Increased Risk of Biochemical Disease Recurrence, Metastasis, Castration-Resistant Prostate Cancer, and Mortality after Radical Prostatectomy: Results from the SEARCH Database." *Cancer* 120 (2): 197–204. doi: 10.1002/cncr.28423.

Moses, Kelvin A., Heather Orom, Alicia Brasel, Jacquelyne Gaddy, and Willie Underwood. 2017. "Racial/Ethnic Disparity in Treatment for Prostate Cancer: Does Cancer Severity Matter?" *Urology* 99 (January): 76–83. https://doi.org/10.1016/J.UROLOGY.2016.07.045.

Myers, L. J. 1998. *Understanding an Afrocentric World View: Introduction to an Optimal Psychology*. Dubuque, IA: Kendall-Hunt.

Nivens, A. S., J. Herman, S. P. Weinrich and M. C. Wenrich. 2001. "Cues to Participation in Prostate Cancer Screening: A Theory for Practice." *Oncol Nurs Forum* 28 (9): 1449–1456.

Nwaneri, A. C., L. McBeth, and T. D. Hinds Jr. 2016. "Prostate Cancer in African American Men: The Effect of Androgens and MicroRNAs on Epidermal Growth Factor Signaling." *Horm Cancer* 7 (5–6): 296–304. https://doi.org/10.1007/s12672-016-0271-4.

Odedina, F. T., T. O. Akinremi, F. Chinegwundoh, R. Roberts, D. Yu, R. R. Reams, M. L. Freedman, B. Rivers, B. L. Green, and N. Kumar. 2009. "Does the Prostate Cancer Disparities Seen in US Black Men Follow the Path of the Transatlantic Slave Trade?" *Infect Agent Cancer* 4: S1–S2.

Odedina, F. T., E. S. Campbell, M. LaRose-Pierre, J. Scrivens, and A. Hill. 2008. "Personal Factors Affecting African-American Men's Prostate Cancer Screening Behavior. *J Natl Med Assoc* 100 (6): 724–733. doi: 10.1016/s0027-9684(15)31350-x.

Odedina, F. T., G. Dagne, S. Pressey, O. Odedina, F. Emanuel, J. Scrivens, R. R. Reams, A. Adams, and M. Larose-Pierre. 2011. "Prostate Cancer Health and Cultural Beliefs of Black Men: The Florida Prostate Cancer Disparity Project." *Infect Agent Cancer* 6 (Suppl. 2): S10. doi: 10.1186/1750-9378-6-S2-S10.

Odedina, F. T., F. Ogunbiyi, F, Ukoli. 2006. "Prostate Cancer Burden in African Americans: Can the Origin Be Traced to Ancestral African Relatives?" *J Natl Med Assoc* 98 (4): 539–543.

Odedina, F. T., J. Scrivens, A. Emanuel, M. LaRose-Pierre, J. Brown, and R. Nash. 2004. "A Focus Group Study of Factors Influencing African-American Men's Prostate Cancer Screening Behavior." *J Natl Med Assoc* 96 (6): 780–788.

Odedina, F. T., J. Scrivens, M. LaRose-Pierre, A, Emanuel, A. A. Adams, G. A. Gagne, S. A. Pressey, and A. O. Odedina. 2011b. "Modifiable Prostate Cancer Risk Reduction and Early Detection Behaviors in Black Men." *Am J Health Behav* 35 (4): 470–484.

Odedina, F. T., J. Scrivens, H. Xiao, A. Massey, and K. Ferrell. 2000. African American Males' Views on Prostate Cancer Screening." *Minority Health Today* 1 (6): 28–34.

Odedina, F. T., M. E. Young, D. Pereira, C. Williams, J, Nguyen, and G. Dagne. 2017a. "Needs of Black Men at the Point of Prostate Cancer Diagnosis (PPCD): The Florida CaPCaS Study." *Int J Cancer Oncol* 4 (1): 1–4.

———. 2017b. "Point of Prostate Cancer Diagnosis (PPCD) Experiences of Black Men: The Florida CaPCaS Study." *J. Comm Support Oncol* 15 (1): 10–19.

Ogunsanya, M. E., C. M. Brown, F. T. Odedina, J. C. Barner, T. B. Adedipe, and B. Corbell. 2017. "Knowledge of Prostate Cancer and Screening among Young Multiethnic Black Men." *Am J Mens Health* 11 (4): 1008–1018. doi: 10.1177/1557988316689497.

Park, S., and M. A. Johnson. 2005. "Living in Low-Latitude Regions in the United States Does Not Prevent Poor Vitamin D Status." *Nutr Rev* 63 (6 Pt 1): 203–209. https://doi.org/10.1301/nr.2005.jun.203-209.

Perczek, R. E., M. A. Burke, C. S. Carver, A. Krongrad, M. K. Terris. 2002. Facing a prostate cancer diagnosis: Who is at risk for increased distress? *Cancer* 94:2923–2929. https://doi.org/10.1002/cncr.10564.

Pierre, C. C., S. M. Hercules, C. Yates, and J. M. Daniel. 2019. "Dancing from Bottoms Up—

Roles of the POZ-ZF Transcription Factor Kaiso in Cancer." *Biochim Biophys Acta Rev Cancer* 1871 (1): 64–74. https://doi.org/10.1016/j.bbcan.2018.10.005.

Powe, B. D. 1995a. "Cancer Fatalism among Elderly Caucasians and African Americans." *Oncol Nurs Forum* 22 (9): 1355–1359.

———. 1995b. "Fatalism among Elderly African Americans: Effects on Colorectal Cancer Screening." *Cancer Nurs* 18: 285–392.

Powe, B. D., and R. Finnie. 2003. "Cancer Fatalism: The State of the Science." *Cancer Nurs* 26: 454–467.

Powell, I. J., G. Dyson, S. R. Chinni, and A. Bollig-Fischer. 2014. "Considering Race and the Potential for ERG Expression as a Biomarker for Prostate Cancer." *Per Med* 11 (4): 409–412. https://doi.org/10.2217/pme.14.26.

Powell, I. J., F. D. Vigneau, C. H. Bock, J. Ruterbusch, and L. K. Heilbrun. 2014. "Reducing Prostate Cancer Racial Disparity: Evidence for Aggressive Early Prostate Cancer PSA Testing of African American Men." *Cancer Epidemiol Biomarkers Prev* 23 (8): 1505–1511.

Prueitt, R. L., T. A. Wallace, S. A. Glynn, M. Yi, W. Tang, J. Luo, T. H. Dorsey, K. A. Stagliano, J. W. Gillespie, et al. 2016. "An Immune-Inflammation Gene Expression Signature in Prostate Tumors of Smokers." *Cancer Res* 76 (5): 1055–1065. https://doi.org/10.1158 /0008-5472.CAN-14-3630.

Pruthi, R. S., C. Tornehl, K. Gaston, K. Lee, D. Moore, C. C. Carson, and E. M. Wallen. 2006. "Impact of Race, Age, Income, and Residence on Prostate Cancer Knowledge, Screening Behavior, and Health Maintenance in Siblings of Patients with Prostate Cancer." *Eur Urol* 50 (1): 64–69.

Reams, R. R., D. Agrawal, M. B. Davis, S. Yoder, F. T. Odedina, N. Kumar, J. M. Higgin-botham, T. Akinremi, S. Suther, et al. 2009. "Microarray Comparison of Prostate Tumor Gene Expression in African-American and Caucasian American Males: A Pilot Project Study." *Infect Agent Cancer* 4 (Suppl. 1): S3. https://doi.org/10.1186/1750-9378-4-S1-S3.

Richardson J. T., J. D. Webster, and N. J. Fields. 2004. "Uncovering Myths and Transforming Realities among Low-SES African-American Men: Implications for Reducing Prostate Cancer Disparities." *J Natl Med Assoc* 96 (10): 1295–1302.

Rieken, M., S. F. Shariat, L. A. Kluth, H. Fajkovic, M. Rink, P. I. Karakiewicz, C. Seitz, A. Briganti, M. Rouprêt, et al. 2015. "Association of Cigarette Smoking and Smoking Cessation with Biochemical Recurrence of Prostate Cancer in Patients Treated with Radical Prostatectomy." *Eur Urol* 68 (6): 949–956. doi: 10.1016/j.eururo.2015.05.038.

Rodríguez, C., E. E. Calle, L. M. Tatham, P. A. Wingo, H. L. Miracle-McMahill, M. J. Thun, and C. W. Heath Jr. 1998. "Family History of Breast Cancer as a Predictor for Fatal Prostate Cancer." *Epidemiology* 9 (5): 525–529.

Rosenberg, A., O. S. Nettey, P. Gogana, U. Sheikh, V. Macias, A. Kajdacsy-Balla, R. Sharifi, R. A. Kittles, and A. B. Murphy. 2019. "Physiologic Serum 1,25 Dihydroxyvitamin D Is Inversely Associated with Prostatic Ki67 Staining in a Diverse Sample of Radical Pros-tatectomy Patients." *Cancer Causes Control* 30 (2): 207–214. https://doi.org/10.1007 /s10552-019-1128-2.

Ross, L. E., R. J. Uhler, and K. N. Williams. 2005. "Awareness and Use of Prostate-Specific Antigen Test among African-American Men." *J Natl Med Assoc* 97 (7): 963–971.

Roy, Satyajeet, Shirisha Vallepu, Cristian Barrios, and Krystal Hunter. 2018. "Comparison of Comorbid Conditions between Cancer Survivors and Age-Matched Patients without Cancer." *Journal of Clinical Med Res* 10 (12): 911. https://doi.org/10.14740/JOCMR 3617W.

Rubicz, R., S. Zhao, M. Geybels, J. L. Wright, S. Kolb, B. Klotzle, M. Bibikova, D. Troyer, R. Lance, et al. 2019. "DNA Methylation Profiles in African American Prostate Cancer Patients in Relation to Disease Progression." *Genomics* 111 (1): 10–16. https://doi.org /10.1016/j.ygeno.2016.02.004.

Sajo, E. A., K. S. Okunade, G. Olorunfemi, K. A. Rabiu, and R. I. Anorlu. 2020. "Serum Vitamin D Deficiency and Risk of Epithelial Ovarian Cancer in Lagos, Nigeria." *Ecancermedicalscience* 14: 1078. https://doi.org/10.3332/ecancer.2020.1078.

Saltzman, A. F., S. Luo, J. F. Scherrer, K. D. Carson, R. L. Grubb 3rd, and M. A. Hudson. 2015. "Earlier Prostate-Specific Antigen Testing in African American Men—Clinical Support for the Recommendation." *Urol Oncol* 33 (7): 330.e9–17.

Satoh, J., and H. Tabunoki. 2013. "A Comprehensive Profile of ChIP-Seq-Based STAT1 Target Genes Suggests the Complexity of STAT1-Mediated Gene Regulatory Mechanisms." *Gene Regul Syst Bio* 7: 41–56. https://doi.org/10.4137/GRSB.S11433.

Shelton, P., S. Weinrich, and W. A. Reynolds Jr. 1999. "Barriers to Prostate Cancer Screening in African American Men." *J Natl Black Nurses Assoc* 10 (2): 14–28.

Shuch, B., M. Mikhail, J. Satagopan, P. Lee, H. Yee, C. Chang, C. Cordon-Cardo, S. S. Taneja, and I. Osman. 2004. "Racial Disparity of Epidermal Growth Factor Receptor Expression in Prostate Cancer." *J Clin Oncol* 22 (23): 4725–4729. https://doi.org/10.1200/JCO .2004.06.134.

Siegel, R. L., K. D. Miller and A. Jemal. 2017. "Cancer Statistics, 2017." *CA Cancer J Clin* 67 (1): 7–30.

Sinfield, P., R. Baker, S. Agarwal, and C. Tarrant. 2008. "Patient-Centred Care: What Are the Experiences of Prostate Cancer Patients and Their Partners?" *Patient Educ Couns* 73 (1): 91–26. doi: 10.1016/j.pec.2008.05.001.

Sinfield, P., R. Baker, J. Camosso-Stefinovic, A. M. Colman, C. Tarrant, J. K. Mellon, W. Steward, R. Kockelbergh, S. Agarwal. 2009. "Men's and Carers' Experiences of Care for Prostate Cancer: A Narrative Literature Review." *Health Expect* 12 (3): 301–312. doi: 10.1111 /j.1369-7625.2009.00546.x.

Singh, G. K., and A. Jemal. 2017. "Socioeconomic and Racial/Ethnic Disparities in Cancer Mortality, Incidence, and Survival in the United States, 1950–2014: Over Six Decades of Changing Patterns and Widening Inequalities." *J Environ Public Health* 2017: 2819372. doi: 10.1155/2017/2819372.

Smedley, B. D., A. Y. Stith, and A. R. Nelson, eds. 2003. *Unequal Treatment: Confronting Racial and Ethnic Disparities in Healthcare*. Washington, DC: National Academy Press.

Smith, Cheryl J., Tiffany H. Dorsey, Wei Tang, Symone V. Jordan, Christopher A. Loffredo, and Stefan Ambs. 2017. "Aspirin Use Reduces the Risk of Aggressive Prostate Cancer and Disease Recurrence in African-American Men." *Cancer Epidemiology, Biomarkers & Prevention* 26 (6): 845–853. https://doi.org/10.1158/1055-9965.EPI-16-1027.

Smith, G. E., M. J. DeHaven, J. P. Grundig, and G. R. Wilson. 1997. "African-American Males and Prostate Cancer: Assessing Knowledge Levels in the Community." *J Natl Med Assoc* 89: 387–391.

Smith, Z. L., S. E. Eggener, and A. B. Murphy. 2017. "African-American Prostate Cancer Disparities." *Curr Urol Rep* 18 (10): 81. doi: 10.1007/s11934-017-0724-5.

Steele, C. B., D. S. Miller, C. Maylahn, R. J. Uhler, and C. T. Baker. 2000. "Knowledge, Attitudes, and Screening among Older Men Regarding Prostate Cancer." *Am J Public Health* 90: 1595–1600.

Surveillance, Epidemiology, and End Results Program. 2021. "Cancer Stat Facts: Prostate Cancer." National Cancer Institute. https://seer.cancer.gov/statfacts/html/prost.html.

Tamir, Christine. 2021. "The Growing Diversity of Black America | Pew Research Center." Pew Research Center. March 25. https://www.pewresearch.org/social-trends/2021/03 /25/the-growing-diversity-of-black-america/.

———. 2022. Key Findings about Black Immigrants in the U.S. Pew Research Center, January 27. Accessed May 24, 2022. https://pewrsr.ch/3u1VIxT.

Tang, W., J. H. Fowke, L. M. Hurwitz, M. Steinwandel, W. J. Blot, and S. Ambs. 2021. "Aspirin Use and Prostate Cancer among African-American Men in the Southern Community Cohort Study." *Cancer Epidemiol Biomarkers Prev* 30 (3): 539–544. https://doi.org /10.1158/1055-9965.EPI-19-0792.

Taylor, B. S., N. Schultz, H. Hieronymus, A. Gopalan, Y. Xiao, B. S. Carver, V. K. Arora, P. Kaushik, E. Cerami, et al. 2010. "Integrative Genomic Profiling of Human Prostate Cancer." *Cancer Cell* 18 (1): 11–22. https://doi.org/10.1016/j.ccr.2010.05.026.

Theodore, S. C., M. Davis, F. Zhao, H. Wang, D. Chen, J. Rhim, W. Dean-Colomb, T. Turner, W. Ji, et al. 2014. "MicroRNA Profiling of Novel African American and Caucasian Prostate Cancer Cell Lines Reveals a Reciprocal Regulatory Relationship of MiR–152 and DNA Methyltranferase 1." *Oncotarget* 5 (11): 3512–3525. https://doi.org/10.18632/onco target.1953.

Underwood, W., S. De Monner, P. Ubel, A. Fagerlin, M. G. Sanda, and J. T. Wei. 2004. "Racial/Ethnic Disparities in the Treatment of Localized/Regional Prostate Cancer." *J Urology* 171 (4): 1504–1507. https://doi.org/10.1097/01.JU.0000118907.64125.E0.

United States Bureau of the Census. 1994. "Statistical Groupings of the States and Counties." In *Geographic Areas Reference Manual*, 6-1–6-25. Accessed August 8, 2021. https:// www2.census.gov/geo/pdfs/reference/GARM/Ch6GARM.pdf.

United States Cancer Statistics Working Group. 2021. "Leading Cancer Cases and Deaths, All Races and Ethnicities, Male and Female, 2018." Accessed August 7, 2021. https://gis .cdc.gov/Cancer/USCS/#/AtAGlance/.

Wallace, Tiffany A., Robyn L. Prueitt, Ming Yi, Tiffany M. Howe, John W. Gillespie, Harris G. Yfantis, Robert M. Stephens, Neil E. Caporaso, Christopher A. Loffredo, and et al. 2008. "Tumor Immunobiological Differences in Prostate Cancer between African-American and European-American Men." *Cancer Research* 68 (3): 927–936. https://doi .org/10.1158/0008-5472.CAN-07-2608.

Wang, H., W. Liu, S. Black, O. Turner, J. M. Daniel, W. Dean-Colomb, Q. P. He, M. Davis, and C. Yates. 2016. "Kaiso, a Transcriptional Repressor, Promotes Cell Migration and Invasion of Prostate Cancer Cells through Regulation of MiR–31 Expression." *Oncotarget* 7 (5): 5677–5689. https://doi.org/10.18632/oncotarget.6801.

Wang, S., D. Huo, S. Kupfer, D. Alleyne, T. O. Ogundiran, O. Ojengbede, W. Zheng, K. L. Nathanson, B. Nemesure, et al. 2018. "Genetic Variation in the Vitamin D Related Pathway and Breast Cancer Risk in Women of African Ancestry in the Root Consortium." *Int J Cancer* 142 (1): 36–43. https://doi.org/10.1002/ijc.31038.

Weinrich, S., D. Holdford, M. Boyd, D. Creanga, K. Cover, A. Johnson, M. Frank-Stromborg, and M. Weinrich 1998. "Prostate Cancer Education in African American Churches." *Public Health Nurs* 15 (3): 188–195. doi: 10.1111/j.1525-1446.1998.tb00338.x.

Welton, Michael, Sara W. Robb, Ye Shen, Paul Guillebeau, and John Vena. 2015. "Prostate Cancer Incidence and Agriculture Practices in Georgia, 2000–2010." *Int J Occup Env Heal* 21 (3): 251–257. https://doi.org/10.1179/2049396714y.0000000106.

Whittemore, A. S., A. H. Wu, L. N. Kolonel, E. M. John, R. P. Gallagher, G. R. Howe, D. W. West, C. Z. Teh, and T. Stamey. 1995. "Family History and Prostate Cancer Risk in Black, White, and Asian Men in the United States and Canada." *Am J Epidemiol* 141 (8): 732–740. doi: 10.1093/oxfordjournals.aje.a117495.

Williams, Vonetta L., Shivanshu Awasthi, Angelina K. Fink, Julio M. Pow-Sang, Jong Y. Park, Travis Gerke, and Kosj Yamoah. 2018. "African-American Men and Prostate Cancer-Specific Mortality: A Competing Risk Analysis of a Large Institutional Cohort, 1989–2015." *Cancer Medicine* 7 (5): 1–12. https://doi.org/10.1002/cam4.1451.

Woods, V. D., S. B. Montgomery, J. C. Belliard, J. Ramirez-Johnson, and C. M. Wilson. 2004. "Culture, Black Men, and Prostate Cancer: What Is Reality?" *Cancer Control* 11 (6): 388–396.

World Cancer Research Fund and American Institute for Cancer Research. 2018. *Diet, Nutrition, Physical Activity and Cancer: A Global Perspective*. Continuous Update Project Expert Report. Accessed July 28, 2021. https://www.wcrf.org/wp-content/uploads/2021/02/Summary-of-Third-Expert-Report-2018.pdf.

Yamoah, K., M. H. Johnson, V. Choeurng, F. A. Faisal, K. Yousefi, Z. Haddad, A. E. Ross, M. Alshalafa, R. Den, et al. 2015. "Novel Biomarker Signature that May Predict Aggressive Disease in African American Men with Prostate Cancer." *J Clin Oncol* 33 (25): 2789–2796. https://doi.org/10.1200/JCO.2014.59.8912.

Yates, C., M. D. Long, M. J. Campbell, and L. Sucheston-Campbell. 2017. "MiRNAs as Drivers of TMPRSS2-ERG Negative Prostate Tumors in African American Men." *Front Biosci (Landmark Ed)* 22: 212–229. https://doi.org/10.2741/4482.

Zane, N., and W. Mak. 2003. "Major Approaches to the Measurement of Acculturation among Ethnic Minority Populations: A Content Analysis and an Alternative Empirical Strategy." In *Acculturation: Advances in Theory, Measurement, and Applied Research*, ed. K. M. Chun, P. B. Organista, and G. Marin, 39–60. Washington, DC: American Psychological Association.

15

Colorectal Cancer

SIDDHARTHA ROY, DrPH, MPH,
STACY N. DAVIS, PhD, MPH,
JOHN S. LUQUE, PhD, MPH,
and CLEMENT K. GWEDE, PhD, MPH, RN, FAAN

It is well established that African Americans experience a higher colorectal cancer (CRC) burden than other racial/ethnic groups.[1,2] The health status of African Americans cannot be discussed without noting the impact of CRC on the African American population (especially those living in the southern United States). What can be done to reduce the burden of CRC on African Americans? Social determinants of health such as access to care, health literacy, education, poverty, neighborhood disadvantage, and social support influence the impact of CRC on African Americans. Many of these factors are prominent issues in the South. Interventions that take into account these and other social determinants of health are needed to reduce the burden of CRC on African Americans.

This chapter will begin by discussing the overall trends associated with CRC and the racial and geographic disparities that exist, including a comparison of CRC incidence and mortality rates for African Americans and whites over time and a comparison of CRC mortality rates for African Americans and whites in the South to those in other regions of the United States. Next, the chapter identifies the types of risk factors for CRC and their prevalence among African Americans in the South. The chapter then highlights the screening tests used to detect and prevent CRC. The chapter will also address individual and structural barriers to CRC screening that affect African Americans, lack of access to CRC screening and treatment in rural areas in the South, various community venues and strategies for implementing effective CRC screening interventions in these venues for African Americans in the South, additional recommendations to increase CRC screening among African Americans, and current CRC research or programs that address CRC.

Given the number of African Americans that are impacted by CRC, especially in the South, addressing the CRC burden within this population needs to be prioritized in order to impact disparities associated with CRC health outcomes. The purpose of this chapter is to provide an overview of the burden of CRC on African Americans highlighting the significant burden on African Americans living in the South and to provide recommendations for developing effective interventions that will reduce the burden of CRC among African Americans in the region.

The CRC Burden

CRC is the third most common cause of cancer death in both men and women in the United States and ranks second when men and women are combined.[1] It is estimated that there will be approximately 106,000 new cases in 2022. It was estimated that close to 53,000 deaths would be attributable to CRC in 2022. Despite this burden, over the past several decades, CRC incidence and mortality rates have steadily improved for individuals 50 years of age and older. CRC incidence has declined in the range of 2.0 to 3.5% annually, and CRC mortality has declined in the range of 1.0 to 2.6%.[1] These declines are thought to be primarily the result of improved screening and advancements in multimodal therapy.[1,3] Unfortunately, marked declines in CRC incidence and mortality have not been equally distributed across all population groups.[1,4] Racial and geographic disparities in CRC incidence, mortality, and survival still persist. There is a cluster of higher CRC incidence and mortality rates in the South (e.g., Alabama, Louisiana, Mississippi) for all Americans, and the higher populations of African Americans in these states contribute to the overall higher rates observed.[5]

National studies have demonstrated profound disparities in CRC incidence and mortality by geographic region and population characteristics.[6–8] A 2015 epidemiologic study that used advanced spatial mapping identified distinct spatial clusters of counties within the US South that had significantly elevated CRC mortality rates.[6] CRC incidence and mortality rates are lowest in the West and highest in Appalachia and in parts of the South (including the lower Mississippi Delta region, southeastern Virginia, and northeastern North Carolina) and Midwest.[1,6] From 2009 to 2011, CRC death rates in these hotspot regions were between 9 to 40% higher than regions outside the hotspots.[6] A cluster of 94 Delta counties has been designated as the nation's largest hotspot for CRC mortality. Many of these counties have also been found to be hotspots for early-onset CRC.[6,9]

The highest CRC mortality rates, including mortality hotspots, are concentrated in the southern United States. The profile of counties designated as CRC hotspots are vastly different from the rest of the country[10] in terms of widespread poverty,[11-13] rurality,[14] higher proportion of African Americans,[15] and shortage of health care professionals.[14,16] Individuals living in poverty, especially African Americans, often have worse CRC outcomes than those not living in poverty.[17] Poverty has been associated with a greater incidence of, mortality from, and late-stage diagnosis of CRC. Poverty is a major issue in the South; almost 84% of counties in poverty are located in the US South.[18] In addition, CRC incidence rates are consistently higher among rural populations (where poverty is greater) than among urban populations. While both rural and urban populations have both seen improvements in CRC incidence rates over time, the rates have improved more slowly among rural populations.[19] Further, a significant disparity in rural and urban settings persists for CRC incidence rates within the Northeast (43.2 vs. 41.8, respectively), the Midwest (44.6 vs. 41.9), and the South (45.5 vs. 39.7). The largest disparity is observed in the South.[19]

CRC Burden among African Americans

In the period 2012 through 2016, CRC incidence rates were 20% higher among African Americans than among non-Hispanic whites.[1] The percentage difference for CRC mortality rates is double that of the incidence rates.[1] Figures 15.1 and 15.2 illustrate the racial disparities associated with CRC incidence and mortality rates over time.[20] Both the overall CRC incidence and mortality rates have decreased among African Americans and non-Hispanic whites, and the disparity gap has decreased over time due to a renewed focus on improving CRC rates among African Americans.

The reasons for the disparities in CRC incidence and mortality are complex, but research has pointed to differences in stage of diagnosis, tumor biology, and socioeconomic status.[21-25] Compared to all racial/ethnic groups, African Americans are more likely to be diagnosed with distant-stage CRC.[1] Although African Americans are consistently diagnosed at a more advanced stage than non-Hispanic whites, adjusting for stage alone does not explain all disparities in their CRC burden.[3,21,23,25]

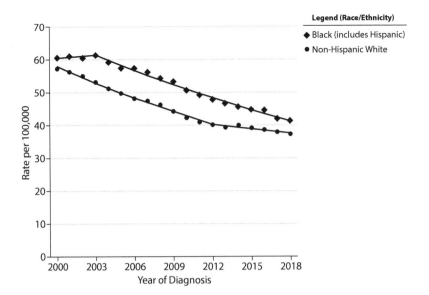

Figure 15.1. Trends in age-adjusted incidence rates of colon and rectal cancer incidence rates by race/ethnicity, 2000–2018. National Cancer Institute, Surveillance, Epidemiology, and End Results (SEER)*Explorer database, seer.cancer .gov.

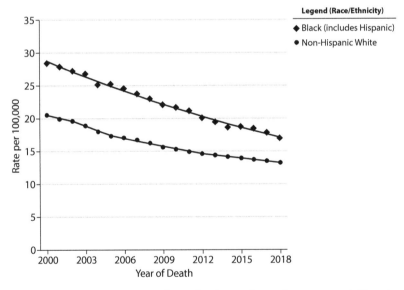

Figure 15.2. Trends in US age-adjusted colon and rectal cancer mortality rates, by race/ethnicity, both sexes, all ages, 2000–2018. National Cancer Institute, Surveillance, Epidemiology, and End Results (SEER)*Explorer database, seer .cancer.gov.

Table 15.1. CRC mortality per 100,000 for US whites and African Americans by state, 2018

	White	AA		White	AA
Total US	12.9	16.8	Missouri	14.6	18.2
Alabama	14.2	19.3	Montana	11.2	—
Alaska	13.1	—[1]	Nebraska	15.2	14.4
Arizona	12.5	15.5	Nevada	12.8	19.0
Arkansas	13.1	18.6	New Hampshire	12.6	—
California	12.3	16.6	New Jersey	12.9	17.2
Colorado	11.0	16.5	New Mexico	13.0	—
Connecticut	9.8	12.5	New York	11.7	13.5
Delaware	13.5	12.4	North Carolina	12.0	15.3
Washington, DC	4.9	17.8	North Dakota	12.6	—
Florida	12.5	15.4	Ohio	14.4	17.6
Georgia	13.4	16.3	Oklahoma	15.3	18.1
Hawaii	12.2	—	Oregon	12.6	16.0
Idaho	13.4	—	Pennsylvania	13.8	16.9
Illinois	13.7	19.6	Rhode Island	12.5	—
Indiana	13.8	20.4	South Carolina	12.3	16.1
Iowa	14.2	25.5	South Dakota	14.6	—
Kansas	14.3	16.5	Tennessee	13.7	20.4
Kentucky	16.3	19.7	Texas	13.4	18.6
Louisiana	14.0	19.3	Utah	9.7	—
Maine	12.8	—	Vermont	13.2	—
Maryland	12.7	17.5	Virginia	12.6	17.0
Massachusetts	11.5	9.0	Washington	11.8	10.4
Michigan	12.6	17.2	West Virginia	17.9	16.1
Minnesota	11.9	11.5	Wisconsin	12.1	18.9
Mississippi	16.4	20.3	Wyoming	13.1	—

Source: Surveillance, Epidemiology, and End Results (SEER) Program, "U.S. Mortality (by State)—AA Rates for White/Black/Other, 1969–2019," SEER*Stat Database, National Cancer Institute, DCCPS, Surveillance Research Program, Surveillance Systems Branch, released April 2022. https://canques.seer.cancer.gov/cgi-bin/cq_submit?dir=usmort2019&db=13&rpt=TAB&sel=1%5E0%5E%5E17%5E33%5E1,2%5E0%5E0&y=Race%5E1,2&x=State%5E0,1,2,3,4,5,6,7,8,9,10,11,12,13,14,15,16,17,18,19,20,21,22,23,24,25,26,27,28,29,30,31,32,33,34,35,36,37,38,39,40,41,42,43,44,45,46,47,48,49,50,51&dec=1,1,1&template=null. Underlying mortality data provided by NCHS (www.cdc.gov/nchs).
Note: AA = African American.
1. A dash indicates that a statistic was suppressed because a state had fewer than 10 cases.

CRC Mortality Rates for African Americans in the Southern United States

Table 15.1 illustrates how African American mortality rates from CRC compare to white mortality rates by state.[26] CRC mortality rates are often highest for African Americans living in southern states, and the gaps between rates for non-Hispanic whites and African Americans are greater in southern states with larger populations of African Americans.

CRC Risk Factors

Many factors contribute to the development and growth of CRC. These can be split into nonmodifiable and modifiable factors, both of which contribute greatly to the development of CRC. African Americans are greatly impacted by these risk factors, especially those living in the US South.

Nonmodifiable factors are associated with heredity and medical history, including a personal or family history of CRC.[27] As many as 30% of individuals who are diagnosed with CRC have a family history of CRC.[27] Individuals with a first-degree relative (parent, sibling, or child) who have been diagnosed with CRC have a 2 to 4 times greater risk of developing CRC than individuals without a family history of CRC. Genetic risk factors also contribute to the burden of early-onset CRC.[28] For the period 1995–2015, Kentucky reported the highest incidence of early-onset CRC: 14.3 per 100,000 for individuals aged 20 to 49.[28] A study of the National Cancer Database for the period 1998–2007 found that early-onset CRC was more prevalent in the southern states for adults above the age of 50.[29]

Modifiable risk factors for CRC include behavioral factors such as obesity, sedentary behavior, red meat consumption, alcohol consumption, and tobacco use, all of which are more prevalent in the US South.[27] Since more than half of all CRCs (55%) are attributable to these factors, they play a key role in addressing CRC in the South.[27] Many of these risk factors are very prevalent among African Americans. According to data from the Behavioral Risk Factor Surveillance System, the majority of states with obesity rates greater than or equal to 35% are located in the South.[30] In addition, 100% of the states in the US South have an obesity prevalence of 35 percent or higher among African Americans.[30] Obese men have a 50% higher risk of developing colon cancer and a 25% higher risk of rectal cancer than men of normal weight.[27] Obese women have a 10% increased risk of colon cancer.[27] Physical inactivity also contributes to obesity and is strongly associated with an increased risk of colon cancer. Studies show that physically active individuals have approximately a 25% lower risk of developing colon cancer than the least active individuals.[27] Consumption of red and processed meats, smoking, and alcohol consumption, factors that contribute to CRC, are also risk factors for obesity. The World Cancer Research Fund reported a 27% increase in risk of colorectal adenomas for every 50 grams/day of processed meat consumed.[27] Twelve percent of CRCs can also be attributed to smoking cigarettes; smokers have a 50% higher risk than people who have never smoked. Additionally, approximately 13% of CRCs in the United States can be attributed to alcohol consumption.[27]

CRC Screening Modalities

In order to reduce health disparities in CRC outcomes and reduce overall CRC incidence and mortality rates, screening for CRC is highly recommended. Various screening tests for CRC have been shown to be effective tools for detecting CRC early.[31-32] Some of these tests include home-based tests that may be easier for African Americans to complete due to their lower cost, convenience, and accessibility.[33] One popular home-based stool test is the fecal immunochemical test (FIT), which uses antibodies to detect hidden blood in the stool.[31-32] Individuals receive a test kit and use a brush to collect the stool sample. The sample can then be mailed to a lab for testing. This test is recommended once every year. The guaiac-based fecal occult blood test (gFOBT) is another home-based screening test and is similar to the FIT except it requires three different bowel samples instead of the one that FIT requires.[32] Cologuard[R] is another home-based test that is increasing in popularity. This screening test looks for abnormal DNA associated with CRC or polyps and is recommended every three years.[31-32] Two invasive screening tests that cannot be done at home are sigmoidoscopy and colonoscopy. During a sigmoidoscopy, a doctor places a short, thin, flexible, lighted tube into the rectum to check for polyps or cancer inside the rectum and the lower third of the colon. This test is recommended every five years. A colonoscopy, the most thorough test available, is considered the gold standard for CRC screening. It is similar to a sigmoidoscopy but uses a longer tube to probe the entire colon to search and remove polyps. It is recommended every ten years.[31-32] New CRC screening guidelines recommend that screening begin at age 45 for average-risk adults.[34] Individuals at increased risk—for example, due to family history of CRC—should start screening earlier after consultation with their health care provider.

Barriers to CRC Screening

African Americans have lower screening rates because of individual-level and society-level barriers. Individual barriers to CRC screening among African Americans include lack of knowledge about the various types of tests, low socioeconomic status, limited health literacy,[35] negative attitudes toward the test,[36] and behavioral characteristics such as low self-efficacy, low perceived susceptibility, cancer fatalism, and fear of positive results.[37] Individual risk factors associated with CRC mortality include nonadherence to CRC screening that meets guidelines, lack of access to timely treatment, poverty, obesity, and unhealthy diets.[38] Recent articles have explained how the COVID-19 pandemic has led to patients having less contact with primary care and delays in recommended cancer screenings, especially for the medically underserved.[39–41] When barriers to CRC screening are compounded by individual behavioral risk factors and systemic barriers, individuals are less likely to receive timely screening and diagnosis. Structural barriers for African Americans associated with lower rates of CRC screening include lack of health insurance, lack of transportation, lack of a primary health care provider, and lack of physician referral for CRC screening due to unconscious bias or other systemic problems in health care such as structural racism and medical mistrust.[42–43] People of low socioeconomic status are likely to encounter both individual and structural barriers to health care, thus diminishing the likelihood that they will have a regular health care provider and will have received a screening recommendation.[44]

Access to CRC Screening and Treatment

African Americans constitute the majority in many rural regions in the South, including Alabama, Mississippi, and Louisiana. Studies have reported that rural areas have less access to CRC screening and treatment such as colonoscopy and less access to adjuvant therapy and tumor resection, which in turn leads to a higher likelihood of late-stage detection.[45] While some studies have examined CRC disparities between African Americans and whites, after adjustment for race in these types of epidemiological studies, differences are better explained by differences in socioeconomic status and in receipt of surgical treatment in stage 1 and stage 4 disease.[46]

Recommendations for Increasing CRC Screening among African Americans

Community Outreach

Community outreach and community-based interventions to increase CRC screening are potentially effective methods for increasing screening among African Americans. Community outreach may include strategies such as health fairs or participation in other community events to feature opportunities for cancer screening.[47] For example, the use of community health workers or patient navigators to educate patients either in person or through technology increases screening participation.[48–50] A Texas study that compared outreach for colonoscopy and FIT to usual care in a large safety-net hospital reported 28% higher completion rates using outreach strategies than with usual care for completion of both screening modalities.[51] In one randomized controlled trial with older African American men recruited from barbershops in New York City, participants in the telephone-based patient navigation arm were more likely to receive CRC screening.[52] In another randomized controlled study in a community health center in Philadelphia with a large African American patient population, serial text messaging with an opt-out mailed FIT kit improved the kit return rate by 17% over the rate for patients with usual care.[53]

The implementation of a comprehensive CRC screening program in Delaware was successful in reducing CRC disparities by instituting a cancer treatment program for the uninsured with an emphasis on the African American population and with locally tailored programs that used nurse navigators and partnerships with community organizations.[54] The result of the Delaware program was an elimination of CRC screening disparities, a leveling off of incidence rates, a reduction in late-stage diagnoses, and a narrowing of mortality differences.[54] These types of cancer control programs could be instituted in other states in the South that have not expanded Medicaid coverage provided by the Affordable Care Act (ACA) if the political will existed to expand coverage for cancer treatment using other sources of state funding. For example, there have been statewide efforts in South Carolina to provide colonoscopy screening opportunities for uninsured patients using patient navigation in partnership with gastroenterologists and community-based health centers.[55] The South Carolina program reported favorable outcomes in terms of low no-show rates, positive colonoscopy quality metrics, capacity building evidenced by collaborations with clinics and gastroenterologists, and early detection success with colonoscopy screening.[55] The South Carolina program screened 1,391 individuals, one-third of whom lived in rural areas and 53% of whom were African American. The study findings did not identify disparities by race for the presence of adenomas or polyps, but it did report differences by sex; more males tested positive for cancer outcomes in adjusted models.

Church-Based Interventions

Churches and other faith-based organizations have frequently been used as both recruitment sites and as partners for the delivery of health promotion interventions in African American communities in the United States.[56-61] An analysis of Health Information National Trends Survey data from the National Cancer Institute reported a significant positive association between church attendance and both recent CRC screening and social support.[62] In one region of the US South, often referred to as the Bible Belt, African Americans are more likely to belong to a church than other racial/ethnic groups.[56] For community-based research, churches have certain advantages because of the characteristics of their members and the availability of meeting facilities.[63-64] First, church members may remain members of the same church over many years and have strong social networks in the church. Thus, researchers can leverage these networks to recruit additional participants for their studies. Second, the church pastor, a trusted leader, can spread the word about a research project through church bulletins or announcement times during a regular church service or through a health ministry group at the church. Third, research activities may occur after regular church member meeting times such as Sunday service or Wednesday prayer meetings. Finally, churches frequently have meeting rooms with kitchens or other facilities that are convenient meeting areas for research activities such as education classes or focus groups.[65]

Many different types of approaches for colorectal cancer education might be implemented in faith-based settings. A unique example in South Carolina was reported by Friedman and colleagues, who described how a community-developed play titled *Rise Up, Get Tested, and Live* was performed in a church for an African American audience.[66] The survey findings demonstrated that audience members increased their knowledge of CRC and their intentions to participate in CRC screening. In Alabama, the Healthy Congregations Healthy Communities program was a community-based research project focused on educating African American participants about diabetes and CRC.[67] The analysis of pre- and post-test scores for 35 participants demonstrated an increased knowledge of CRC, wellness, nutrition, and lifestyle. The researchers stressed that involvement of church pastors was a key to the success of the project.[67]

Broad-Based Strategies

Recognizing the increased risk for African Americans, some leading policy organizations have long recommended that routine screening begin at an earlier age for this racial/ethnic group, a distinction from the historical average risk screening age of 50 for the general population. This includes a recommendation by the American College of Gastroenterology that screening for African Americans begin at age 45.[68-69] Some policy groups have advocated colonoscopy as a primary screening modality for African Americans, considering the differences in early-onset CRC and location of tumors (e.g., a higher propensity for proximal lesions on the right side) for this group.[68-69] However, given the barriers and impediments to access to and completion of CRC screening among African Americans, it is important to implement broad-based strategies that increase access to and use of all available screening modalities. To effectively improve health equity, it is important to recognize that the best test for screening and early detection of CRC is the test that will get done. Thus, home stool tests and colonoscopy screening must be considered comparable options in comprehensive community-based and/or initiatives from health care systems to increase CRC screening among African Americans.

The Centers for Disease Control and Prevention's (CDC) Community Preventive Services Task Force publishes the Community Guide, which recommends multicomponent interventions to increase CRC screening.[70] Specifically, it suggests that multicomponent interventions lead to greater effects when they combine strategies for increasing community demand for and access to cancer screening, particularly in the context of a strong provider recommendation. Although the studies included in the Community Guide were not limited to the southern United States and did not focus primarily on African Americans, the recommended strategies are widely implemented nationally with diverse populations in both community and health care system settings. Such interventions can increase both initial and repeated screening among underserved populations such as African Americans, as reflected in the examples summarized above (e.g., community outreach or faith-based interventions). It is critically important in both community and health care system settings to provide links to care for all patients/participants—that is, to remove barriers to access and provide appropriate follow-up care and treatment when cancer is found. Culturally appropriate engagement strategies would help reduce and eliminate barriers access and engender trust among historically underserved African American populations.

Multicomponent interventions that combine two or more evidence-based intervention approaches[70] are grouped into three strategies: (1) increasing community demand (e.g., with client reminders, client incentives, small media, mass media, group education, and one-on-one education); (2) increasing community access (e.g., by reducing structural barriers and reducing client out-of-pocket costs); and (3) increasing provider education and delivery of screening services (e.g., provider assessment and feedback, provider incentives, and provider reminders). The National Cancer Institute's Evidence-Based Cancer Control Program[71] also lists effective CRC screening interventions aimed at reducing structural barriers that include reducing administrative barriers, assisting with appointment scheduling, setting up alternative screening sites, adding screening hours, addressing transportation barriers, providing language translation services, and offering child care. Similarly, evidence-based reports by the American Cancer Society and the National Colorectal Cancer Roundtable have identified similar effective strategies for health system- and community-based interventions involving diverse populations.[72-73]

One outreach/community-based intervention study called Increasing Access to Colorectal Cancer Testing in Florida recruited 330 average-risk African American men and women aged 50–75 years who were not up to date with CRC screening and were asymptomatic.[74] Participants were recruited in various community settings outside health care systems, including historically African American neighborhoods, cultural centers or programs, faith-based organizations, barbershops and beauty salons, and shopping outlets through historically black media (e.g., ethnic newspapers and radio programs).[74] Participants (52% male, 7% born outside the United States) were provided either education with a traditional CDC brochure on CRC screening or a culturally targeted photonovella booklet. Both groups received FIT tests at three time points (annually for three years). Individuals who had an abnormal FIT test result were linked or navigated to access follow-up colonoscopy and subsequent cancer care. Both study groups had high initial uptake (87% for the combined sample), demonstrating that education combined with access to screening test and follow-up care was an effective strategy in a community population. The type of educational information made little difference.

Findings from comparable studies implemented in health systems (e.g., federally qualified health centers) with diverse racial/ethnic samples that included sizable numbers of African Americans (~28%) corroborate the high uptake of CRC screening.[75-76] In the Florida study,[75] there was no differential effect of African American race, suggesting that these strategies work effectively when access to screening is actualized. On the other hand, a 2016 study by Rawl et al.[76] involving multiple sites in southern states reported that a one-time computer-tailored intervention improved CRC screening rates among low-income African American patients. A greater effect of the intervention was observed for stool-based testing, although the effect of intervention on colonoscopy screening was also strong. These findings support the general observation that clinic patients and the public need test options and that provision of stool test kits and ensured follow-up care after abnormal stool testing is important.[74-77] The American Gastroenterological Association white paper "Roadmap for the Future of Colorectal Cancer Screening in the United States" provides a critical appraisal of current efforts and offers several strategic modifications designed to improve CRC screening uptake and outcomes.[77] Many of these approaches are relevant to racial/ethnic minorities such as African Americans and populations experiencing geographic and socioeconomic disparities. These strategies include (but are not limited to) integration of stool testing options and other noninvasive testing instead of focusing solely on colonoscopy.[77]

Policy Implications

It is important to examine the impact of the ACA and Medicaid expansion on reducing CRC screening disparities among African Americans.[78] In many states, the ACA increased insurance coverage through health exchanges alone or with Medicaid expansion. Some southern states have not expanded Medicaid to date, including North Carolina, South Carolina, Tennessee, Mississippi, Alabama, Georgia, Florida, and Texas. Powell et al.[78] analyzed and reported on the CRC outcomes and economic costs using individual-based simulation models to estimate the impact of the ACA on three CRC outcomes (screening, stage-specific incidence, and deaths) and the economic costs among African American and white males in North Carolina aged 50–75 during the study period of 2013–2023.[78] This study found that health exchanges and Medicaid expansion improved simulated CRC outcomes overall, although the impact was more substantial among African American males. The findings also demonstrated that relative to health exchanges alone, Medicaid expansion would prevent 7.1 to 25.5 CRC cases among African American men and 4.1 to 16.4 per 100,000 cases among white men. The study authors concluded that policies that expand affordable quality health care coverage could have a demonstrable cost-saving impact while reducing cancer disparities.[78]

More analysis in other southern states that did not expand Medicaid is needed to assess the broader impact of the ACA on CRC outcomes in the South. It is also important to examine and compare the incidence of CRC among the thirty-seven states plus the District of Columbia that have expanded Medicaid eligibility with the incidence for those that did not expand Medicaid, especially in the South. There is growing evidence that expanded eligibility has a disproportionately positive impact on adult men because men have historically been less often eligible for Medicaid or other government subsidized coverage. As evidence of prospective studies accumulates, it is important to ascertain whether these gains will translate into demonstrable benefits for CRC screening and outcomes among African American males.

Current Research and Programs on CRC: What Is Being Done to Address CRC?

There is mounting evidence that nationwide implementation of targeted CRC screening initiatives, including in many southern states, is effective. Here we summarize three recent or ongoing initiatives that have recruited diverse samples including African Americans in different regions of the country. These initiatives have used evidence-based CRC screening interventions and components approved by the Community Guide and/or are included in National Cancer Institute's Evidence-Based Cancer Control Program.[70-71]

First, since 2004, the CDC has funded the Colorectal Cancer Screening Demonstration Program to address the burden of CRC and the low uptake of CRC screening tests among populations that traditionally have had limited access to health care services.[79] On the basis of the success of the Colorectal Cancer Screening Demonstration Program and lessons learned from both the demonstration program and the National Breast and Cervical Cancer Early Detection Program, the CDC launched a five-year Colorectal Cancer Control Program to provide CRC screening tests to low-income, uninsured, and underinsured populations and to promote the importance of screening with the ambitious goal of increasing screening rates to 80% in twenty-five states and with four tribal organizations.[80] The components of the Colorectal Cancer Control Program include (1) screening promotion, which involved activities to increase awareness and uptake of CRC screening among underserved pre-Medicare populations aged 50–64 (uninsured, underinsured, and those with an annual household income less than or equal to 250% of the federal poverty level); and (2) CRC screening tests for people with low incomes and no or limited health insurance using 2008 United States Preventive Services Task Force guidelines/modalities (FOBT, FIT, flexible sigmoidoscopy, or colonoscopy). Evidence-based strategies in the Colorectal Cancer Control Program included patient outreach and awareness, patient navigation, client and provider reminders, provider assessment and feedback, reduction of structural barriers, and small media education[81] as identified in the Community Guide[70] to increase population-level CRC screening.

Second, the CDC and the American Cancer Society launched collaborative national or multistate efforts to increase CRC screening including programs or campaigns.[82–83] The CDC's Screen for Life: National Colorectal Cancer Action Campaign is a national mass media and small media campaign that informs adults about the importance of getting screened for CRC.[84] In 2014, the National Colorectal Cancer Roundtable, an organization the CDC and the American Cancer Society founded to bring organizations together to coordinate efforts to address the burden of CRC, launched the 80% by 2018 campaign, which focused on interventions to increase CRC screening rates.[72] After 2018, the National Colorectal Cancer Roundtable focused its efforts on a new health equity targeted goal of achieving 80% CRC screening in every community.[73] Finally, the CDC's National Comprehensive Cancer Control Program supports the development and implementation of cancer control plans and partners with state, tribal, and territorial cancer coalitions to leverage resources to address cancer prevention and control, including efforts to increase use of CRC screening tests.[85] Results from the evaluation of the CDC's 2009–2015 multistate Colorectal Cancer Control Program, including its design, implementation, outcomes, and costs, were published in a collection of five articles in the journal *Preventing Chronic Disease* in 2019.[87–92]

Third, the National Cancer Institute's Center to Reduce Cancer Health Disparities (CRCHD) implemented a nationwide CRC outreach education and screening initiative titled Screen to Save with 42 sites across the country.[86] Its purpose was to promote awareness and knowledge of CRC in racial/ethnic and rural populations using evidence-based approaches through the robust infrastructure of the CRCHD's National Outreach Network, a national network of National Cancer Institute–designated community health educators aligned with cancer centers across the nation. A total of 3,183 pre and post surveys were obtained from a sample of male and female participants aged 50 to 74 years from diverse racial/ethnic backgrounds that included 27.4% African Americans. The study found increases in knowledge and behavioral intentions (e.g., to obtain CRC screening and increase physical activity) across all racial/ethnic groups. The study also provided links to CRC screening through the Connections to Care component of the initiative and reported that 82% of the participants who obtained CRC screening during the three-month follow-up period obtained their screening results.[86] These results suggest that a nationwide culturally tailored educational intervention using evidence-based components ("standardized" educational outreach, use of promotoras / community health workers, navigation, and linkage to care) is effective for increasing CRC awareness, knowledge, intentions, and screening behavior.

More expanded and intensified initiatives are needed in high-burden regions such as the southern United States and for African American communities experiencing disparate burdens of CRC incidence and mortality and underutilization of CRC screening modalities in order to reach or exceed the 80% goal in every community.[73] A critical element is the implementation of effective models of connections to care, beginning with community-based access to follow-up colonoscopies after abnormal FIT results and ready access to treatments and survivorship care locally. While these nationwide examples were not restricted to the southern United States or to people of African ancestry, they demonstrate the value of culturally and linguistically targeted efforts based in community and health systems for addressing health equity for people with CRC and increasing screening and early detection of CRC among underserved populations. African American communities in the southern United States could benefit from targeted and evidence-based strategies that address barriers to achieving health equity in CRC screening. As many states have expanded Medicaid and are engaged in ACA-funded programs, the positive impact on CRC-related outcomes might be further illuminated.

Conclusion

Despite marked declines in CRC incidence and mortality rates (including among African Americans) due to increased screening, racial and geographic disparities associated with CRC outcomes that impact African Americans living in the southern United States persist. A multitude of educational interventions and strategies are being used to increase CRC screening among African Americans. In order to be effective, these interventions need to address individual and structural barriers that contribute to lower rates of screening among African Americans. Culturally tailored, evidence-based, multicomponent interventions implemented in both community and clinic settings are necessary to address CRC screening barriers for African Americans and facilitate linkages to care. These interventions should use evidence-based strategies such as the use of community health workers or patient navigators to increase access to and utilization of all available screening modalities (including home stool tests and colonoscopy screening). African Americans in the South can benefit greatly from these interventions, especially those who have risk factors for CRC such as obesity. Screening strategies focused on developing interventions that target both those who have risk factors for CRC and those with average risk will help to reduce late-stage diagnoses and lead to improved cancer outcomes. The accumulation of evidence-based interventions addressing the CRC burden will significantly improve the overall health and quality of life of African Americans in the US South. Current and future policies (or their absence) will also play a significant role in impacting CRC disparities. Given the unpredictable and uncertain nature of political leadership and health policy priorities, it is imperative for researchers, community leaders, and clinics to work together with the goals of implementing evidence-based interventions that focus on increasing CRC screening, eliminating racial and geographic disparities associated with CRC outcomes, and achieving health equity.

REFERENCES

1. Siegel, Rebecca L., Kimberly D. Miller, Ann Goding Sauer, Stacey A. Fedewa, Lynn F. Butterly, Joseph C. Anderson, Andrea Cercek, Robert A. Smith, and Ahmedin Jemal. "Colorectal Cancer Statistics, 2020." *CA: A Cancer Journal for Clinicians* 70, no. 3 (2020): 145–164.

2. DeSantis, Carol E., Kimberly D. Miller, Ann Goding Sauer, Ahmedin Jemal, and Rebecca L. Siegel. "Cancer Statistics for African Americans, 2019." *CA: A Cancer Journal for Clinicians* 69, no. 3 (2019): 211–233.

3. Murphy, Caitlin C., Robert S. Sandler, Hanna K. Sanoff, Y. Claire Yang, Jennifer L. Lund, and John A. Baron. "Decrease in Incidence of Colorectal Cancer among Individuals 50 Years or Older after Recommendations for Population-Based Screening." *Clinical Gastroenterology and Hepatology* 15, no. 6 (2017): 903–909.

4. Jackson, Christian S., Matthew Oman, Aatish M. Patel, and Kenneth J. Vega. "Health Disparities in Colorectal Cancer among Racial and Ethnic Minorities in the United States." *Journal of Gastrointestinal Oncology* 7, Suppl. 1 (2016): S32–S43.

5. National Cancer Institute and Centers for Disease Control and Prevention. State Cancer Profiles. https://statecancerprofiles.cancer.gov/map/map.noimage.php.

6. Siegel, Rebecca L., Liora Sahar, Anthony Robbins, and Ahmedin Jemal. "Where Can Colorectal Cancer Screening Interventions Have the Most Impact?" *Cancer Epidemiology and Prevention Biomarkers* 24, no. 8 (2015): 1151–1156.

7. Perdue, David G., Donald Haverkamp, Carin Perkins, Christine Makosky Daley, and Ellen Provost. "Geographic Variation in Colorectal Cancer Incidence and Mortality, Age of Onset, and Stage at Diagnosis among American Indian and Alaska Native People, 1990–2009." *American Journal of Public Health* 104, no. S3 (2014): S404–S414.

8. Naishadham, Deepa, Iris Lansdorp-Vogelaar, Rebecca Siegel, Vilma Cokkinides, and Ahmedin Jemal. "State Disparities in Colorectal Cancer Mortality Patterns in the United States." *Cancer Epidemiology and Prevention Biomarkers* 20, no. 7 (2011): 1296–1302.

9. Rogers, Charles R., Justin X. Moore, Fares Qeadan, Lily Y. Gu, Matthew S. Huntington, and Andreana N. Holowatyj. "Examining Factors Underlying Geographic Disparities in Early-Onset Colorectal Cancer Survival among Men in the United States." *American Journal of Cancer Research* 10, no. 5 (2020): 1592–1607.

10. Gennuso, Keith P., Amanda Jovaag, Bridget B. Catlin, Matthew Rodock, and Hyojun Park. "Peer Reviewed: Assessment of Factors Contributing to Health Outcomes in the Eight States of the Mississippi Delta Region." *Preventing Chronic Disease* 13 (2016): E33.

11. Behringer, Bruce, and Gilbert H. Friedell. "Appalachia: Where Place Matters in Health." *Preventing Chronic Disease* 3, no. 4 (2006): A113.

12. Cosby, Arthur G., and Diana M. Bowser. "The Health of the Delta Region: A Story of Increasing Disparities." *Journal of Health and Human Services Administration* 31, no. 1 (2008): 58–71.

13. United States Census Bureau. "Small Area Income and Poverty Estimates (SAIPE): 2011 Highlights." December 1, 2012. Last revised October 8, 2021. https://www.census.gov/library/publications/2012/demo/SAIPE-highlights-2011.html.

14. Meilleur, Ashley, S. V. Subramanian, Jesse J. Plascak, James L. Fisher, Electra D. Paskett, and Elizabeth B. Lamont. "Rural Residence and Cancer Outcomes in the United States: Issues and Challenges." *Cancer Epidemiology and Prevention Biomarkers* 22, no. 10 (2013): 1657–1667.

15. Zahnd, Whitney E., Wiley D. Jenkins, and Georgia S. Mueller-Luckey. "Cancer Mortality in the Mississippi Delta Region: Descriptive Epidemiology and Needed Future Re-

search and Interventions." *Journal of Health Care for the Poor and Underserved* 28, no. 1 (2017): 315–328.

16. Foutz, Julia, Samantha Artiga, and Rachel Garfield. "The Role of Medicaid in Rural America." Kaiser Family Foundation, April 25, 2017. https://www.kff.org/medicaid/issue-brief/the-role-of-medicaid-in-rural-america/.

17. Mitka, Mike. "Poverty and Colon Cancer." *JAMA* 287, no. 20 (2002): 2645–2645.

18. Lavalley, Megan. "Out of the Loop: Rural Schools Are Largely Left out of Research and Policy Discussions, Exacerbating Poverty, Inequity, and Isolation." Center for Public Education, 2018.

19. Zahnd, Whitney E., Aimee S. James, Wiley D. Jenkins, Sonya R. Izadi, Amanda J. Fogleman, David E. Steward, Graham A. Colditz, and Laurent Brard. "Rural–Urban Differences in Cancer Incidence and Trends in the United States." *Cancer Epidemiology, Biomarkers & Prevention* 27, no. 11(2018): 1265–1274.

20. National Cancer Institute, NCI Surveillance, Epidemiology, and End Results Program. "All Cancer Sites Combined: Recent Trends in SEER Age-Adjusted Incidence Rates, 2000-2019, By Sex, Delay-Adjusted SEER Incidence Rate, All Races, All Ages." SEER*Explorer. https://seer.cancer.gov/explorer/application.html?site=1&data_type=1&graph_type=2&compareBy=sex&chk_sex_3=3&chk_sex_2=2&rate_type=2&race=1&age_range=1&hdn_stage=101&advopt_precision=1&advopt_show_ci=on&advopt_display=2.

21. Sineshaw, Helmneh M., Kimmie Ng, W. Dana Flanders, Otis W. Brawley, and Ahmedin Jemal. "Factors that Contribute to Differences in Survival of Black vs White Patients with Colorectal Cancer." *Gastroenterology* 154, no. 4 (2018): 906–915.

22. Lansdorp-Vogelaar, Iris, Karen M. Kuntz, Amy B. Knudsen, Marjolein Van Ballegooijen, Ann G. Zauber, and Ahmedin Jemal. "Contribution of Screening and Survival Differences to Racial Disparities in Colorectal Cancer Rates." *Cancer Epidemiology and Prevention Biomarkers* 21, no. 5 (2012): 728–736.

23. May, Folasade P., Beth A. Glenn, Catherine M. Crespi, Ninez Ponce, Brennan M. R. Spiegel, and Roshan Bastani. "Decreasing Black-White Disparities in Colorectal Cancer Incidence and Stage at Presentation in the United States." *Cancer Epidemiology and Prevention Biomarkers* 26, no. 5 (2017): 762–768.

24. Silber, Jeffrey H., Paul R. Rosenbaum, Richard N. Ross, Bijan A. Niknam, Justin M. Ludwig, Wei Wang, Amy S. Clark, Kevin R. Fox, and Min Wang. "Racial Disparities in Colon Cancer Survival: A Matched Cohort Study." *Annals of Internal Medicine* 161, no. 12 (2014): 845–854.

25. Lai, Yinzhi, Chun Wang, Jesse M. Civan, Juan P. Palazzo, Zhong Ye, Terry Hyslop, Jianqing Lin, Ronald E. Myers, Bingshan Li, et al. "Effects of Cancer Stage and Treatment Differences on Racial Disparities in Survival from Colon Cancer: A United States Population-Based Study." *Gastroenterology* 150, no. 5 (2016): 1135–1146.

26. Surveillance, Epidemiology, and End Results (SEER) Program, "U.S. Mortality (by State)—AA Rates for White/Black/Other, 1969–2019." SEER*Stat Database, National Cancer Institute, DCCPS, Surveillance Research Program, Surveillance Systems Branch. Released April 2022. https://canques.seer.cancer.gov/cgi-bin/cq_submit?dir=usmort2019&db=13&rpt=TAB&sel=1%5E0%5E%5E17%5E33%5E1,2%5E0%5E0&y=Race%5E1,2&x=State%5E

E0,1,2,3,4,5,6,7,8,9,10,11,12,13,14,15,16,17,18,19,20,21,22,23,24,25,26,27,28,29,30,31,32,33, 34,35,36,37,38,39,40,41,42,43,44,45,46,47,48,49,50,51&dec=1,1,1&template=null.

27. American Cancer Society. *Colorectal Cancer Facts & Figures 2020–2022*. Atlanta: American Cancer Society, 2020. https://www.cancer.org/content/dam/cancer-org/research/cancer -facts-and-statistics/colorectal-cancer-facts-and-figures/colorectal-cancer-facts-and-figures -2020-2022.pdf.

28. Muller, Charles, Ehizokha Ihionkhan, Elena M. Stoffel, and Sonia S. Kupfer. "Disparities in Early-Onset Colorectal Cancer." *Cells* 10, no. 5 (2021): 1018.

29. You, Y. Nancy, Yan Xing, Barry W. Feig, George J. Chang, and Janice N. Cormier. "Young-Onset Colorectal Cancer: Is It Time to Pay Attention?" *Archives of Internal Medicine* 172, no. 3 (2012): 287–289.

30. CDC. "Adult Obesity Prevalence Maps." Last reviewed September 27, 2021. https:// www.cdc.gov/obesity/data/prevalence-maps.html.

31. CDC. "Colorectal Cancer Screening Tests." Last reviewed February 17, 2022. https:// www.cdc.gov/cancer/colorectal/basic_info/screening/tests.htm.

32. American Cancer Society. "Colorectal Cancer Screening Tests." Last reviewed June 29, 2020. https://www.cancer.org/cancer/colon-rectal-cancer/detection-diagnosis-staging /screening-tests-used.html.

33. Roy, Siddhartha, Sabrina Dickey, Hsiao-Lan Wang, Alexandria Washington, Randy Polo, Clement K. Gwede, and John S. Luque. "Systematic Review of Interventions to Increase Stool Blood Colorectal Cancer Screening in African Americans." *Journal of Community Health* 46, no. 1 (2021): 232–244.

34. U.S. Preventive Services Task Force. "Screening for Colorectal Cancer: US Preventive Services Task Force Recommendation Statement." *JAMA* 325, no. 19 (2021): 1965–1977.

35. Davis, Stacy N., Jonathan W. Wischhusen, Steven K. Sutton, Shannon M. Christy, Enmanuel A. Chavarria, Megan E. Sutter, Siddhartha Roy, Cathy D. Meade, and Clement K. Gwede. "Demographic and Psychosocial Factors Associated with Limited Health Literacy in a Community-Based Sample of Older Black Americans." *Patient Education and Counseling* 103, no. 2 (2020): 385–391.

36. Smith, Selina A., Ernest Alema-Mensah, Wonsuk Yoo, Benjamin E. Ansa, and Daniel S. Blumenthal. "Persons Who Failed to Obtain Colorectal Cancer Screening Despite Participation in an Evidence-Based Intervention." *Journal of Community Health* 42, no. 1 (2017): 30–34.

37. May, Folasade P., Cynthia B. Whitman, Ksenia Varlyguina, Erica G. Bromley, and Brennan M. R. Spiegel. "Addressing Low Colorectal Cancer Screening in African Americans: Using Focus Groups to Inform the Development of Effective Interventions." *Journal of Cancer Education* 31, no. 3 (2016): 567–574.

38. Doubeni, Chyke A., Jacqueline M. Major, Adeyinka O. Laiyemo, Mario Schootman, Ann G. Zauber, Albert R. Hollenbeck, Rashmi Sinha, and Jeroan Allison. "Contribution of Behavioral Risk Factors and Obesity to Socioeconomic Differences in Colorectal Cancer Incidence." *Journal of the National Cancer Institute* 104, no. 18 (2012): 1353–1362.

39. Nodora, Jesse N., Samir Gupta, Nicole Howard, Kelly Motadel, Tobe Propst, Javier Rodriguez, James Schultz, Sharon Velasquez, Sheila F. Castañeda, et al. "The COVID-19

Pandemic: Identifying Adaptive Solutions for Colorectal Cancer Screening in Underserved Communities." *JNCI: Journal of the National Cancer Institute* 113, no. 8 (2021): 962–968.

40. Issaka, Rachel B., Lauren D. Feld, Jason Kao, Erin Hegarty, Brandon Snailer, Gorav Kalra, Yutaka Tomizawa, and Lisa Strate. "Real-World Data on the Impact of COVID-19 on Endoscopic Procedural Delays." *Clinical and Translational Gastroenterology* 12, no. 6 (2021): e00365.

41. Hooper, M. Webb, A. M. Nápoles and E. J. Pérez-Stable. "COVID-19 and Racial/ Ethnic Disparities." *JAMA* 323, no. 24 (2020): 2466–2467.

42. Davis, Terry C., Connie L. Arnold, Alfred W. Rademaker, Daci J. Platt, Julia Esparza, Dachao Liu, and Michael S. Wolf. "FOBT Completion in FQHCs: Impact of Physician Recommendation, FOBT Information, or Receipt of the FOBT Kit." *Journal of Rural Health* 28, no. 3 (2012): 306–311.

43. Adams, Leslie B., Jennifer Richmond, Giselle Corbie-Smith, and Wizdom Powell. "Medical Mistrust and Colorectal Cancer Screening among African Americans." *Journal of Community Health* 42, no. 5 (2017): 1044–1061.

44. Carethers, John M., and Chyke A. Doubeni. "Causes of Socioeconomic Disparities in Colorectal Cancer and Intervention Framework and Strategies." *Gastroenterology* 158, no. 2 (2020): 354–367.

45. Hines, Robert, Talar Markossian, Asal Johnson, Frank Dong, and Rana Bayakly. "Geographic Residency Status and Census Tract Socioeconomic Status as Determinants of Colorectal Cancer Outcomes." *American Journal of Public Health* 104, no. 3 (2014): e63–e71.

46. Le, Hoa, Argyrios Ziogas, Steven M. Lipkin, and Jason A. Zell. "Effects of Socioeconomic Status and Treatment Disparities in Colorectal Cancer Survival." *Cancer Epidemiology and Prevention Biomarkers* 17, no. 8 (2008): 1950–1962.

47. Boutsicaris, Andrew S., James L. Fisher, Darrell M. Gray, Toyin Adeyanju, Jacquelin S. Holland, and Electra D. Paskett. "Changes in Colorectal Cancer Knowledge and Screening Intention among Ohio African American and Appalachian Participants: The Screen to Save Initiative." *Cancer Causes & Control* (2021): 1–11.

48. Farr, Deeonna E., Venice E. Haynes, Cheryl A. Armstead, and Heather M. Brandt. "Stakeholder Perspectives on Colonoscopy Navigation and Colorectal Cancer Screening Inequities." *Journal of Cancer Education* 36, no. 4 (2021): 670–676.

49. Lasser, Karen E., Jennifer Murillo, Sandra Lisboa, A. Naomie Casimir, Lisa Valley-Shah, Karen M. Emmons, Robert H. Fletcher, and John Z. Ayanian. "Colorectal Cancer Screening among Ethnically Diverse, Low-Income Patients: A Randomized Controlled Trial." *Archives of Internal Medicine* 171, no. 10 (2011): 906–912.

50. Percac-Lima, Sanja, Richard W. Grant, Alexander R. Green, Jeffrey M. Ashburner, Gloria Gamba, Sarah Oo, James M. Richter, and Steven J. Atlas. "A Culturally Tailored Navigator Program for Colorectal Cancer Screening in a Community Health Center: A Randomized, Controlled Trial." *Journal of General Internal Medicine* 24, no. 2 (2009): 211–217.

51. Singal, Amit G., Samir Gupta, Celette Sugg Skinner, Chul Ahn, Noel O. Santini, Deepak Agrawal, Christian A. Mayorga, Caitlin Murphy, Jasmin A. Tiro, et al. "Effect of Colonoscopy Outreach vs Fecal Immunochemical Test Outreach on Colorectal Cancer Screening Completion: A Randomized Clinical Trial." *JAMA* 318, no. 9 (2017): 806–815.

52. Cole, Helen, Hayley S. Thompson, Marilyn White, Ruth Browne, Chau Trinh-Shevrin, Scott Braithwaite, Kevin Fiscella, Carla Boutin-Foster, and Joseph Ravenell. "Community-Based, Preclinical Patient Navigation for Colorectal Cancer Screening among Older Black Men Recruited from Barbershops: The MISTER B Trial." *American Journal of Public Health* 107, no. 9 (2017): 1433–1440.

53. Huf, Sarah W., David A. Asch, Kevin G. Volpp, Catherine Reitz, and Shivan J. Mehta. "Text Messaging and Opt-Out Mailed Outreach in Colorectal Cancer Screening: A Randomized Clinical Trial." *Journal of General Internal Medicine* 36, no. 7 (2021): 1–7.

54. Grubbs, Stephen S., Blase N. Polite, John Carney Jr., William Bowser, Jill Rogers, Nora Katurakes, Paula Hess, and Electra D. Paskett. "Eliminating Racial Disparities in Colorectal Cancer in the Real World: It Took a Village." *Journal of Clinical Oncology* 31, no. 16 (2013): 1928–1930.

55. Eberth, Jan M., Annie Thibault, Renay Caldwell, Michele J. Josey, Beidi Qiang, Edsel Peña, Delecia LaFrance, and Franklin G. Berger. "A Statewide Program Providing Colorectal Cancer Screening to the Uninsured of South Carolina." *Cancer* 124, no. 9 (2018): 1912–1920.

56. Campbell, Marci Kramish, Marlyn Allicock Hudson, Ken Resnicow, Natasha Blakeney, Amy Paxton, and Monica Baskin. "Church-Based Health Promotion Interventions: Evidence and Lessons Learned." *Annual Review of Public Health* 28 (2007): 213–234.

57. Berkley-Patton, Jannette, Carole Bowe Thompson, Alexandria G. Bauer, Marcie Berman, Andrea Bradley-Ewing, Kathy Goggin, Delwyn Catley, and Jenifer E. Allsworth. "A Multilevel Diabetes and CVD Risk Reduction Intervention in African American Churches: Project Faith Influencing Transformation (FIT) Feasibility and Outcomes." *Journal of Racial and Ethnic Health Disparities* 7, no. 6 (2020): 1160–1171.

58. Gross, Tyra Toston, Chandra R. Story, Idethia Shevon Harvey, Marie Allsopp, and Melicia Whitt-Glover. "'As a Community, We Need to Be More Health Conscious': Pastors' Perceptions on the Health Status of the Black Church and African-American Communities." *Journal of Racial and Ethnic Health Disparities* 5, no. 3 (2018): 570–579.

59. Leone, Lucia A., Marlyn Allicock, Michael P. Pignone, Joan F. Walsh, La-Shell Johnson, Janelle Armstrong-Brown, Carol C. Carr, Aisha Langford, Andy Ni, et al. "Cluster Randomized Trial of a Church-Based Peer Counselor and Tailored Newsletter Intervention to Promote Colorectal Cancer Screening and Physical Activity among Older African Americans." *Health Education & Behavior* 43, no. 5 (2016): 568–576.

60. Lumpkins, Crystal Y., Priya Vanchy, Tamara A. Baker, Christine Daley, Florence Ndikum-Moffer, and K. Allen Greiner. "Marketing a Healthy Mind, Body, and Soul: An Analysis of How African American Men View the Church as a Social Marketer and Health Promoter of Colorectal Cancer Risk and Prevention." *Health Education & Behavior* 43, no. 4 (2016): 452–460.

61. Ralston, Penny A., Jennifer L. Lemacks, Kandauda K. A. S. Wickrama, Iris Young-Clark, Catherine Coccia, Jasminka Z. Ilich, Cynthia M. Harris, Celeste B. Hart, Arrie M. Battle, and Catherine Walker O'Neal. "Reducing Cardiovascular Disease Risk in Mid-Life and Older African Americans: A Church-Based Longitudinal Intervention Project at Baseline." *Contemporary Clinical Trials* 38, no. 1 (2014): 69–81.

62. Leyva, Bryan, Anh B. Nguyen, Jennifer D. Allen, Stephen H. Taplin, and Richard P.

Moser. "Is Religiosity Associated with Cancer Screening? Results from a National Survey." *Journal of Religion and Health* 54, no. 3 (2015): 998–1013.

63. DeHaven, Mark J., Irby B. Hunter, Laura Wilder, James W. Walton, and Jarett Berry. "Health Programs in Faith-Based Organizations: Are They Effective?" *American Journal of Public Health* 94, no. 6 (2004): 1030–1036.

64. Lancaster, K. J., Lori Carter-Edwards, Stephanie Grilo, C. Shen, and A. M. Schoenthaler. "Obesity Interventions in African American Faith-Based Organizations: A Systematic Review." *Obesity Reviews* 15 (2014): 159–176.

65. Luque, John S., Matthew Vargas, Kristin Wallace, Olayemi O. Matthew, Rima Tawk, Askal A. Ali, Gebre-Egziabher Kiros, Cynthia M. Harris, and Clement K. Gwede. "Engaging the Community on Colorectal Cancer Screening Education: Focus Group Discussions among African Americans." *Journal of Cancer Education* 37, no. 2 (2022): 251–262.

66. Friedman, Daniela B., Swann Arp Adams, Heather M. Brandt, Sue P. Heiney, James R. Hébert, John R. Ureda, Jessica S. Seel, Courtney S. Schrock, Wilhelmenia Mathias, et al. "Rise Up, Get Tested, and Live: An Arts-Based Colorectal Cancer Educational Program in a Faith-Based Setting." *Journal of Cancer Education* 34, no. 3 (2019): 550–555.

67. Morales-Aleman, Mercedes M., Artisha Moore, and Isabel C. Scarinci. "Development of a Participatory Capacity-Building Program for Congregational Health Leaders in African American Churches in the US South." *Ethnicity & Disease* 28, no. 1 (2018): 11–18.

68. Williams, Renee, Pascale White, Jose Nieto, Dorice Vieira, Fritz Francois, and Frank Hamilton. "Colorectal Cancer in African Americans: An Update." *Clinical and Translational Gastroenterology* 7, no. 7 (2016): e185.

69. Waghray, Abhijeet, Alok Jain, and Nisheet Waghray. "Colorectal Cancer Screening in African Americans: Practice Patterns in the United States. Are We Doing Enough?" *Gastroenterology Report* 4, no. 2 (2016): 136–140.

70. CDC, The Community Guide. "Cancer." Accessed July 1, 2021. https://www.thecommunityguide.org/topic/cancer.

71. National Cancer Institute, Evidence-Based Cancer Control Programs (EBCCP). "Colorectal Cancer Screening Evidence-Based Programs Listing." Accessed July 1, 2021. https://ebccp.cancercontrol.cancer.gov/topicPrograms.do?topicId=102265&choice=default.

72. Wender, Richard C., Mary Doroshenk, Durado Brooks, James Hotz, and Robert A. Smith. "Creating and Implementing a National Public Health Campaign: The American Cancer Society's and National Colorectal Cancer Roundtable's 80% by 2018 Initiative." *American Journal of Gastroenterology* 113, no. 12 (2018): 1739–1741.

73. National Colorectal Cancer Roundtable. "80% In Every Community." Accessed July 1, 2021. https://nccrt.org/80-in-every-community/.

74. Christy, Shannon M., Stacy N. Davis, Kimberly R. Williams, Xiuhua Zhao, Swapomthi K. Govindaraju, Gwendolyn P. Quinn, Susan T. Vadaparampil, Hui-Li Lin, Steven K. Sutton, et al. "A Community-Based Trial of Educational Interventions with Fecal Immunochemical Tests for Colorectal Cancer Screening Uptake among Blacks in Community Settings." *Cancer* 122, no. 21 (2016): 3288–3296.

75. Davis, Stacy N., Shannon M. Christy, Enmanuel A. Chavarria, Rania Abdulla, Steven K. Sutton, Alyssa R. Schmidt, Susan T. Vadaparampil, Gwendolyn P. Quinn, Vani M. Simmons, et al. "A Randomized Controlled Trial of a Multicomponent, Targeted, Low-

Literacy Educational Intervention Compared with a Nontargeted Intervention to Boost Colorectal Cancer Screening with Fecal Immunochemical Testing in Community Clinics." *Cancer* 123, no. 8 (2017): 1390–1400.

76. Rawl, Susan M., Shannon M. Christy, Susan M. Perkins, Yan Tong, Connie Krier, Hsiao-Lan Wang, Amelia M. Huang, Esther Laury, Broderick Rhyant, et al. "Computer-Tailored Intervention Increases Colorectal Cancer Screening among Low-Income African Americans in Primary Care: Results of a Randomized Trial." *Preventive Medicine* 145 (2021): 106449.

77. Melson, Joshua E., Thomas F. Imperiale, Steven H. Itzkowitz, Xavier Llor, Michael L. Kochman, William M. Grady, Robert E. Schoen, Carol A. Burke, Aasma Shaukat, et al. "AGA White Paper: Roadmap for the Future of Colorectal Cancer Screening in the United States." *Clinical Gastroenterology and Hepatology* 18, no. 12 (2020): 2667–2678.

78. Powell, Wizdom, Leah Frerichs, Rachel Townsley, Maria Mayorga, Jennifer Richmond, Giselle Corbie-Smith, Stephanie Wheeler, and Kristen Hassmiller Lich. "The Potential Impact of the Affordable Care Act and Medicaid Expansion on Reducing Colorectal Cancer Screening Disparities in African American Males." *PLOS One* 15, no. 1 (2020): e0226942.

79. Seeff, Laura C., and Elizabeth A. Rohan. "Lessons Learned from the CDC's Colorectal Cancer Screening Demonstration Program." *Cancer* 119 (2013): 2817–2819.

80. CDC, Colorectal Cancer Control Program. "About the Program." Last reviewed February 15, 2022. Accessed July 1, 2021. https://www.cdc.gov/cancer/crccp/about.htm.

81. Joseph, Djenaba A., Amy S. DeGroff, Nikki S. Hayes, Faye L. Wong, and Marcus Plescia. "The Colorectal Cancer Control Program: Partnering to Increase Population Level Screening." *Gastrointestinal Endoscopy* 73, no. 3 (2011): 429–434.

82. Verma, Manisha, Mona Sarfaty, Durado Brooks, and Richard C. Wender. "Population-Based Programs for Increasing Colorectal Cancer Screening in the United States." *CA: A Cancer Journal for Clinicians* 65, no. 6 (2015): 496–510.

83. Riehman, Kara S., Robert L. Stephens, Joenell Henry-Tanner, and Durado Brooks. "Evaluation of Colorectal Cancer Screening in Federally Qualified Health Centers." *American Journal of Preventive Medicine* 54, no. 2 (2018): 190–196.

84. CDC. "Screen for Life: National Colorectal Cancer Action Campaign." Last reviewed February 3, 2022. Accessed July 1, 2021. https://www.cdc.gov/cancer/colorectal/sfl/index .htm.

85. Pyron, Trina, Jamila Fonseka, Monique Young, LaTisha Zimmerman, Angela R. Moore, and Nikki Hayes. "Examining Comprehensive Cancer Control Partnerships, Plans, and Program Interventions: Successes and Lessons Learned from a Utilization-Focused Evaluation." *Cancer Causes & Control* 29, no. 12 (2018): 1163–1171.

86. Whitaker, Damiya E., Frederick R. Snyder, Sandra L. San Miguel-Majors, LeeAnn O. Bailey, and Sanya A. Springfield. "Screen to Save: Results from NCI's Colorectal Cancer Outreach and Screening Initiative to Promote Awareness and Knowledge of Colorectal Cancer in Racial/Ethnic and Rural Populations." *Cancer Epidemiology and Prevention Biomarkers* 29, no. 5 (2020): 910–917.

87. Joseph, D. A., and A. DeGroff. "The Colorectal Cancer Control Program, 2009–2015." *Preventing Chronic Disease* 16 (2019): 190336.

88. Nadel, M. R., J. Royalty, D. Joseph, T. Rockwell, W. Helsel, W. Kammerer, et al.

"Variations in Screening Quality in a Federal Colorectal Cancer Screening Program for the Uninsured." *Preventing Chronic Disease* 16 (2019): 180452.

89. Hannon, P. A., A. E. Maxwell, C. Escoffery, T. Vu, M. J. Kohn, L. Gressard, et al. "Adoption and Implementation of Evidence-Based Colorectal Cancer Screening Interventions Among Cancer Control Program Grantees, 2009–2015." *Preventing Chronic Disease* 16 (2019): 180682.

90. Hoover, S., S. Subramanian, and F. Tangka. "Developing a Web-Based Cost Assessment Tool for Colorectal Cancer Screening Programs." *Preventing Chronic Disease* 16 (2019): 180336.

91. Subramanian, S., F. K. Tangka, S. Hoover, M. Cole-Beebe, D. Joseph, and A. DeGroff. "Comparison of Program Resources Required for Colonoscopy and Fecal Screening: Findings from 5 Years of the Colorectal Cancer Control Program." *Preventing Chronic Disease* 16 (2019): 180338.

92. Tangka, F. K., S. Subramanian, S. Hoover, M. Cole-Beebe, A. DeGroff, D. Joseph, et al. "Expenditures on Screening Promotion Activities in CDC's Colorectal Cancer Control Program, 2009–2014." *Preventing Chronic Disease* 16 (2019): 180337.

16

Lung Cancer

STEVEN S. COUGHLIN, PhD, MPH

Lung cancer is the leading cause of cancer-related death among both men and women in the United States and many other countries.[1] In 2021, there were an estimated 235,760 cases of lung cancer in the United States and 131,880 deaths from the disease.[2] Non-small-cell lung cancer (NSCLC) accounts for about 85% of lung cancer cases in the United States. Race and socioeconomic status are well known to influence lung cancer incidence and mortality patterns in the United States.[3,4] Stage is one of the most important predictors of survival. Blacks are less likely than whites to be diagnosed with localized disease.[5] Although survival from lung cancer has improved since the early 1990s, racial differences in lung cancer survival persist such that Blacks experience poorer five-year survival rates for lung cancer than whites do.[5] Populations living in the southern United States experience the highest mortality for lung cancer, especially among men.[5]

In the period 1975–2016, lung cancer incidence rates in the United States were higher among Blacks than whites.[6] Black males have the highest rates of age-adjusted lung cancer incidence among all racial/ethnic groups in the United States (73.5 per 100,000 vs. 63.5 per 100,000 for white males).[6] Compared with other racial/ethnic groups, Black males also have the highest lung cancer mortality.[6]

The challenges economically disadvantaged African Americans experience while receiving lung cancer services include diagnostic and treatment facilities that are located outside the patient's neighborhood, lack of transportation, the patient's lack of understanding of lung cancer, unavailability of support resources for them to access lung cancer treatment services, lack of access to primary care, and lack of familiarity with resources available from cancer support organizations.[1] Factors that likely contribute to the relatively high lung cancer death rates for African Americans include the roles played by low health literacy, lack of knowledge about lung cancer, attitudes, beliefs, cultural factors, and lack of access to health services. Other barriers to receiving lung cancer services include fear and mistrust, uncertainty, lack of information, lack of a primary care provider, and unfamiliarity with providers. These challenges are made worse by the disjointed, fragmented nature of service provision and the lack of a coordinated effort to address lung cancer treatment challenges in many communities.

This chapter discusses disparities in lung cancer incidence, mortality, and survivorship among African Americans. First, advances in the early detection and treatment of lung cancer are discussed. Then, Black-white disparities in lung cancer treatment are discussed, including factors that may contribute to such disparities. This is followed by a discussion of smoking cessation interventions for patients with or without a lung cancer diagnosis; the important roles cultural competency, patient trust in their physician, and health literacy play in addressing lung cancer disparities; and remaining challenges in this area.

Advances in the Early Detection and Treatment of Lung Cancer

The prognosis for NSCLC is poor. Five-year survival rates range from 49% for patients with stage 1A disease to about 1% for those with stage 4.[7] Receipt of timely, stage-appropriate care for patients with NSCLC can increase the length of survival.[7,8] Once a patient has been staged, timely receipt of surgical resection has an important impact on survival outcomes among those with early-stage NSCLC. Surgical resection remains the primary and preferred approach to the treatment of stages 1 and 2 NSCLC.[9,10] The use of adjuvant chemotherapy for stage 2 NSCLC is recommended and has shown benefit. Every patient should have systematic mediastinal lymph node sampling at the time of curative-intent surgical resection. Perioperative morbidity and mortality are reduced and long-term survival is improved when surgical resection is performed by a board-certified thoracic surgeon.[9] In the United States, about 30% of pulmonary resections are performed by general surgeons. Recommended treatment for patients with late-stage disease ranges from chemotherapy and radiation with or without surgery (stage 3A) to chemotherapy and radiation without surgery or chemotherapy alone (stage 3B) to chemotherapy alone for patients with metastatic disease (stage 4).

Epidermal growth factor receptor (EGFR) mutation testing is increasingly performed using biopsy material from lung cancer patients because targeted tyrosine kinase inhibitor drugs have been introduced for the treatment of patients with advanced NSCLC. These targeted therapies have been shown to improve progression-free survival and quality of life in patients with high EGFR expression in their tumors compared to platinum-based chemotherapy.[11]

In the National Lung Screening Trial (NLST), 53,454 older current or former heavy smokers were randomized to receive low-dose computed tomography (LDCT) or chest radiography for three annual screens.[12] LDCT detected more than twice the number of early-stage lung cancers and resulted in a stage shift from advanced to early-stage disease. Persons screened with LDCT had a 20% greater reduction in lung cancer mortality than those screened with annual chest X-rays. Most of the individuals randomized to the trial (48,549, or 91%) were white; only 2,378 (4.4%) were Black.

In a secondary analysis of data from the NLST, Tanner et al.[13] found that screening with LDCT reduced lung cancer mortality in all racial groups but more so in Black individuals (hazard ratio [HR] = 0.61 vs. 0.86). Smoking increased the likelihood of death from lung cancer and Black smokers were twice as likely to die as white smokers (HR = 4.10 vs. 2.25). After adjustment for sociodemographic and behavioral characteristics, Black individuals experienced higher all-cause mortality than white individuals (HR = 1.35, 95% CI 1.22–1.49). However, Black individuals screened with LDCT had a reduction in all-cause mortality.

The NLST results were confirmed in the NELSON (Dutch-Belgian Lung Cancer Screening) trial. Preliminary reports from the NELSON trial suggest a 26% relative reduction in lung cancer mortality with LDCT screening at 10 years in men and a greater mortality benefit (39%) among women.[14]

The probability of cancer in screen-detected nodules depends on their size and whether the nodules are detected on prevalence or incidence screens.[15] Management strategies for screen-detected nodules include serial CT imaging and CT-guided biopsy for larger nodules and those that demonstrate growth on follow-up.

Guidelines have been developed to help identify appropriate screening populations and to develop standards for radiological testing. Challenges with routine lung cancer screening include the potential for overdiagnosis and the large number of false positive results. In the NLST, 24.2% of the screens were positive, but 96.4% of these proved to be false positive results.[16] Although some questions remain about LDCT screening, a comprehensive lung cancer screening program aimed at higher-risk persons can increase the detection of potentially curable disease.[12] The National Comprehensive Cancer Network, the American Cancer Society, and the United States Preventive Services Taskforce have published guidelines for LDCT screening.[17,18] The Preventive Services Taskforce recommends lung cancer screening with LDCT annually for individuals aged 50 to 80 years with a reasonable life expectancy and at least a 20-pack-per-year smoking history who either currently smoke or have quit within the previous 15 years.[18]

Current uptake of lung cancer screening is low across the United States.[14] Reasons include limited access to screening, limited patient acceptance, and lack of physician knowledge about screening guidelines.[14,19] African American smokers have lower rates of lung cancer screening than white smokers.[14]

Black-White Disparities in Lung Cancer Treatment

The survival of patients with stage 1 or 2 lung cancer differs significantly based on race/ethnicity and socioeconomic status. Racial differences in cancer outcomes may be due to several factors, including decreased access to quality care, differences in tumor biology resulting in increased aggressiveness or resistance to treatment, socioeconomic factors influencing treatment options, increased comorbid conditions among African Americans, and suboptimal patient-physician interactions.[20,21] Several studies have identified racial disparities in the quality of care among NSCLC patients that may contribute to racial differences in outcomes.[7] Racial disparities in the timeliness of care for lung cancer patients have also been observed.[22] Numerous studies have shown that African American patients are less likely to receive surgical resection than whites.[8,23–26] African Americans appear to have the lowest survival for early-stage NSCLC.[7]

Aldrich et al.[5] conducted a prospective study among 81,697 racially diverse and medically underserved adults enrolled in the Southern Community Cohort Study in 11 states of the Southeast. Using linkages with state cancer registries, 501 incident NSCLC cases were identified. More African Americans were diagnosed at the distant stage than whites (57% vs. 45%, $p = 0.03$). After adjustment for pack-years of smoking, age, body mass index, health insurance, socioeconomic status, and disease stage, the lung cancer HR was similar for African Americans and whites (HR = 0.99, 95% confidence interval 0.74–1.32).

Shugarman et al.[25] evaluated the relationship between race and sex with timely and appropriate treatment for NSCLC treatment using Surveillance Epidemiology and End Results data linked to Medicare claims data over the period 1995 to 1999 (N = 22,145). Blacks were 66% less likely to receive timely and appropriate treatment than whites. Black men were least likely to receive resection (22% vs. 43.7% for white men). Blacks were 34% less likely to receive timely surgery, chemotherapy, or radiation for stage 3 disease and were 51% less likely to receive chemotherapy in a timely fashion for stage 4 disease than whites.[25] Similar findings were reported by Hardy et al. (2009), who examined racial disparities in treatment for NSCLC using Surveillance Epidemiology and End Results data linked to Medicare claims data for the period 1991 to 2002 (N = 83,101 patients aged ≥ 65 years). Steele et al.[26] linked data from the Alabama State Cancer Registry with state Medicare data to examine urban/rural patterns in receipt of treatment for NSCLC among Black and white Medicare beneficiaries. They identified 3,481 cases of stages 1–4 and unknown-stage NSCLC diagnosed in 2000–2002. Among those with resectable NSCLC (stages 1–3A), urban whites were more likely to undergo surgical resection than urban Blacks (49.3% and 33.0%, respectively) and more rural whites than rural Blacks (49.8% and 23.9%, respectively) underwent surgery. There was less variation by race and urban/rural residence in the receipt of chemotherapy and radiation therapy.

The causes of these racial differences are complex and include patient, environmental, and health system factors.[7] The data show that when patients receive appropriate care at the right time, few racial differences in NSCLC survival rates exist. Studies of NSCLC patients who received treatment at Veterans Affairs facilities, a single-payer, accessible health care system, have demonstrated few Black-white disparities in lung cancer outcomes.[7,27] Nevertheless there is ample evidence that pronounced lung cancer disparities persist in the United States. Black-white differences in patient refusal rates and in patient attitudes, beliefs, and knowledge about lung cancer may contribute to racial differences in receipt of appropriate treatment for NSCLC.[24] Patient attitudes such as fatalism and denial can lead to delays in presenting for medical evaluation when symptoms occur.[12] In addition, important differences have been identified in the understanding of lung cancer among different racial/ethnic and socioeconomic groups. Individuals from disadvantaged backgrounds are more likely to have misperceptions about their risk of lung cancer, the benefits of surgical resection, and lung cancer mortality.[12,28]

Cigarette Smoking and Other Risk Factors for Lung Cancer

Cigarette smoking is the most important preventable cause of lung cancer, although secondhand smoke, exposure to environmental/occupational hazards (e.g., asbestos, chromium, diesel exhaust, some forms of silica), ionizing radiation, and genetic factors also contribute to lung cancer morbidity and mortality.[29] Low socioeconomic status populations and minority populations experience greater exposure to environmental and occupational hazards.[14] For example, in the NLST, about 28% of participants reported at least one occupational exposure, including 6.5% exposed to silica and 4.7% to asbestos. African Americans reported occupational exposure more frequently than white participants, including exposures to asbestos and silica.[30] Exposure to radon gas is a leading cause of lung cancer in nonsmokers.

In the United States, cigarette smoking causes about 90% of lung cancers. African Americans are more likely to die from smoking-related diseases than whites, although they usually smoke fewer cigarettes and start smoking cigarettes at an older age. African American smokers have greater exposure to tobacco carcinogens at lower amounts of cigarette consumption than white smokers as a result of increased intensity of smoking and slower nicotine metabolism.[14] African Americans are more likely to smoke mentholated cigarettes. Using other tobacco products such as cigars or pipes also increases the risk of lung cancer. The Centers for Disease Control and Prevention (CDC) reports that tobacco smoke is a toxic mix of more than 7,000 chemicals, of which at least 70 are known to cause cancer. Individuals who smoke are 15–30 times more likely to get lung cancer or die from lung cancer than people who do not smoke. The risk of lung cancer increases with a greater number of years a person smokes and a higher number of cigarettes smoked each day.[45]

Following a cancer diagnosis, continued tobacco use increases cancer treatment toxicity, cancer recurrence, second primary tumors, and mortality and impairs quality of life.[31] For the major cancer treatment modalities (surgery, chemotherapy, and radiation therapy), smoking has been found to diminish treatment effectiveness, increase side effects, and interfere with wound healing.[31] Cigarette smoking is an established risk factor for a variety of pulmonary, cardiovascular, and infectious complications.[32] Nevertheless, studies have shown that 50–83% of cancer patients continue to smoke after a diagnosis.[33] Some cancer patients may accept the negative consequences of smoking or not see the point in quitting smoking. There is a need to increase access to tobacco cessation support for cancer patients and to study ways to increase the efficacy of tobacco cessation after a cancer diagnosis.[34] Few studies have combined provider training on tobacco cessation with training for cultural competency and patient-provider communication.

Cultural Competency, Patient Trust in Their Physician, and Health Literacy

A patient's trust in their physician is essential for desirable treatment outcomes such as satisfaction and adherence to treatment recommendations.[35] This is especially true in oncology because of the life-threatening nature of cancer. Studies have shown that patient trust is enhanced by a physician's technical competence, honesty, and patient-centered behavior. A trusting relationship between a patient and their physician can improve communication and medical decision-making, decrease patient fear, and improve treatment adherence.[35] Perceived quality of lung cancer communication has been associated with receiving potentially curative surgery for early-stage disease.[36] Gordon et al.[37] examined Black-white differences in patient trust associated with physician-patient communication about lung cancer treatment. Data were obtained from 103 patients seen at thoracic surgery or oncology clinics in a large Veterans Affairs hospital in the southern United States for initial treatment recommendations for suspicious pulmonary nodules or lung cancer. Black patients had lower post-visit trust in their physician than white patients ($p = 0.02$). Compared with white patients, Black patients judged the physicians' communication as less informative, less supportive, and less partnering. These findings raise concern that Black patients may have lower trust in their physician in part because of poorer physician-patient communication.[37] Improving patient communication with their provider is essential for ensuring that patients receive optimal care for NSCLC.[36] Studies have shown that effective patient-physician communication is related to improved adherence to medical regimens, better decision-making, and increased satisfaction with the patient-physician relationship.[38] Cultural competency skills can improve patient-provider communication.

Cultural competency influences how health messages are transmitted and perceived, how illness is defined, how symptoms are described, when and where care is obtained, and how treatment options are considered.[1] Cultural competency, which can be taught as part of medical education and continuing professional education programs, includes the acquisition and integration of knowledge, awareness, and skills about culture and cultural differences. This competency enables health care professionals to provide optimal care to patients from different racial, ethnic, socioeconomic, and cultural backgrounds.

Patient health literacy is also important. Low health literacy has been associated with decreased use of smoking cessation programs, increased risk of having cancer, poorer treatment adherence, and poorer health outcomes.[39] Low health literacy is associated with a decreased likelihood that a person will seek cancer information from a health care professional, an increased sense of fatalism about cancer, and later stage at diagnosis.[40] Health literacy also influences patient-provider communication. Individuals with low health literacy are more passive when interacting with providers, less likely to engage in shared decision making, and less likely to ask questions.[41] The ability to effectively communicate with providers is particularly important because of the complexity of cancer care. Furthermore, health professionals often overestimate the health literacy skills of patients, have inadequate awareness about health literacy issues, and do not routinely use recommended communication strategies.[42] Although studies have suggested that African Americans in the United States have lower health literacy than their white counterparts, racial differences in health literacy may be due to uncontrolled confounding factors such as age and education.

Discussion

Several studies have shown that after a lung cancer diagnosis, many men and women, particularly African Americans, do not receive treatment consistent with clinical guidelines for lung cancer staging and treatment. People who are least likely to navigate the health care system for lung cancer often have a low level of education, less health literacy, belong to a minority racial/ethnic group, are uninsured/underinsured and poor, and live in a medically underserved community. Cancer care is often fragmented, inadequately coordinated, and not always organized around the needs of the patient. Culturally competent patient navigation programs are needed that support lung cancer patients—especially socioeconomically disadvantaged patients—from the point of diagnosis to the initiation and completion of treatment.

Health care providers have an important role to play in both the primary prevention of lung cancer and other smoking-related diseases and the tertiary prevention of lung cancer recurrence and other tobacco-related malignancies among lung cancer patients. Such efforts can help address disparities in lung cancer among African Americans. Resources are available such as "A Clinical Practice Guideline for the Treatment of Tobacco Dependence" (United States Public Health Service)[43] and "How to Help Your Patients Stop Smoking" (National Cancer Institute).[44]

Providers who want to help African American patients stop smoke should acquire cultural competency education and train to improve patient-provider communication. Providers should inform their patients abut resources such as the 1-800-QUIT-NOW national telephone quit line. First-line pharmocotherapies for smoking cessation include nicotine (patch, gum, inhaler, spray, and lozenge) and buproprion.

As lung cancer and other diseases become more preventable due to advances in medical knowledge, individuals with greater access to resources tend to benefit more, which can lead to the worsening of health disparities. Public health interventions are therefore needed to facilitate a more equitable distribution of medical advances and the improved uptake and utilization of lung cancer treatment among lower socioeconomic groups such as economically disadvantaged African Americans.

REFERENCES

1. Coughlin, S. S., P. Matthews-Juarez, P. D. Juarez, C. E. Melton, and M. King. "Opportunities to Address Lung Cancer Disparities among African Americans." *Cancer Medicine* 3, no. 6 (2014): 1467–1476.

2. Siegel, R. L., K. D. Miller, H. E. Fuchs, and A. Jemal. "Cancer Statistics, 2021." *CA: A Cancer Journal for Clinicians* 71, no. 1 (2021): 7–33.

3. Albano, J. D., E. Ward, A. Jemal, A., R. Anderson, V. E. Cokkinides, T. Murray, J. Henley, J. Liff, and M. J. Thun. "Cancer Mortality in the United States by Education Level and Race." *Journal of the National Cancer Institute* 99, no. 18 (2007): 1384–1394.

4. Howlader, N., A. M. Noone, M. Krapcho, M. Garshell, J. Miller, S. F. Altekruse, C. L. Kosary, M. Yu, J. Ruhl, et al. *SEER Cancer Statistics Review, 1975–2011*. Bethesda, MD: National Cancer Institute, 2014. https://seer.cancer.gov/archive/csr/1975_2011/.

5. Aldrich, M. C., E. L. Grogan, H. M. Munro, L. B. Signorello, and W. J. Blot. "Stage-

Adjusted Lung Cancer Survival Does Not Differ between Low-Income Blacks and Whites." *Journal of Thoracic Oncology* 8, no. 10 (2013): 1248–1254.

6. Howlader, N., A. M. Noone, M. Krapcho, D. Miller, A. Brest, M. Yu, J. Ruhl, Z. Tatalovich et al., eds. *SEER Cancer Statistics Review, 1975–2016.* Bethesda, MD: National Cancer Institute, 2019.

7. Zullig, L. L., W. R. Carpenter, D. T. Provenzale, M. Weinberger, B. B. Reeve, C. D. Williams, and G. L. Jackson. "The Association of Race with Timeliness of Care and Survival among Veterans Affairs Health Care System Patients with Late-Stage Non-Small Cell Lung Cancer." *Cancer Management and Research* 5 (July 24, 2013): 157–163.

8. Hardy, D., C. C. Liu, R. Xia, J. N. Cormier, W. Chan, A. White, K. Burau, and X. L. Du. "Racial Disparities and Treatment Trends in a Large Cohort of Elderly Black and White Patients with Nonsmall Cell Lung Cancer." *Cancer* 115, no. 10 (2009): 2199–2211.

9. Howington, J. A., M. G. Blum, A. C. Chang, A. A. Balekian, and S. C. Murthy. "Treatment of Stage I and II Non-Small Cell Lung Cancer: Diagnosis and Management of Lung Cancer, 3rd ed: American College of Chest Physicians Evidence-Based Clinical Practice Guidelines." *Chest* 143, Suppl. 5 (2013): e278S–e313S.

10. Lackey, A., and J. S. Donington. "Surgical Management of Lung Cancer." *Seminars in Interventional Radiology* 30, no. 2 (2013): 133–140.

11. Pirker, R. "Novel Drugs against Nonsmall-Cell Lung Cancer." *Current Opinion in Oncology* 26, no. 2 (2014): 145–151.

12. Aberle, D. R., F. Abtin, and K. Brown. "Computed Tomography Screening for Lung Cancer: Has it Finally Arrived? Implications of the National Lung Screening Trial." *Journal of Clinical Oncology* 31, no. 8 (2013): 1002–1008.

13. Tanner, N. T., M. Gebregziabher, C. H. Halbert, E. Payne, L. A. Egede, and G. A. Sylvestri. "Racial Differences in Outcomes within the National Lung Screening Trial." *American Journal of Respiratory and Critical Care Medicine* 192, no. 2 (2015): 200–208.

14. Haddad, D. N., K. L. Sandler, L. M. Henderson, M. P. Rivera, and M. C. Aldrich. "Disparities in Lung Cancer Screening: A Review." *Annals of the American Thoracic Society* 17, no. 4 (2020): 399–405.

15. Grosu, H. B., G. A. Eapen, A. Jimenez, R. C. Morice, and D. Ost. "Lung Cancer Screening: Making the Transition from Research to Clinical Practice." *Current Opinion in Pulmonary Medicine* 18, no. 4 (2012): 295–303.

16. Prosch, H., and C. Schaefer-Prokop. "Screening for Lung Cancer." *Current Opinion in Oncology* 26 (2014): 131–137.

17. Wender, R., E. T. H. Fontham, E. Barrera Jr., G. A. Colditz, T. R. Church, D. S. Ettinger, R. Etzioni, C. R. Flowers, G. S. Gazelle, et al. "American Cancer Society Lung Cancer Screening Guidelines." *CA: A Cancer Journal for Clinicians* 63, no. 2 (2013): 107–117.

18. US Preventive Services Task Force. "Screening for Lung Cancer: US Preventive Services Task Force Recommendation Statement." *Journal of the American Medical Association* 325, no. 10 (2021): 962–970.

19. Lewis, J. A., H. Chen, K. E. Weaver, L. B. Spalluto, K. L. Sandler, L. Horn, R. S. Dittus, P. P. Massion, C. L. Roumie, et al. "Low Provider Knowledge Is Associated with Less Evidence-Based Lung Cancer Screening." *Journal of the National Comprehensive Cancer Network* 17, no. 4 (2019): 339–346.

20. King, T. E., Jr., and P. Brunetta. "Racial Disparity in Rates of Surgery for Lung Cancer." *New England Journal of Medicine* 341 (1999): 1231–1233.

21. Albain, K. S., J. M. Unger, J. J. Crowley, C. A. Coltman Jr., and D. L. Hershman. "Racial Disparities in Cancer Survival among Randomized Clinical Trials Patients of the Southwest Oncology Group." *Journal of the National Cancer Institute* 101, no. 14 (2009): 984–992.

22. Olsson, J. K., E. M. Schultz, and M. K. Gould. "Timeliness of Care in Patients with Lung Cancer: A Systematic Review." *Thorax* 64, no. 9 (2009): 749–756.

23. Margolis, M. L., J. K. Christie, G. A. Silvestri, L. Kaiser, S. Santiago, and J. Hansen-Flaschen. "Racial Differences Pertaining to a Belief about Lung Cancer Surgery: Results from a Multicenter Survey." *Annals of Internal Medicine* 139, no. 7 (2003): 558–563.

24. Farjah, F., D. E. Wood, N. D. Yanez 3rd, T. L. Vaughan, L. G. Symons, B. Krishnadasan, and D. R. Flum. "Racial Disparities among Patients with Lung Cancer Who Were Recommended Operative Therapy." *Archives of Surgery* 144, no. 1 (2009): 14–18.

25. Shugarman, L. R., K. Mack, M. E. Sorbero, H. Tian, A. K. Jain, J. S. Ashwood, and S. M. Asch. "Race and Sex Differences in the Receipt of Timely and Appropriate Lung Cancer Treatment." *Medical Care* 47, no. 7 (2009): 774–781.

26. Steele, C. B., M. Pisu, and L. C. Richardson. "Urban/Rural Patterns in Receipt of Treatment for Non-Small Cell Lung Cancer among Black and White Medicare Beneficiaries, 2000–2003." *Journal of the National Medical Association* 103, no. 8 (2011): 711–718.

27. Ganti, A. K., Subbiah, S. P., Kessinger, A., W. I. Gonsalves, P. T. Silberstein, and F. R. Loberiza Jr. "Association between Race and Survival of Patients with Non-small-cell Lung Cancer in the United States Veterans Affairs Population." *Clinical Lung Cancer* 15, no. 8 (2013): 152–158.

28. Rutten, L. F., B. W. Hesse, R. P. Moser, K. D. McCaul, and A. J. Rothman. "Public Perceptions of Cancer Prevention, Screening, and Survival: Comparison with State-of-Science Evidence for Colon, Skin, and Lung Cancer." *Journal of Cancer Education* 24, no. 1 (2009): 40–48.

29. Ridge, C. A., A. M. McErlean, and M. S. Ginsberg. "Epidemiology of Lung Cancer." *Seminars in Interventional Radiology* 30, no. 2 (2013): 93–98.

30. Juon, H. S., A. Hong, M. Pimpinelli, M. Rojulpote, and J. A. Barta. "Racial Disparities in Occupational Risks and Lung Cancer Incidence: Analysis of the National Lung Screening Trial." *Preventive Medicine* 143 (2021): 106355.

31. Gritz, E. R., M. C. Fingeret, D. J. Vidrine, A. B. Lazev, N. V. Mehta, and G. P. Reece. "Successes and Failures of the Teachable Moment. Smoking Cessation in Cancer Patients." *Cancer* 106, no. 1 (2006): 17–27.

32. Møller, A. M., T. Pedersen, N. Villebro, M. Haas, and R. Tønneson. "A Study of the Impact of Long-Term Tobacco Smoking on Postoperative Intensive Care Admission." *Anaesthesia* 58, no. 1 (2003): 55–59.

33. Duffy, S. A., S. A. Louzon, and E. Gritz. "Why Do Cancer Patients Smoke and What Can Providers Do about It?" *Community Oncology* 9, no. 11 (2012): 344–352.

34. Gritz, E. B., B. A. Toll, and G. W. Warren. "Tobacco Use in the Oncology Setting: Advancing Clinical Practice and Research." *Cancer Epidemiology Biomarkers and Prevention* 23 (2014): 3–9.

35. Hillen, M. A., H. C. de Haes, and E. M. Smets. "Cancer Patients' Trust in Their Physician—A Review." *Psychooncology* 20, no. 3 (2011): 227–241.

36. Dalton, A. F., A. J. Bunton, S. Cykert, G. Corbie-Smith, P. Dilworth-Anderson, F. R. McGuire, M. H. Monroe, P. Walker, and L. J. Edwards. "Patient Characteristics Associated with Favorable Perceptions of Patient-Provider Communication in Early-Stage Lung Cancer Treatment." *Journal of Health Communication* 19, no. 5 (2014): 532–544.

37. Gordon, H. S., R. L. Street Jr., B. F. Sharf, P. A. Kelly, and J. Souchek. "Racial Differences in Trust and Lung Cancer Patients' Perceptions of Physician Communication." *Journal of Clinical Oncology* 20, no. 6 (2006): 904–909.

38. Diefenbach, M., G. Turner, K. M. Carpenter, L. Kennedy Sheldon, K. M. Mustian, M. A. Gerend, C. Rini, C. von Wagner, E. R. Gritz, et al. "Cancer and Patient-Physician Communication." *Journal of Health Communication* 14, Suppl. 1 (2009): 57–65.

39. Berkman, N. D., S. L. Sheridan, K. E. Donahue, D. J. Halpern, and K. Crotty. "Low Health Literacy and Health Outcomes: An Updated Systematic Review." *Annals of Internal Medicine* 155, no. 2 (2011): 97–107.

40. Davis, T. C., M. V. Williams, E. Marin, R. M. Parker, and J. Glass. "Health Literacy and Cancer Communication." *CA: A Cancer Journal for Clinicians* 52, no. 3 (2002): 134–149.

41. Paasche-Orlow, M. K., and M. S. Wolf. "The Causal Pathways Linking Health Literacy to Health Outcomes." *American Journal of Health Behavior* 31, Suppl. 1 (2007): S19–S26.

42. Coleman, C. "Teaching Health Care Professionals about Health Literacy: A Review of the Literature." *Nursing Outlook* 59, no. 2 (2011): 70–78.

43. Fiore, M. C., C. R. Jaen, T. B. Baker, et al. *Treating Tobacco Use and Dependence: 2008 Update. Clinical Practice Guideline*. Rockville, MD: U.S. Department of Health and Human Services, Public Health Service, 2009. https://www.ncbi.nlm.nih.gov/books/NBK63952/.

44. Epps, R. P., and M. W. Manley. "How to Help Your Patients Stop Smoking: A National Cancer Institute Program for Physicians." *Journal of the Florida Medical Association* 77, no. 4 (1990): 454–456.

45. CDC. "What Are the Risk Factors for Lung Cancer?" Division of Cancer Prevention and Control, CDC. Last reviewed October 18, 2021. https://www.cdc.gov/cancer/lung/basic_info/risk_factors.htm.

17

Sexual and Reproductive Health

LUCY A. INGRAM, PhD, MPH,

FAITH E. FLETCHER, PhD, MA,

TIFFANY BYRD, MPH, CHES,

and ANTONIKA KADIRI, MPH

In this chapter, we present key topics in sexual and reproductive health (SRH) as it relates to African Americans in the southern United States. In addition to defining SRH terms and concepts, we will present context for the current state of SRH among African Americans in the American South. We focus on the challenges and experiences of African American cisgender women. We acknowledge that SRH and associated inequities also disproportionately affect others, including men, transgender women, and gender-nonconforming and nonbinary individuals. Although dedicated conversations about those lived experiences are essential, they are beyond the scope of this chapter.

What Is Sexual and Reproductive Health?

Sexual health is the "state of physical, mental, and social well-being in relation to sexuality" (World Health Organization 2020). Reproductive health "addresses the reproductive processes, functions and system at all stages of life. Reproductive health, therefore, implies that people are able to have a responsible, satisfying and safe sex life and that they have the capability to reproduce and the freedom to decide if, when and how often to do so" (World Health Organization 2020). These definitions explain the significance of SRH to the overall health and well-being of individuals. Although the terms "sexual health" and "reproductive health" are intertwined and at times are used interchangeably, they are not synonymous. Sexual health and reproductive health are each vitally important to forming overall health and well-being.

For many people, seeking services for SRH is a gateway into the health care system. Examples include family planning, prenatal care, testing and treatment for human immunodeficiency virus (HIV) and sexually transmitted infections (STIs), as well as screening for reproductive cancers, substance abuse, and intimate partner violence. Increasing awareness of and attention to health services and research in this arena is essential for understanding and addressing a number of health outcomes (e.g., reducing rates of infectious disease, unintended pregnancy, and infertility) and social challenges (e.g., increasing public health education, career opportunities, and financial stability) (Healthy People 2022a).

We include the important and related concepts of reproductive justice and reproductive autonomy in our definition of SRH. They are essential for understanding and optimizing SRH among African American women.

Reproductive Justice

According to Ross and Solinger (2017, 9), reproductive justice necessitates sexual autonomy and gender freedom for every human being and has three primary principles: the right not to have a child, the right to have a child, and the right to parent children in safe and healthy environments. Realizing reproductive justice equity in clinical and research settings calls for partnering with reproductive health and justice organizations that are engaged in research, education, outreach, practice, advocacy, and policy efforts. Some of these entities include Sister Song, Black Mamas Matter Alliance, ROOTT (Restoring Our Own Through Transformation n.d.), the National Black Women's Reproductive Justice Agenda (In Our Voice 2022), Black Women's Health Imperative (2022), the International Center for Traditional Childbearing (Healing Hands Community Doula Project n.d.), and the Center for Reproductive Health Research in the Southeast (Rollins School of Public Health n.d.). As Ross and Solinger (2017, 57) note, "acting collectively, reproductive justice organizations and their allies have refocused and redefined the basic elements of sexual and reproductive dignity for all." It is important to illuminate the work of pioneers and innovators in discussions about SRH, particularly among African American women.

The notion of reproductive justice and reproductive justice movement concepts are not new. In the United States, reproduction has been central to wealth and power and as such has been a target of governmental control. For example, in 1976, the Hyde Amendment prohibited federal support for poor women seeking abortions. It stated that only women with the financial means to control their fertility could have access to abortion (Ross and Solinger 2017, 47). This amendment was one of the first major anti-abortion federal laws. In addition, legislators in at least thirteen states have attempted to pass laws mandating sterilization for female Medicaid recipients or recipients using housing assistance who have had "too many" children (Ross and Solinger 2017, 50). In addition to equitable access to contraception and abortion, reproductive justice also requires access to community resources such as high-quality health care, education, housing, living wages, and the resources necessary to enable safe childbirth and parenting (Ross and Solinger 2017, 9). It also means the right to refuse sterilization, to end long-acting contraceptive use at will, and to give birth in the way a person chooses. Access to these resources is often limited by federal policies. Today, limitations remain in access to reproductive health care services. For example, some states' insurance plans refuse contraceptives to dependents covered by a parent's insurance plan without special medical preauthorization. Only nine states prohibit such practices (Guttmacher 2022). People continue to have difficulty obtaining equitable access to doula care services, even when they have access to public or private health care coverage (Maryland State Doulas n.d.). As this text is being written, the United States is on the precipice of a decision to overturn *Roe v. Wade*, the case that legalized abortion in the United States (Planned Parenthood 2022; Gerstein and Ward 2022). While the extent of the effect of overturning this legislation is unknown, it will undoubtedly undermine and compromise notions of reproductive justice, and underserved and minoritized groups will suffer the most detrimental impacts.

Reproductive Autonomy

Reproductive autonomy is integral to achieving SRH equity among African American women in the South. Respect for autonomy is a moral principle that has particular salience for discussions about SRH within the contexts of research, medicine, and health care (Fletcher et al. 2021). Autonomy, derived from the Greek words *autos* ("self") and *nomos* ("rule"), refers to the "capacity to be one's own person, to live one's life according to reasons and motives that are taken as one's own and not the product of manipulative or distorting external forces" (Beauchamp and Childress 1994). Both liberty (independence from controlling influences) and agency (capacity for

intentional action) are essential conditions of autonomy. By extension, reproductive autonomy is the "power to decide when, if at all, to have children"
(Purdy 2006, 287). At the optimal level, women should be able to exercise
autonomy in their reproductive decision-making free of bias, pressure, and
coercion. Anyone or any system that hinders a person's autonomous rights
is a threat. Examples of threats to reproductive autonomy include policies
that restrict safe access to reproductive health services, including abortion
services (White and Rice, 2022), implicit or explicit bias in reproductive or
contraceptive counseling, directive advice to abstain from reproductive interests, and a lack of patient centeredness in SRH preferences that ultimately
violates the reproductive choices and moral agency of women (Fletcher,
Ingram, Kerr, Buchberg, Bogdan-Lovis et al. 2021; Fletcher, Ingram, Kerr,
Buchberg, Richter et al. 2016; Gomez and Wapman 2017).

One last foundational concept that is pertinent to this discussion is intersectionality. Understanding and addressing the SRH of African American
women living in the South requires an intersectional lens that considers the
unique vulnerabilities of African American women that may lead to differences in SRH health outcomes.

Intersectionality

Bowleg defines intersectionality as a "theoretical framework for understanding how multiple social identities such as race, gender, sexual orientation, and disability intersect at the micro level of individual experience
to reflect interlocking systems of privilege and oppression (i.e., racism, sexism, heterosexism, classism) at the macro social-structural level" (Bowleg
2012, 1267). Originally coined by Kimberlé Crenshaw, the term intersectionality was designed to "denote the various ways in which race and gender
interact to shape the multiple dimensions of Black women's employment
experience" (Crenshaw 1989, 139). African American women may face heightened health disadvantages related to their geographic location, racial minority group membership, and other social statuses (Walcott et al. 2015). These
coexisting statuses are structurally embedded within social, economic, and
other hierarchies that create, compound, and perpetuate health inequities
in various locales (Watkins-Hayes 2014), including research and health care
settings (Fletcher et al. 2019; Fletcher et al. 2016; Kerr et al. 2021; Rice et al.
2019). Research suggests that health consequences are exacerbated for groups

that experience coexisting stigmas (e.g., racism, sexism, transphobia, and mental health stigma) (Rice et al. 2018). The term "intersectional stigma" refers to the intersection and interaction of these multiple stigmatized identities (Turan et al. 2019). The intersectionality framework offers an important lens for addressing health inequities in SRH. In this chapter, we draw on the intersectionality framework to describe health disparities and vulnerabilities that African American women living in the South experience and the resilience they demonstrate.

Racial Health Disparities in STIs and HIV

STIs continue to persist as a major public health issue in the United States. Each year an estimated 19 million new cases occur (CDC 2019). Case rates are persistently high in the southern United States, and racially and ethnically minoritized groups, African American women in particular, are disproportionately affected (CDC 2019). STIs can have numerous lifelong health consequences that can prove much more deleterious for women than for men (CDC 2019; Cates et al. 2004; Fleming and Wasserheit 1999). When STIs are not detected, the reproductive health effects for women can include infertility, cervical cancer, pelvic inflammatory disease, or possible STI transmission from mother to child during childbirth (Cates et al. 2004; Mills et al. 2006).

The southern United States has the highest rates of reported chlamydia and gonorrhea in the country (CDC 2019). African American infection rates lead in both disease categories. The reported chlamydia rate among African American females is five times the rate of white females, and the rate among African American males is almost seven times the rate of white males (CDC 2019). The rate of reported cases of gonorrhea for African American females is 6.9 times the rate of white females, and for African American men it is 8.5 times that of white males (CDC 2019). Reported rates of HIV infection maintain this trend; the rates of HIV are highest in the South and among African Americans (CDC 2020). Seven of the 10 states with the highest rate of HIV infection among females are in the South (CDC 2020). Although African American females make up only 13% of the female population, they account for 58% of HIV diagnoses among women (CDC 2020). The South ranks second in the nation in syphilis cases, and African Americans have the highest infection rates of adult and congenital syphilis cases in the South (CDC 2019).

Racial Health Disparities in Reproductive Health

MATERNAL MORTALITY

Each year, approximately 700 women in the United States die from pregnancy-related causes, also termed maternal mortality (CDC 2022). While maternal mortality rates have declined worldwide by almost 50%, African American maternal mortality rates in the United States rank as the second highest among developed nations (Owens and Fett 2019). In the United States, southern states bear the burden of the disparity (Moore 2019). This disparity worsens with age; pregnancy-related deaths are four to five times higher for African American women over the age of 30 (CDC 2022). Unlike the trend seen among white women, higher income and education are not protective factors against maternal mortality risk; African American women with a college degree are five times more likely to die from pregnancy-related causes than white women with a high school diploma (CDC 2022).

INFANT MORTALITY AND LOW BIRTH WEIGHT

Infant mortality is defined as the death of an infant before their first birthday (CDC 2021). Low birth weight, a leading cause of infant mortality, refers to babies who weigh less than 2,500 grams (5.5 pounds) at birth (CDC 2021; World Health Organization 2010; Burton, Hernandez-Reif, and Lian 2017). Other complications of low birth weight include respiratory distress, cognitive development challenges, and heart disease. Tracking infant mortality and low birth weight rates provides insight into the health not only of mothers and children but also of the surrounding society. These rates can be markers of the effectiveness of public health interventions to promote optimal reproductive outcomes for women. In the United States, infant mortality rates among African Americans are more than twice those of non-Hispanic whites and Hispanic/Latinos and three times those of Asians (Mathewson et al. 2017; Al Hazzani et al. 2011; Chang et al. 2015; Fitzgibbons et al. 2009; Fan, Portuguez, and Nunes 2013). African American infants are almost twice as likely as white infants to be born at a low birthweight (March of Dimes 2022). The infant mortality rates in the American South are the highest in the nation. The reasons for these disparities are varied and include social determinants of health and chronic stressors such as racism.

UNINTENDED PREGNANCY

Unintended pregnancy refers to pregnancies that are either mis-timed or unwanted (Kost 2015, 4). Unintended pregnancy rates tend to be higher in the southern United States than in other regions of the country (Kost 2015; Finer and Kost 2011). Rates are highest among women who are low income, women aged 18–24, women who are cohabitating, and women of color (Finer and Zolna 2016). The unintended pregnancy rate for African American women is more than twice that of white women (Finer and Zolna 2016).

CONTRIBUTORS TO RACIAL DISPARITIES IN SRH

Disparities in SRH are linked to social determinants of health, which are defined as the "conditions in the environments in which people are born, live, learn, work, play, worship, and age that affect a wide range of health, functioning, and quality-of-life outcomes and risks" (Office of Disease Prevention and Health Promotion 2020). These factors are shaped by the distribution of power, money, and resources, which influence the availability of employment opportunities, the safety and affordability of housing and transportation, and access to high-quality health care coverage.

Structural racism is a significant contributor to SRH inequities. It is defined as racism that is "pervasively and deeply embedded in and throughout systems, laws, written or unwritten policies, entrenched practices, and established beliefs and attitudes that produce, condone, and perpetuate widespread unfair treatment of people of color" (Braveman et al. 2022). Structural racism in health care provision for African American women equates to a poorer quality of health care service delivery, refusal to help when an African American woman is experiencing pain, and failure to treat African American women with dignity and respect (Taylor et al. 2019). Childbirth is one of the most vulnerable, dangerous, and painful life experiences, and discrimination and racial bias during this sensitive period can be detrimental to the health of both the woman and her baby. Studies as recent as 2016 about perceptions of medical students showed that half believed that African Americans had shorter nerve endings and therefore are less sensitive to pain (Hoffman et al. 2016). In other words, half of the future providers in this study had unfounded beliefs about the pain tolerance levels of African Americans that will undoubtedly impact how they deliver health care services. To promote equity in health and health care delivery, leading academic medical organizations have determined that dismantling racism in medical education and health care practices is a national priority (American Medical Association and American Association of Medical Colleges Center for Health Justice 2021).

The SRH of African Americans and Unethical Medical Research

Among African Americans, particularly in the American South, SRH has a harrowing historical context. During slavery, the female Black body was controlled, used for experimentation, and exploited. In fact, the value of a Black woman's body was determined by how much value it could provide to a white person. The value of slaveholders' life insurance policies for enslaved women and girls was determined by the childbearing potential of enslaved women and girls (Owens and Fett 2019). Even in death, Black bodies were often commodified and used as teaching material for white medical school students (Owens and Fett 2019). In the mid-1800s, Dr. J. Marion Sims, known by some as the "father of modern gynecology", repeatedly experimented on enslaved women in Alabama to develop a procedure to repair vaginal fistulas (Mohatt et al. 2014). It was not until the procedure was proven successful that he began using anesthesia—on white women volunteers (Mohatt et al. 2014). Unfortunately, the abolishment of slavery did not erase deeply ingrained societal beliefs about African American women's pain tolerance or humanity (Hoffman et al. 2016; Taylor et al. 2019). Today, these beliefs are embedded in the infrastructure of the institutions and ideologies that dominate American culture (Gee and Ford 2011). Well-documented medical research on the harms imposed on African American women underscore the need for a focus on addressing anti-Black racism in research and health care settings (Goodwin 2020; Roberts 1997; Sederstrom and Lasege 2022; Washington 2006), particularly in the context of African American women and SRH.

The U.S. Public Health Service Syphilis Study at Tuskegee (1932–1972) provides an important framework for understanding African Americans' loss of confidence in U.S. medical and public health systems (Jones 1981; Thomas and Quinn 1991) and serves as a reminder that building and sustaining trusting relationships and equity in health care is a goal that has not been realized (Best et al. 2021). The outrage over the 40-year government study involving

600 poor African American men from Macon County, Alabama, prompted the passage of the National Research Act of 1974 and the establishment of a federal policy to protect human research subjects. All US research involving human subjects must now be approved by an institutional review board (Department of Health, Education, and Welfare 2014). In addition to the morbidity and mortality the men in the study experienced, some of their wives acquired syphilis, and some of their children suffered complications from congenital syphilis (Washington 2011, 193). While the women who were affected are less discussed, this infamous study had serious implications for the SRH of African American women, particularly as it related to restricted agency and autonomy related to health care decisions. The lack of attention to African American women affected by the Tuskegee study also underscores the marginalization and invisibility of African American women in US society.

While the U.S. Public Health Service Syphilis Study at Tuskegee is one of the most well-known accounts of unethical medical research in the United States and for some, symbolizes "racism in medicine, misconduct in human research, the arrogance of physicians, and government abuse of Black people" (Gamble 1997), Dr. Vanessa Northington Gamble emphasizes that it is important to understand the broader historical and social contexts that influence African Americans' attitudes towards the biomedical community. Other scholarly works present additional information that illuminates the historical and contemporary context of African American women's health (James 2022; Thomas 2022; Washington 2006; Wilson 2022;). This section describes just a few examples of countless atrocities against African American female bodies that have a direct impact today on women's perspectives, perceptions, and well-being related to SRH.

Interventions to Address SRH Disparities

Ecological Frameworks

Understanding the SRH of African Americans in the American South requires a recognition that the lived experience of this group is multilayered and complex. Because of this, interventions to optimize the SRH of southern African American women should also be multidimensional and should be tailored to the unique needs of this population. The socio-ecological model, which emphasizes the complex interplay between individual behavior and environmental factors, is a useful framework for conceptualizing intervention approaches and key components of intervention (Glanz and Rimer

2002). This model enables researchers and practitioners to take into account the multiple levels of factors that may influence SRH that may ultimately be used to guide interventions at appropriate levels. First introduced by Bronfenbrenner (1977, 1986, 1989), the socio-ecological model has been adapted over the years to expand how the different levels of influence are identified. McLeroy and colleagues categorize the levels of influence according to intrapersonal, interpersonal, and community-level factors (McLeroy et al. 1988). The intrapersonal refers to individual characteristics that influence behavior such as knowledge, attitudes, beliefs, and personality traits. The interpersonal level consists of interpersonal processes such as social networks and social support that may inhibit or promote behavior change. The community level includes institutional factors, public policy factors, and the broader social system.

Traditional public health research focuses on changing individual-level risk factors such as behavior (e.g., sexual abstinence, wearing condoms, engaging in reproductive health care). These factors can be easier to modify than macro-level factors such as structural racism. However, focusing on individual-level factors while ignoring broader contextual factors can have unintended consequences such as characterizing certain populations as risk-taking and irresponsible. Ecological frameworks support the notion that individuals who live in socially disadvantaged environments are not inherently risk-taking but live in risk as a result of complex, integrated, and overlapping social, economic, and political systems (Fletcher, Jiang, and Best 2021; Phelan, Link, and Tehranifar 2010). This perspective is particularly relevant when discussing the lived experiences of women in the environment of the US South. Other useful ecological and justice-oriented theoretical frameworks to consider for interventions that seek to address SRH disparities include the PEN-3 cultural model, critical race theory, the life course perspective, Black feminist thought, and the reproductive justice framework (DiClemente, Salazar, and Crosby 2019).

Patient-Centered Care

Typically, decisions about health and health care are driven by health care providers with little or no input from patients. More innovative and engaged models of care are needed to address persistent health inequities. Patient-centered care is a method of care that takes into account the medical, financial, social, spiritual needs and desired health outcomes of a patient when making health care decisions (NEJM Catalyst 2007). In this framework, providers view patients as partners in a shared decision-making process for developing a comprehensive plan that is tailored to their needs. "Patient-centered care is a method of care that relies upon effective communication, empathy, and a feeling of partnership between doctor and patient to improve patient care outcomes and satisfaction, to lessen patient symptoms, and to reduce unnecessary costs" (Rickert 2012). The need to prioritize patient preferences is even more pronounced when African American women are making decisions about their SRH (Centering Healthcare Institute n.d.). Centering patient preferences acknowledges that evidence-based recommendations must be carefully balanced with the patient's expressed needs to maximize the health and well-being of patients and to minimize harms (Fletcher et al. 2021).

Community Engagement

Community engagement is a multidisciplinary approach to working with communities to inform programs and interventions. Israel et al. (2005, 1464) define community-based participatory research as "a partnership approach to research that equitably involves, for example, community members, organizational representatives, and researchers in all aspects of the research process, in which all partners contribute expertise and share decision making and responsibilities" (see also Israel et al. 1998; Israel et al. 2003). The ultimate goal of community-based participatory research is to "increase knowledge and understanding of a given phenomenon and integrate the knowledge gained . . . to improve health and quality of life of community members" (Israel et al. 2005, 1464). Although some interventions address the SRH needs of African Americans, few programs incorporate the expressed perspectives and insight of the populations that are most impacted by disparities in sexual and reproductive health care (Annang et al. 2011). Direct input or formal participation from members of the affected communities in the intervention planning, implementation, and evaluation stages of a research study can improve the effectiveness of programs that are known to positively influence the SRH of African Americans, particularly those in the South. Active community involvement, especially in the formative phase of a study, can strengthen program development capacity and ensure that the community of interest has a substantial voice (Israel et al. 1998).

Methods and approaches used in community-based participatory research include stakeholder interviews, community advisory boards, focus groups, the nominal group technique, and photovoice. These approaches can be used at different phases of program development and implementation in order to better capture insights from the intended audience (Annang et al. 2016; Annang et al. 2011; Ingram et al. 2018; Ingram et al. 2016; Ingram et al. 2020; McCabe et al. 2022; Molina et al. 2019).

Stakeholder interviews are typically performed one-on-one with a trained interviewer using a standardized, semi-structured discussion guide. Stakeholders are persons who are knowledgeable about a particular topic and who represent a particular community of interest. Their experiences of living in their community often provide useful insights about community issues, concerns, strengths, and assets that can lead to the most relevant and informed intervention approaches (McCabe et al. 2022; Wallerstein and Duran 2010).

Community advisory boards are usually partnerships between community members and academic researchers (Yuan et al. 2020). These boards should represent a diverse cross-section of the community of interest. Drawing on the diversity of its members, a community advisory board is connected to the opinions and attitudes of the larger community and is able to discuss community experiences, activities, and relevant local social networks and cultural practices (Yuan et al. 2020).

Focus groups are groups with a trained moderator to facilitate discussion (Morgan and Krueger 1997). The moderator relies on a standardized discussion guide and implements a carefully planned strategy for recruiting members to the group. Typically, they are conducted at a location with some level of privacy so that discussions cannot be overheard by others not involved in the project or the discussion, and a recording device is used to document the discussion. Focus group methodology has been reimagined due to social distancing guidelines during the COVID-19 pandemic. While face-to-face meetings can be modified to accommodate physical distancing recommendations, some researchers have elected to move to virtual focus groups using teleconferencing or videoconferencing technologies.

The nominal group technique is a tool that allows individuals to present their ideas and then prioritize them within a group with the goal of building consensus around a topic of interest. The technique promotes group participation and consensus as opposed to domination by a vocal minority. Ideally, the process results in a list of solutions, recommendations, or responses to the moderator's questions that represent the priorities and preferences of the entire group. If the nominal group technique is used in the formative research phase, data generated from it can be used to develop culturally and regionally appropriate interventions tailored to the population of interest based on the expertise of the nominal group (Annang et al. 2011).

Photovoice is a qualitative method of inquiry that is based on the idea that a photograph can provide a researcher with valuable insights into the cultural practices and lived experiences of individuals and communities (Nykiforuk, Vallianatos, and Nieuwendyk 2011; Wang 2006; Wang et al. 2004). Through a participatory framework, the process promotes dialogue and issue selection with the goal of engaging social change and action (Braithwaite et al. 2007; Gee and Payne-Sturges 2004; Jack and Glied 2002; North et al. 2008; Shore, Tatum, and Vollmer 1986; Wang et al. 2000). Through photovoice, a group of people is asked to express their thoughts about a particular issue or phenomenon through pictures. The individuals are asked to take or present photos in response to the phenomenon of interest and then discuss how their image is responsive to the issue at hand. Discussions are facilitated by five guiding questions known as the SHOWeD method (Wang and Burris 1994, 1997): (1) What do you See in the photograph?, (2) What is Happening in the photograph?, (3) How does this photograph relate to Our lives or other members in the community?, (4) Why do these issues currently exist within the community?, and (5) What can we Do about these issues? The methodology is grounded in Paulo Freire's education for critical consciousness and feminist theory (Freire 1970). These theories and key elements of documentary photography are the framework from which the photovoice concept was developed.

Interventions in Sexual and Reproductive Health
MOBILE TECHNOLOGY

One avenue for promoting SRH uses mobile technology. Because the majority of the US population has access to a smartphone, mobile technology can play a significant role in optimizing the SRH of African American women (Perrin and Turner 2019; Smith 2014; Pew Research Center 2019). The primary advantages of this platform are an increase in reach and engagement, ease of scalability, and greater cost effectiveness (Muessig et al. 2015; James and Harville 2018). mHealth (using mobile devices for health) and mobile technology programs focused on SRH have been developed based on characteristics of interest such as age/developmental stage (e.g., adolescence), health outcome (e.g., HIV), or subpopulation (e.g., men who have sex with men). However, mobile interventions that target African American women are less prevalent, even though that population has exhibited increasing interest in participating in mHealth studies (Steinberg et al. 2018; Bonnet Rivera and Garcia Perez 2014; Jones 2014; Jones, Hoover, and Lacroix 2013; Phillips et al. 2013; Schnall et al. 2014; Goldenburg et al. 2014; Abara et al. 2014; Chandler et al. 2020; Muessig et al. 2013; Jones and Lacroix 2012; Gonzalez Gladstein 2018; Browne et al. 2018; Tufts et al. 2015; Simoni, Kutner, and Horvath 2015; James et al. 2017). Findings from the literature on mHealth suggest that if mobile technology is to be an effective method of promoting the SRH of African American women, the programs and interventions should have the needs, preferences, and lived experience relating to SRH of the end user in mind (Ingram et al. 2020; Chandler et al. 2020; Jackson et al. 2016; Guse et al. 2012; Boyar, Levine, and Zensius 2011; Cornelius et al. 2011; Cole-Lewis and Kershaw 2010). Promising developments in this area include gamification, virtual reality, and ecological momentary assessment platforms (Muessig et al. 2015).

BREASTFEEDING

Breastfeeding is considered the gold standard for nourishing babies. Thus, leading public health and medical organizations such as the World Health Organization and American Academy of Pediatrics encourage exclusive breastfeeding for the first six months of life. Breast milk contains antibodies, hormones, and nutrients that protect infants against infections and diseases (Ballard and Morrow 2013). Breastfed children also experience lower rates of asthma, respiratory infections, sudden infant death syndrome, and later-life obesity and diabetes (Marseglia et al. 2015). For mothers, breastfeeding lowers the risk of ovarian cancer and breast cancer (CDC 2018) and aids in returning to pre-pregnancy weight. Despite these widely expressed benefits, research indicates that African American mothers are less likely to breastfeed than mothers of other racial/ethnic groups. On average, 10% to 20% fewer African American women initiate breastfeeding than white women (Beauregard et al. 2019). Several factors, many beyond a woman's mere desire to breastfeed, impact this behavior, including knowledge about the practice, cultural and social norms, the woman's concerns about her breast milk supply, level of social support, and degree of support in work and child-care environments (Office of the Surgeon General, Centers for Disease Control and Prevention, and Office on Women's Health 2011). African American women face disproportionate barriers that influence their breastfeeding decisions and capacity (e.g., returning to work early, inadequate receipt of breastfeeding information from providers, and lack of access to professional support). These barriers place African American mothers and babies at higher risk for poor health outcomes and could be substantial contributors to the origins of other health disparities between African Americans and other racial/ethnic groups (Johnson et al. 2015). The United States is currently experiencing a national infant formula shortage, primarily due to global supply chain challenges exacerbated by the COVID-19 pandemic (Assistant Secretary for Public Affairs 2022). This crisis presents an opportunity for employers, health care providers, and others to increase their support for African American women who wish to breastfeed but who face substantial barriers. Such efforts could help alleviate the current disparity we see in breastfeeding uptake.

Driven by a desire to encourage broader acceptance, numerous national organizations have encouraged the implementation of policies and programs designed to protect, promote, and support breastfeeding. For example, the United Nations Children's Fund and the World Health Organization collaborated to establish the Baby-Friendly Hospital Initiative, which consists of a 10-step approach to improving breastfeeding outcomes that is widely accepted by birthing facilities (Healthy People 2020b). Public health leaders have also implemented interventions focused on improving breastfeeding rates among African American women including psychotherapy and parenting education programs for mothers experiencing depression, peer support initiatives, media and social marketing projects, and support for employer incentives (Pennsylvania Department of Health 2018; Segura-Pérez et al. 2021; Spinelli, Endicott, and Goetz 2013).

DOULA CARE

Research demonstrates that doulas have the potential to improve African American women's birth experiences through greater satisfaction with care, higher rates of spontaneous vaginal birth, higher Apgar scores for newborns, shorter labors, lower rates of the use of regional anesthesia (e.g., epidurals) and forceps or vacuum deliveries, and fewer cesarean deliveries.

Doulas are trained childbirth professionals who provide continuous personal, emotional, and physical support during the perinatal period. Despite the benefits of having doulas throughout the birthing experience and a general increase in doula care in the United States, the rate of use remains low within communities of color.

Many health insurance plans do not cover the cost of doula services, which average from $300 to $1,200. This situation has made the service and its benefits largely inaccessible to persons who cannot afford this expense. Racially minoritized persons who can afford the service rarely find doulas who share their cultural, racial, or ethnic background, as the profession consists of mostly white upper-middle-class women (Kozhimannil et al. 2014). As a result, African American women, who face an increased risk for adverse birth outcomes and poor obstetric care, rarely benefit from what could be a promising strategy for reducing disparate birthing outcomes.

Conclusion

In this chapter, we introduced key terms related to SRH, identified areas where SRH disparities are most prominent, and discussed the determinants of these disparities. We also exposed historical injustices that impact the present-day SRH of African Americans in the South and described intervention approaches that have been particularly successful in valuing the multidimensionality of southern African American women and discussed the need to tailor intervention efforts to the needs of this population. Through this process, we identified numerous organizations and scholars, many of which are led by African American women who are on the front lines of the work to optimize the SRH of African Americans. These individuals and groups should be more widely publicized and elevated in discussions about achieving SRH equity.

We also noted that the SRH of African American women in the American South is greatly impacted by the historical and contemporary contexts that shape their lived experiences. At the writing of this chapter, several present-day challenges are occurring, namely the COVID-19 pandemic, anti-abortion legislation, and the infant formula shortage. These crises will undoubtedly have a grave impact on future SRH and on the social determinants of health outcomes.

As public health professionals, we should be committed to social justice and advocate for and provide resources to optimize SRH. A vital component of bettering the overall health status of African Americans is to achieve and maintain optimal SRH. While racial disparities in SRH abound that compromise the overall health and well-being of African American women, we are optimistic that improved awareness about these issues and continued advancements in health care, health care policies, and the social determinants of health can aid in disrupting those disparities and inequities.

REFERENCES

Abara, Winston, Lucy Annang, Melinda Spencer, Amanda Jane Fairchild, and Debbie Billings. 2014. "Understanding Internet Sex-Seeking Behavior and Sexual Risk among Young Men Who Have Sex with Men: Evidence from a Cross-Sectional Study." *Sexually Transmitted Infections* 90 (8): 596–601.

Al Hazzani, Fahad, Saleh Al-Alaiyan, Jihan Hassanein, and Emad Khadawardi. 2011. "Short-Term Outcome of Very Low-Birth-Weight Infants in a Tertiary Care Hospital in Saudia Arabia." *Annals of Saudi Medicine* 31 (6): 581–585. doi: 10.4103/0256-4947.87093.

American Medical Association and American Association of Medical Colleges Center for Health Justice. 2021. *Advancing Health Equity: A Guide to Language, Narrative and Concepts*. American Medical Association. https://www.ama-assn.org/system/files/ama-aamc -equity-guide.pdf.

Annang, Lucy, Lonnie Hannon 3rd, Faith Fletcher, Wendy Skyes Horn, and Disa Cornish. 2011. "Using Nominal Technique to Inform a Sexual Health Program for Black Youth." *American Journal Health Behavior* 35 (6): 664–673. https://doi.org/10.5993/ajhb.35.6.3.

Annang, Lucy, Sacoby Wilson, Chiwoneso Tinago, Louisiana Wright Sanders, Tina Bevington, Bethany Carlos, Evangeline Cornelius, and Erik Svendsen. 2016. "Photovoice: Assessing the Long-Term Impact of a Disaster on a Community's Quality of Life." *Qualitative Health Research* 26 (2): 241–251. https://doi.org/10.1177/1049732315576495.

Assistant Secretary for Public Affairs. 2022. "Information for Families During the Formula Shortage." HHS.gov, July 1. https://www.hhs.gov/formula/index.html.

Ballard, Olivia, and Ardythe L. Morrow. 2013. "Human Milk Composition: Nutrients and Bioactive Factors." *Pediatric Clinics of North America* 60 (1): 49–74. https://doi.org/10 .1016/j.pcl.2012.10.002.

Beauchamp, Tom, and James F. Childress. 1994. *Principles of Biomedical Ethics*. New York: Oxford University Press.

Beauregard, Jennifer, Heather C. Hamner, Jian Chen, Wendy Avila-Rodriguez, Laurie D. Elam-Evans, and Cria G. Perrine. 2019. "Racial Disparities in Breastfeeding Initiation and Duration Among U.S. Infants Born in 2015." *Morbidity and Mortality Weekly Report* 68 (34): 745–748. https://www.cdc.gov/mmwr/volumes/68/wr/mm6834a3.htm.

Best, Alicia L., Faith E. Fletcher, Mika Kadono, and Rueben C. Warren. 2021. "Institutional Distrust among African Americans and Building Trustworthiness in the COVID-19 Response: Implications for Ethical Public Health Practice." *Journal of Health Care for the Poor and Underserved* 32(1). doi: 10.1353/hpu.2021.0010.

Black Women's Health Imperative. 2022. "Eliminating Barriers to Wellness for Black Women and Girls." https://bwhi.org/.

Bonnet Rivera, A. M., and W. G. Garcia Perez. 2014. "Innovative Strategies to Expand Access to HIV Testing, Increase Linkage to Care among High-Risk Latino Young Men Who Have Sex with Men (YMSM) in Puerto Rico." Paper presented at United States Conference on AIDS, San Diego, CA, October 2–5.

Bowleg, Lisa. 2012. "The Problem with the Phrase Women and Minorities: Intersectionality—an Important Theoretical Framework for Public Health." *American Journal of Public Health* 102 (7): 1267–1273. https://dx.doi.org/10.2105%2FAJPH.2012.300750.

Boyar, Robin, Deb Levine, and Natalie Zensius. 2011. *TECHsex USA: Youth Sexuality and Reproductive Health in the Digital Age.* [Oakland, CA]: ISIS, Inc. https://www.yth.org/wp-content/uploads/YTH-youth-health-digital-age.pdf.

Braithwaite, Rhonda, Sarah Cockwill, Martin O'Neill, and Deanne Rebane. 2007. "Insider Participatory Action Research in Disadvantaged Post-Industrial Areas." *Action Research* 51 (1): 61–74. doi: 10.1177/1476750307072876.

Braveman, Paula A., Elaine Arkin, Dwayne Proctor, Tina Kauh, and Nicole Holm. 2022. "Systemic and Structural Racism: Definitions, Examples, Health Damages, and Approaches to Dismantling." *Health Affairs* 41 (2). https://doi.org/10.1377/hlthaff.2021.01394.

Bronfenbrenner, Urie. 1977. "Toward an Experimental Ecology of Human Development." *Am Psychologist* 32: 513–531. doi: 10.1037/0003-066X.32.7.513.

———. 1986. "Ecology of the Family as a Context for Human Development: Research Perspectives." *Developmental Psychology Journal* 22 (6): 723–742. doi: 10.1037/0012-1649.22.6.723.

———. 1989. "Ecological Systems Theory." In *Annals of Child Development*, ed. R. Vasta, 187–249. London: Jessica Kingsley Publishers.

Brosh, Joanne, and Monica K. Miller. 2008. "Regulating Pregnancy Behaviors: How the Constitutional Rights of Minority Women are Disproportionately Compromised." *American University Journal of Gender, Social Policy & the Law* 16 (4): 437–457.

Browne, Felicia A., Wendee M. Wechsberg, Paul N. Kizakevich, William A. Zule, Courtney P. Bonner, Ashton N. Madison, Brittni N. Howard, and Leslie B. Turner. 2018. "mHealth versus Face-to-Face: Study Protocol for a Randomized Trial to Test a Gender-Focused Intervention for Young African American Women at Risk for HIV in North Carolina." *BMC Public Health* 18 (1): article 982. doi: 10.1186/s12889-018-5796-8.

Burton, Wanda M., Maria Hernandez-Reif, and Brad Lian. 2017. "Addressing the Racial Disparity in Birth Outcomes: Implications for Maternal Racial Identity on Birth Weight." *Journal of Health Disparities Research and Practice* 10 (2): 142–155.

Cates, Willard, Nancy L. Herndon, Susan L. Schulz, Jacqueline E. Darroch. 2004. *Our Voices, Our Lives, Our Futures: Youth and Sexually Transmitted Diseases.* Chapel Hill: University of North Carolina at Chapel Hill, School of Journalism and Mass Communication.

Centering Healthcare Institute. N.d. "Centering Pregnancy." Accessed March 10, 2021. https://www.centeringhealthcare.org/what-we-do/centering-pregnancy.

CDC (Centers for Disease Control and Prevention). 2018. "CDC Releases 2018 Breastfeeding Report Card." Press release, CDC Newsroom, August 20. https://www.cdc.gov/media/releases/2018/p0820-breastfeeding-report-card.html.

———. 2019. *Sexually Transmitted Disease Surveillance 2018.* Atlanta, GA: Centers for Disease Control and Prevention. https://stacks.cdc.gov/view/cdc/79370.

———. 2020. *HIV Surveillance Report, 2018.* Vol. 31. https://www.cdc.gov/hiv/library/reports
/hiv-surveillance/vol-31/index.html.

———. 2021. "Infant Mortality." Reviewed September 8, 2021. https://www.cdc.gov/repro
ductivehealth/maternalinfanthealth/infantmortality.html.

———. 2022. "Pregnancy Mortality Surveillance System." Centers for Disease Control and
Prevention. https://www.cdc.gov/reproductivehealth/maternal-mortality/pregnancy
-mortality-surveillance-system.htm#how.

Chandler, Rasheeta, Natalie Hernandez, Dominique Guillaume, Shanaika Grandoit, Desiré
Branch-Ellis, and Marguerita Lightfoot. 2020. "A Community-Engaged Approach to
Creating a Mobile HIV Prevention App for Black Women: Focus Group Study to Determine Preferences via Prototype Demos." *JMIR Mhealth Uhealth* 8 (7): article e18437. doi:
10.2196/18437.

Chang, Hung-Yang, Yi-Hsiang Sung, Shwu-Meei Want, Hou-Ling Lung, Jui-Hsing Chang,
Chyong-Hsin Hsu, Wai-Tim Jim, Ching-Hsiao Lee, and Hsiao-Fang Hung. 2015. "Short-
and Long-Term Outcomes in Very Low Birth Weight Infants with Admission Hypo-
thermia." *PLOS One* 10 (7): e0131976. doi: 10.1371/journal.pone.0131976.

Cole-Lewis, Heather, and Trace Kershaw. 2010. "Text Messaging as a Tool for Behavior
Change in Disease Prevention and Management." *Epidemiologic Reviews* 32 (1): 56–69.
https://doi.org/10.1093/epirev/mxq004.

Cornelius, Judith B., Michael Cato, Janet St. Lawrence, Cherrie B. Boyer, and Marguerita
Lightfoot. 2011. "Development and Pretesting Multimedia HIV-Prevention Text Messages for Mobile Cell Phone Delivery." *Journal of the Association of Nurses in AIDS Care*
22 (5): 407–413. doi: 10.1016/j.jana.2010.11.007.

Crenshaw, Kimberlé. 1989. "Demarginalizing the Intersection of Race and Sex: A Black Feminist Critique of Antidiscrimination Doctrine, Feminist Theory and Antiracist Politics."
University of Chicago Legal Forum 1989 (1): 139–167.

Department of Health, Education, and Welfare. 2014. "The Belmont Report. Ethical Principles and Guidelines for the Protection of Human Subjects of Research." *The Journal of
the American College of Dentist* 81 (3): 4–13.

DiClemente, Ralph, Laura Salazar, and Richard Crosby. 2019. *Health Behavior Theory for Public Health: Principles, Foundations, and Applications.* Atlanta: Jones & Bartlett.

Fan, Rachel G., Mirna Wetters Portuguez, and Magda Lahorgue Nunes. 2013. "Cognition,
Behavior and Social Competence of Preterm Low Birth Weight Children at School Age."
Clinics (Sao Paulo) 68 (7): 915–921. doi: 10.6061/clinics/2013(07)05.

Finer, Lawrence, and Kathryn Kost. 2011. "Unintended Pregnancy Rates at the State Level."
Perspectives on Sexual and Reproductive Health 43 (2): 78–87. doi: 10.1363/4307811.

Finer, Lawrence, and Mia R. Zolna. 2016. "Declines in Unintended Pregnancy in the United
States, 2008–2011." *New England Journal of Medicine* 374 (9): 843–85. doi: 10.1056
/NEJMsa1506575.

Fitzgibbons, Shimae C., Yiming Ching, David Yu, Joe Carpenter, Michael Kenny, Christopher Welcon, Craig Lillehi, Clarissa Valim, Jeffrey D. Horbar, and Tom Jaksic. 2009.
"Mortality of Necrotizing Enterocolitis Expressed by birth weight categories." *Journal
of Pediatric Surgery* 44 no. 6 (2009): 1072–1076. doi: 10.1016/j.jpedsurg.2009.02.013.

Fleming, Douglas, and Judith N. Wasserheit. 1999. "From Epidemiological Synergy to Public Health Policy and Practice: The Contribution of Other Sexually Transmitted Diseases to Sexual Transmission of HIV Infection." *Sexually Transmitted Infections* 75: 3–17.

Fletcher, Faith, Ndidiamaka Amutah-Onukagha, Julie Attys, and Whitney S. Rice. 2021. "How Can the Experiences of Black Women Living with HIV Inform Equitable and Respectful Reproductive Health Care Delivery?" *AMA Journal of Ethics* 23 (2): E150–159.

Fletcher, Faith., Lucy A. Ingram, Jelani Kerr, Meredith Buchberg, Libby Bogdan-Lovis, and Sean Philpott-Jones. 2016. "'She told them, oh that bitch got AIDS': Experiences of Multilevel HIV/AIDS-Related Stigma among African American Women Living with HIV/AIDS in the South." *AIDS Patient Care STDS* 30 (7): 349–356. doi: 10.1089/apc.2016 .0026.

Fletcher, Faith., Lucy A. Ingram, Jelani Kerr, Meredith Buchberg, Donna L. Richter, and Richard Sowell. 2016. "'Out of all of this mess, I got a blessing': Perceptions and Experiences of Reproduction and Motherhood in African American Women Living with HIV." *Journal of the Association of Nurses in AIDS Care* 27 (4): 381–391.

Fletcher, Faith, Wendy Jiang, and Alicia Best. 2021. "Anti-Racist Praxis in Public Health Research: A Call to Address Structural Racism through Ethical Engagement of Health Disparity Populations." *Hastings Center Report* 51 (2): 6–9.

Fletcher, Faith E., Whitney S. Rice, Lucy A. Ingram, and Celia B. Fisher. 2019. "Ethical Challenges and Lessons Learned from Qualitative Research with Low-Income African American Women Living with HIV in the South." *Journal of Health Care for the Poor and Underserved* 30 (4s): 116–129. doi: 10.1353/hpu.2019.0122.

Freire, P. 1970. *Pedagogy of the Oppressed*. New York: Seabury Press.

Gamble, Vanessa N. 1997. "Under the Shadow of Tuskegee: African Americans and Health Care." *American Journal of Public Health* 87 (11): 1773–1778. doi: 10.2105/ajph.87.11.1773.

Gee, Gilbert, and Chandra L. Ford. 2011. "Structural Racism and Health Inequities." *Du Bois Review* 8 (1): 1–18. doi: 10.1017oS1742058X11000130.

Gee, Gilbert, and Devon C. Payne-Sturges. 2004. "Environmental Health Disparities: A Framework Integrating Psychosocial and Environmental Concepts." *Environmental Health Perspectives* 112 (17): 1645–1653.

Gerstein, Josh, and Alexander Ward. 2022. "Supreme Court Has Voted to Overturn Abortion Rights, Draft Opinion Shows." Politico, May 2. Accessed May 30, 2022. https://www .politico.com/news/2022/05/02/supreme-court-abortion-draft-opinion-00029473.

Glanz, Karen, and Barbara K. Rimer. 2002. *Health Behavior and Health Education: Theory, Practice and Research*. 3rd ed. San Francisco: Jossey-Bass.

Goldenburg, Tamar, Sarah J. McDougal, Patrick S. Sullivan, Joanne D. Stekler, and Rob Stephenson. 2014. "Preferences for a Mobile HIV Prevention App for Men Who Have Sex with Men." *JMIR MHealth Uhealth* 2 (4): e47. doi: 10.2196/mhealth.3745.

Gomez, Anu, and Mikaela Wapman. 2017. "Under (Implicit) Pressure: Young Black and Latina Women's Perceptions of Contraceptive Care." *Contraception* 96 (4): 221–226. doi: 10.1016/j.contraception.2017.07.007.

Gonzalez Gladstein, Sonia K. 2017. "Acceptability Study and Pilot RCT of a Guide to Understanding Reproductive Health for Ladeez (Gurhl) Code: An HIV Risk Reduction APP Intervention for Black and Latina Young Women in New York City." PhD diss., City University of New York.

Goodwin, M. 2020. *Policing the Womb: Invisible Women and the Criminalization of Motherhood*. Cambridge: Cambridge University Press.

Guse, K., D. Levine, S. Martins, A. Lira, J. Gaarde, W. Westmorland, and M. Gilliam. 2012. "Interventions Using New Digital Media to Improve Adolescent Sexual Health: A Systematic Review." *Journal of Adolescent Health* 51 (6): 535–543.

Guttmacher Institute. 2022. "Insurance Coverage of Contraceptives." Last reviewed July 1, 2022. https://www.guttmacher.org/state-policy/explore/insurance-coverage-contraceptives.

Healing Hands Community Doula Project. N.d. "The International Center for Traditional Childbearing." https://blackdoulasblackmamas.org/resources/the-international-center-for-traditional-childbearing/.

Healthy People. 2022a. "Reproductive and Sexual Health." Last updated February 6, 2022. https://www.healthypeople.gov/2020/leading-health-indicators/2020-lhi-topics/Reproductive-and-Sexual-Health.

———. 2022b. "Using Law and Policy to Promote Breastfeeding in the United States." Healthy People.gov. Last updated February 6, 2022. https://www.healthypeople.gov/2020/law-and-health-policy/topic/maternal-infant-child-health.

Hoffman, Kelly, Sophie Trawalter, Jordan R. Axt, and M. Norman Oliver. 2016. "Racial Bias in Pain Assessment and Treatment Recommendation, and False Beliefs about Biological Differences between Blacks and Whites." *Proceedings of the National Academy of Sciences of the United States of America* 113 (16): 4296–4301. doi: 10.1073/pnas.1516047113.

In Our Voice: Black Women's Reproductive Justice Agenda. 2022. "Black Reproductive Justice Policy Agenda." https://blackrj.org/blackrjpolicy/.

Ingram, Lucy A., Chiwoneso Tinago, Bo Cai, Louisiana Wright Sanders, Tina Bevington, Sacoby Wilson, Kathryn M. Magruder, and Erik Svendsen. 2018. "Examining Long-Term Mental Health in a Rural Community Post-Disaster: A Mixed Methods Approach." *Journal of Health Care for the Poor and Underserved* 29 (1): 284–302.

Ingram, Lucy A., Chiwoneso Tinaco, Robin Estrada, Sacoby Wilson, Louisiana Wright Sanders, Tina Bevington, Bethany Carlos, Evangeline Cornelius, Erik Svendsen, and Julia Ball. 2016. "Off the Rails in Rural South Carolina: A Qualitative Study of Healthcare Provider Perspectives on the Long-Term Health Impact of the Graniteville Train Disaster." *Rural and Remote Health* 16 (3): 3906.

Ingram, Lucy A., Crystal Stafford, Quentin McCollum, and McKenzie Isreal. 2020. "African American Emerging Adult Perspectives on Unintended Pregnancy and Meeting Their Needs with Mobile Technology: Mixed Methods Qualitative Study." *JMIR mHealth and uHealth* 8 (10): article e21454. doi: 10.2196/21454.

Israel, Barbara A., Edith A. Parker, Zachary Rowe, Alicia Salvatore, Meredith Minkler, Jesús López, Arlene Butz, A. Mosely, L. Coates, et al. 2005. "Community-Based Participatory Research: Lessons Learned from the Centers for Children's Environmental Health and Disease Prevention REsearch." *Environmental Health Perspectives* 113 (10): 1463–1471. doi: 10.1289/ehp.7675.

Israel, Barbara A., Amy J. Shulz, Edith A. Parker, and Adam B. Becker. 1998. "Review of Community-Based Research: Assessing Partnership Approaches to Improve Public

Health." *Annual Review of Public Health* 19: 173–202. https://doi.org/10.1146/annurev .publhealth.19.1.173.

Israel, Barbara A., Amy J. Schulz, Edith A. Parker, Adam B. Becker, and J. R. Guzman. 2003. "Critical Issues in Developing and Following Community-Based Participatory Research Principles." In *Community-Based Participatory Research for Health*, ed. Meredith Minkler and Nina Wallerstein, 56–76. San Francisco: Jossey-Bass.

Jack, Katherine, and Sherry Glied. 2002. "The Public Costs of Mental Health Response: Lessons From the New York City Post–9/11 Needs Assessment." *Journal of Urban Health* 79 (3): 332–339.

Jackson, Dawnyea, Lucy A. Ingram, Cherrie B. Boyer, Alyssa G. Robillard, and Michael Huhns. 2016. "Can Technology Decrease Sexual Risk Behaviors among Young People? The Results of a Pilot Study Examining the Effectiveness of a Mobile Application Intervention." *American Journal of Sexuality Education* 11 (1): 41–60.

James, Delores C. S., and Cedric Harville 2nd. 2018. "Smartphone Usage, Social Media Engagement, and Willingness to Participate in mHealth Weight Management Research among African American Women." *Health Education & Behavior* 45 (3): 315–322. https:// doi.org/10.1177/1090198117714020.

James, Delores C., Cedric Harville 2nd, Cynthia Sears, Orisatalabi Efunbumi, and Irina Bondoc. 2017. "Participation of African Americans in e-Health and m-Health Studies: A Systematic Review." *Telemedicine Journal and e-Health* 23 (5): 351–364. doi: 10.1089/tmj .2016.0067.

James, Jennifer E. 2022. "Black Feminist Bioethics: Centering Community to Ask Better Questions." *Hastings Center Report* 52 (Suppl 1): S21–S23. doi: 10.1002/hast.1363.

Johnson, Angela, Rosalind Kirk, Katherine Lisa Rosenblum, and Maria Muzik. 2015. "Enhancing Breastfeeding Rates among African American Women: A Systematic Review of Current Psychosocial Interventions." *Breastfeeding Medicine* 10 (1): 45–62. doi: 10.1089 /bfm.2014.0023.

Jones, James H. 1981. *Bad Blood: The Tuskegee Syphilis Experiment*. New York: Free Press.

Jones, Rachel, Donald R. Hoover, and Lorraine J. Lacroix. 2013. "A Randomized Controlled Trial of Soap Opera Videos Streamed to Smartphones to Reduce Risk of Sexually Transmitted Human Immunodeficiency Virus (HIV) in Young Urban African American Women." *Nursing Outlook* 61 (4): 205–215.e.3. https://doi.org/10.1016/j.outlook.2013 .03.006.

Jones, Rachel, and Lorraine J. Lacroix. 2012. "Streaming Weekly Soap Opera Video Episodes to Smartphones in a Randomized Controlled Trial to Reduce HIV Risk in Young Urban African American / Black Women." *AIDS and Behavior* 16 (5): 1341–1358. doi: 10.1007 /s10461-012-0170-9.

Jones, Rhondette, and Kathleen Green. 2014. "A Peek into CDC's e-Learning Training Toolkit to Improve Adherence to Antiretroviral Treatment." Paper presented at the 9th International Conference on HIV Treatment and Prevention Adherence, Miami, FL, June 8–10. https://www.iapac.org/AdherenceConference/presentations/ADH9_OA473.pdf.

Kerr, Jelani, Kelsey Burton, Wangari Tharao, Nicole Greenspan, Liviana Calzavara, Orville Browne, Henry Luyombya, Keresa Arnold, Joanita Nakamwa, et al. 2021. "Examining

HIV-Related Stigma among African, Caribbean, and Black Church Congregants from the Black PRAISE study in Ontario, Canada." *AIDS Care* 33 (12)1636–1641. doi: 10.1080 /09540121.2021.1871723.

Kost, Kathryn. 2015. "Unintended Pregnancy Rates at the State Level: Estimates for 2010 and Trends since 2002." Guttmacher Institute, January. http://www.guttmacher.org /pubs/StateUP10.pdf.

Kozhimannil, Katy B., Laura B Attanasio, Judy Jou, Lauren K. Joarnt, Pamela J. Johnson, and Dwenda K. Gjerdingen. 2014. "Potential Benefits of Increased Access to Doula Support During Childbirth." *American Journal of Managed Care* 20, no. 8, e340–e352.

March of Dimes. 2022. "Low Birthweight by Race/Ethnicity: United States, 2018–2020 Average." March of Dimes Peristats. Accessed March 19, 2021. https://www.marchofdimes .org/Peristats/ViewSubtopic.aspx?reg=99&top=4&stop=45&lev=1&slev=1&obj=1.

Marseglia, Lucia, Sara Manti, Gabriella D'Angelo, Caterina Cuppari, Vincenzo Salpietro, Martina Filippelli, Antonio Trovato, Eloisa Gitto, Carmelo Salpietro, and Teresa Arrigo. 2015. "Obesity and Breastfeeding: The Strength of Association." *Women and Birth* 28 (2): 81–86. doi: 10.1016/j.wombi.2014.12.007.

Maryland State Doulas. N.d. "Insurance Reimbursement: Does My Insurance Cover a Doula?" https://www.marylandstatedoulas.com/blog/does-my-insurance-cover-a-doula.

Mathewson, Jaren J., Cheryl H. T. Chow, Kathleen G. Dobson, Eliza I. Pope, Louis A. Schmidt, and Ryan J. Van Lieshout. 2017. "Mental Health of Extremely Low Birth Weight Survivors: A Systematic Review and Meta-Analysis." *Psychological Bulletin* 143 (4): 347–383. doi: 10.1037/bul0000091.

McCabe, K., A. Hotton, A. B. Loyd, B. Floyd, G. Donenberg, and Faith E. Fletcher. 2022. "The Process of Adapting a Sexual Health Intervention for Black Early Adolescents: A Stakeholder Engagement Approach." *Health Education Research* 37 (1): 7–22. doi: 10.1093/her /cyab041.

McLeroy, Kenneth R., Daniel Bibeau, Allan Steckler, and Karen Glanz. 1988. "An Ecological Perspective on Health Promotion Programs." *Health Education Quarterly* 15 (4): 351–377. doi: 10.1177/109019818801500401.

Mills, Nicola, Gavin Daker-White, Anna Graham, and Rona Campbell. 2006. "Population Screening for Chlamydia Trachomatis Infection in the UK: A Qualitative Study of the Experiences of Those Screened." *Family Practice* 23 (5): 550–557. doi: 10.1093/fampra /cmlo31.

Mohatt, Nathaniel Vincent, Azure B. Thompson, Nghi D. Thai, and Jacob Kraemer Tebes. 2014. "Historical Trauma as a Public Narrative: A Conceptual Review of How History Impacts Present-Day Health." *Social Science & Medicine* 106: 128–136. doi: 10.1016/j .socscimed.2014.01.043.

Molina, Y., Karriem S. Watson, Liliana G. San Miguel, Karen Aguirre, Mariana Hernandez-Flores, Titiana B. Giraldo, Araceli Lucio, Nora Coronado, et al. 2019. "Integrating Multiple Community Perspectives in Intervention Development." *Health Education Research* 34 (4): 357–371.

Moore, Sarah. 2019. "Institute Index: Addressing the South's Maternal Mortality Crisis." Institute for Southern Studies. Facing South, June 4. https://www.facingsouth.org/2019 /06/institute-index-addressing-souths-maternal-mortality-crisis.

Morgan, David L. and Richard Krueger. 1997. *The Focus Group Kit*. Thousand Oaks, CA: SAGE Publishing. https://us.sagepub.com/en-us/nam/the-focus-group-kit/book6796.

Muessig, Kathryn, Manali Nekkanti, Jose Bauermeister, Sheana Bull, and Lisa B. Hightow-Weidman. 2015. "A Systematic Review of Recent Smartphone, Internet and Web 2.0 Interventions to Address the HIV Continuum of Care." *Current HIV/AIDS Reports* 12 (1): 173–190. doi: 10.1007/s11904-014-0239-3.

Muessig, Kathryn, Emily C. Pike, Beth Fowler, Sara LeGrand, Jeffrey T. Parsons, Sheana S. Bull, Patrick A. Wilson, David A. Wohl, and Lisa B. Hightow-Weidman. 2013. "Putting Prevention in Their Pockets: Developing Mobile Phone-Based HIV Interventions for Black Men Who Have Sex with Men." *AIDS Patient Care and STDs* 27 (4): 211–222. https://doi.org/10.1089/apc.2012.0404.

NEJM Catalyst. 2007. "What Is Patient-Centered Care?" NEJM Catalyst, January 1. https://catalyst.nejm.org/doi/full/10.1056/CAT.17.0559.

North, Carol, Barry A. Hong, Alina Suris, and Edward L. Spitznagel. 2008. "Distinguishing Distress and Psychopathology among Survivors of the Oakland/Berkeley Firestorm." *Psychiatry* 71 (1): 35–45. https://doi.org/10.1521/psyc.2008.71.1.35.

Nykiforuk, Candace I., Helen Vallianatos, and Laura M. Nieuwendyk. 2011. "Photovoice as a Method for Revealing Community Perceptions of the Built and Social Environment." *International Journal of Qualitative Methods* 10 (2): 103–124. doi: 10.1177/160940691101000201.

Office of Disease Prevention and Health Promotion. 2020. "Social Determinants of Health." HealthyPeople.gov. Last Modified February 6, 2022. https://www.healthypeople.gov/2020/topics-objectives/topic/social-determinants-of-health#:~:text=Social%20deter minants%20of%20health%20are%20conditions%20in%20the,of%20health%2C%20 functioning%2C%20and%20quality-of-life%20outcomes%20and%20risks.

Office of the Surgeon General, Centers for Disease Control and Prevention, and Office on Women's Health. 2011. "Barriers to Breastfeeding in the United States." https://www.ncbi.nlm.nih.gov/books/NBK52688/.

Owens, Deirdre Cooper, and Sharla M. Fett. 2019. "Black Maternal and Infant Health: Historical Legacies of Slavery." *American Journal of Public Health* 109 (10): 1342–1345. doi: 10.2105/AJPH.2019.305243.

Pennsylvania Department of Health. 2018. "Supporting Breastfeeding within African-American Communities: Evidence-Based and Research-Informed Practices." Pennsylvania Department of Health, Bureau of Family Health https://www.health.pa.gov/topics/Documents/Programs/Infant%20and%20Children%20Health/3-18_TA_Breast feeding_FINAL_Updated_BFH.pdf.

Perrin, Andrew, and Erica Turner. 2019. "Smartphones Help Blacks, Hispanics Bridge Some—but Not All—Digital Gaps with Whites." Pew Research Center, August 20. Accessed March 23, 2021. https://www.pewresearch.org/fact-tank/2019/08/20/smartphones-help-blacks-hispanics-bridge-some-but-not-all-digital-gaps-with-whites/.

Phelan, Jo C., Bruce G. Link, and Parisa Tehranifar. 2010. "Social Conditions as Fundamental Causes of Health Inequalities: Theory, Evidence, and Policy Implications." *Journal of Health and Social Behavior* 51 (1 suppl.). doi:10.1177/0022146510383498.

Phillips, Karran A., David H. Epstein, Mustapha Mezghanni, Massoud Vahabzadeh, David

Reamer, Daniel Agage, and Kenzie L. Preston. 2013. "Smartphone Delivery of Mobile HIV Risk Reduction Education." *AIDS Research and Treatment* 2013: article 231956. https://doi.org/10.1155/2013/231956.

Planned Parenthood. 2022. "Roe v. Wade at Risk: Nationwide Legal Abortion May Be a Thing of the Past." Accessed May 30, 2022. https://www.plannedparenthoodaction.org/issues/abortion/roe-v-wade.

Purdy, L. 2006. "Women's Reproductive Autonomy: Medicalisation and Beyond." *Journal of Medical Ethics* 32 (5): 287–291. doi: 10.1136/jme.2004.013193.

Restoring Our Own Through Transformation. N.d. "What We Do." https://www.roottrj.org/what-we-do-3.

Rice, Whitney S., Carmen H. Logie, Tessa M. Napoles, Melonie Walcott, Abigail W. Batchelder, Mirjam-Colette Kempf, Gina M. Wingood, Deborah J. Konkle-Parker, Bulent Turan, et al. 2018. "Perceptions of Intersectional Stigma among Diverse Women Living with HIV in the United States." *Social Science & Medicine* 208: 9–17. doi: 10.1016/j.socscimed.2018.05.001.

Rice, Whitney S., Bulent Turan, Faith E. Fletcher, Tessa M. Nápoles, Melonie Walcott, Abigail Batchelder, Mirjam-Colette Kempf, Deborah J. Konkle-Parker, Tracey E. Wilson, et al. 2019. "A Mixed Methods Study of Anticipated and Experienced Stigma in Health Care Settings Among Women Living with HIV in the United States." *AIDS Patient Care STDS* 33 (4): 184–195. doi: 10.1089/apc.2018.0282.

Rickert, James. 2012. "Patient-Centered Care: What It Means And How To Get There." Health Affairs, January 24. https://www.healthaffairs.org/do/10.1377/hblog20120124.016506/full/.

Roberts, D. 1997. *Killing the Black Body*. New York: Random House.

Rollins School of Public Health, Emory University. N.d. "The Center for Reproductive Health Research in the Southeast." https://rise.emory.edu/.

Rosenthal, Lisa, and Marci Lobel. 2016. "Stereotypes of Black American Women Related to Sexuality and Motherhood." *Psychology of Women Quarterly* 40 (3): 414–427. https://doi.org/10.1177/0361684315627459.

Ross, Jasmine, N. 2012. "Sexual Scripts and African American Women: Empirical Validation of Stephens and Phillips' (2003) Hip-Hop Sexual Scripting Model with African American College Women." PhD diss., University of Houston.

Ross, Loretta, and Rickie Solinger. 2017. *Reproductive Justice: An Introduction*. Oakland, CA: University of California Press.

Schnall, Rebecca, Jasmine Travers, Marlene Rojas, and Alex Carballo-Diéguez. 2014. "eHealth Interventions for HIV Prevention in High-Risk Men Who Have Sex with Men: A Systematic Review." *Journal of Medical Internet Research* 16 (5): e134. doi: 10.2196/jmir.3393.

Sederstrom, Nneka, and Tamika Lasege. 2022. "Anti-Black Racism as a Chronic Condition." *Hastings Center Report* 52 (Suppl 1): S24–S29. doi: 10.1002/hast.1364.

Segura-Pérez, Sofia, Amber Hromi-Fiedler, Misikir Adnew, Kate Nyhan, and Rafael Pérez-Escamilla. 2021 "Impact of Breastfeeding Interventions among United States Minority Women on Breastfeeding Outcomes: A Systematic Review." *International Journal for Equity in Health* 20: article 72. doi.org/10.1186/s12939-021-01388-4.

Shore, James H., Ellie L. Tatum, and William M. Vollmer. 1986. "Psychiatric Reactions to

Disaster: The Mount St. Helens Experience." *American Journal of Psychiatry* 143 (1): 590–595. https://doi.org/10.1176/ajp.143.5.590.

Simoni, Jane M., Bryan A. Kutner, and Keith J. Horvath. 2015. "Opportunities and Challenges of Digital Technology for HIV Treatment and Prevention." *Current HIV/AIDS Reports* 12 (4): 437–440. doi: 10.1007/s11904-015-0289-1.

Smith, Aaron. 2014. "African Americans and Technology Use: A Demographic Portrait." Pew Research Center, January 6. https://www.pewresearch.org/internet/2014/01/06/african-americans-and-technology-use/.

Spinelli, Margaret G., Jean Endicott, and Raymond R. Goetz. 2013. "Increased Breastfeeding Rates in Black Women after a Treatment Intervention." *Breastfeeding Medicine* 8 (6): 479–484. doi: 1089/bfm.2013.0051.

Steinberg, Allyna, Marybec Griffin-Tomas, Desiree Abu-Odeh, and Alzen Whitten. 2018. "Evaluation of a Mobile Phone App for Providing Adolescents with Sexual and Reproductive Health Information, New York City, 2013–2016." *Public Health Reports* 133 (3): 234–239. https://doi.org/10.1177/0033354918769289.

Taylor, Jamila, Christina Novoa, Katie Hamm, and Shilpa Phadke. 2019. "Eliminating Racial Disparities in Maternal and Infant Mortality: A Comprehensive Blueprint." Accessed March 14, 2021. https://www.americanprogress.org/issues/women/reports/2019/05/02/469186/eliminating-racial-disparities-maternal-infant-mortality/.

Thomas, Shameka P. 2022. "Trust Also Means Centering Black Women's Reproductive Health Narratives." *Hastings Center Report* 52 (Suppl 1): S18–S21. doi: 10.1002/hast.1362.

Thomas, Stephen B., and Sandra C. Quinn. 1991. "The Tuskegee Syphilis Study, 1932 to 1972: Implications for HIV Education and AIDS Risk Education Programs in the Black Community." *American Journal of Public Health* 81 (11). doi: 10.2105/ajph.81.11.1498.

Tufts, Kimberly A., Kaprea F. Johnson, Jewel G. Shepherd, Ju-Young Lee, Muna S. Bait Ajzoon, Lauren B. Mahan, and Miyong T. Kim. 2015. "Novel Interventions for HIV Self-Management in African American Women: A Systematic Review of mHealth Interventions." *Journal of the Association of Nurses in AIDS Care* 26 (2): 139–150. doi: 10.1016/j.jana.2014.08.002.

Turan, Janet M., Melissa A. Elafros, Carmen H. Logie, Swagata Banik, Bulent Turan, Kaylee B. Crockett, Bernice Pescosolido, and Sarah M. Murray. 2019. "Challenges and Opportunities in Examining and Addressing Intersectional Stigma and Health." *BMC Medicine* 17 (7): 1–15. https://doi.org/10.1186/s12916-018-1246-9.

Walcott, Melonie, Mirjam-Colette Kempf, Jessica S. Merlin, and Janet M. Turan. 2015. "Structural Community Factors and Sub-optimal Engagement in HIV Care among Low-Income Women in the Deep South of the USA." *Culture, Health, and Sexuality* 18, (6): 682–694. doi: 10.1080/13691058.2015.111025.

Wallerstein, N., and Bonnie Duran. 2010. "Community-Based Participatory Research Contributions to Intervention Research: The Intersection of Science and Practice to Improve Health Equity." *American Journal of Public Health* (April). doi:10.2105/AJPH.2009.184036.

Wang, Caroline C. 2006. "Youth Participation in Photovoice as a Strategy for Community Change." *Journal of Community Practice* 14 (1–2): 147–161.

Wang, Caroline C., and Mary Ann Burris. 1994. "Empowerment through Photo Novella: Portraits of Participation." *Health Education Quarterly* 21: 171–186.

———. 1997. "Photovoice: Concept, Methodology, and Use for Portraits of Participation." *Health Education & Behavior* 24: 369-387.

Wang, Caroline C., Susan Morrel-Samuels, Peter M. Hutchinson, Lee Bell, and Robert M. Pestronk. 2004. "Flint Photovoice: Community Building among Youths, Adults, and Policymakers." *American Journal of Public Health* 94 (6): 911–913. doi: 10.2105/ajph.94 .6.911.

Wang, Xiangdong, Lan Gao, Naotaka Shinfuku, Huabiao Zhang, Chengzhi Zhao, and Yucun Shen. 2000. "Longitudinal Study of Earthquake-Related PTSD in a Randomly Selected Community Sample in North China." *The American Journal of Psychiatry* 157 (8): 1260–1266.

Washington, Delesco A. 2011. "Examining the 'Stick' of Accreditation for Medical Schools through Reproductive Justice Lens: A Transformative Reproductive Lens: A Transformative Remedy for Teaching the Tuskegee Syphilis Study." *Florida A&M University College of Law Scholarly Commons* 26 (1): 153–195.

Washington, Harriet A. 2006. *Medical Apartheid: The Dark History of Medical Experimentation on Black Americans from Colonial Times to the Present*. New York: Harlem Moon Broadway Books.

Watkins-Hayes, Celeste. 2014. "Intersectionality and the Sociology of HIV/AIDS: Past, Present, and Future Research Directions." *Annual Review of Sociology* 7 (40): 431–457. doi: 10.1146/ annurevsoc-071312-14562.

White, Kari, and Whitney Rice. 2022. "Abortion Deserts Could Come with Supreme Court's Next Case." *The Hill*, May 30, 2022. https://thehill.com/opinion/civil-rights/556119 -abortion-deserts-could-come-with-supreme-courts-next-case/.

Wilson, Yolanda. 2022. "Is Trust Enough? Anti-Black Racism and the Perception of Black Vaccine 'Hesitancy.'" *Hastings Center Report* 52 (Suppl 1):S12–S17. doi: 10.1002/hast.1361.

Woodard, J. B., and T. Mastin. 2005. "Black Womanhood: Essence and Its Treatment of Stereotypical Images of Black Women." *Journal of Black Studies* 36: 264–281. https://doi .org/10.1177/0021934704273152.

World Health Organization. 2010. "International Statistical Classification of Diseases and Related Health Problems." *ICD–10* 2. World Health Organization.

———. 2020. "Sexual Health." World Health Organization. Accessed March 7, 2021. https:// www.who.int/health-topics/sexual-health#tab=tab_1.

Yuan, Nicole P., Brian M. Mayer, Lorencita Joshweseoma, Dominic Clichee, and Nicolette I. Teufel-Shone. 2020. "Development of Guidelines to Improve the Effectiveness of Community Advisory Boards in Health Research." *Progress in Community Health Partnerships: Research, Education, and Action* 14 (2): 259–269. doi10.1353/cpr.2020.0026.

18

Infant Mortality

PAUL C. MANN, MD

> The mean rates of infant mortality are, roughly speaking, something like twice as high for the colored population as for the white population in each of the demographic units considered, and at all times. This, again, is a fact in general well known, but here we have precise figures on the point, with probable errors, which show definitely how tremendously poorer the negro baby's chances of surviving the first year of life are than the white baby's.

Raymond Pearl, 1921[1]

It has been recognized for over a century that African American (hereafter Black) infants have higher infant mortality rates than infants of all other races and ethnicities.[1] Although the causes of those disparities have changed over time, one thing has remained consistent decade after decade: the mortality rate for Black infants is roughly double that of their white counterparts. This chapter explores causal factors for divergent outcomes related to infant mortality with a focus on unique drivers of Black infant mortality in the southern United States.

Historical Infant Mortality for Black Infants

Modern attempts to quantify infant mortality in the West first began in the seventeenth century, when the infant mortality rate (IMR) was defined as the number of deaths of young children under the age of 1 per 1,000 live births. This definition began to gain acceptance in the 1880s.[2] The IMR has long been recognized to be substantially impacted by socioeconomic status; poverty is a major contributor.[3] British Minister of Health Arthur Newsholme noted in 1911 that "infant mortality is the most sensitive index we possess of sanitary administration and of social welfare."[4]

In the antebellum South, it is estimated that the IMR of enslaved infants was about 2.5 times that of white infants.[5] Seasonal variations in the nutritional status of mothers, exposure to infectious diseases (e.g., malaria), grueling work expectations throughout pregnancy, and limited access to medical care resulted in excessive numbers of stillborn infants or infants born with very low birth weight. Historical records from cotton, rice, and sugar plantations in South Carolina, Georgia, Alabama, and Louisiana show estimated ranges of Black infant mortality from 176 to a staggering 392 deaths per 1,000 live births.[5]

After the Thirteenth Amendment in 1865 outlawed slavery in the United States, significant health disparities remained between Black and white infants. Although vital statistics did not became available for all 48 states until 1933, records from North Carolina, South Carolina, and New York for the period 1895 to 1940 provide some insights into trends for infant mortality of Black infants during that time period.[6] They reveal a rapid decline in infant mortality for Black infants in New York from 235 deaths per thousand live births in 1900 to 56 in 1940. North Carolina and South Carolina, by comparison, started with a lower IMR (165 per thousand in 1900) but had slower rates of decline to 74 and 86 per thousand by 1940.[6] The more substantive decline in mortality among Black infants in New York State was likely the result of improvements in urban living conditions for Black families; significant advances were made in sanitation during that time period. The more rural southern States lagged behind in decreases in Black infant mortality in part due to disparities in access to health care. Data from Mississippi in 1921 reflects this inequity: 33% of white women received prenatal care and 79% were attended by a physician at delivery, compared to 12% of Black women who received prenatal care and only 8% who were delivered by a physician.[6]

The IMR in the United States has consistently lagged behind those of its industrialized peers. One of the earliest reports to compare international IMRs was written by Newmayer in 1911.[7] The US rate, 165 deaths per 1000 live births, ranked 18th out of the 31 countries listed. The US rate was more the double that of the leader at that time, New Zealand, which reported 76 deaths per 1,000 live births. Notably, even at that time, the value of organized and practical public health interventions, such as home visits by nurses in at-risk communities and educational campaigns encouraging breastfeeding, were recognized to have substantial benefits in reducing infant mortality.[7]

Current Drivers of Excessive Black Infant Mortality

Although US infant mortality decreased 71% from 1961 to 2010, it remains a significant public health concern.[8] Despite higher overall per capita spending on health care for children than in other wealthy developed nations, infants in the United States have a 76% greater risk of death than infants in other developed countries.[8] The United States currently ranks 54th out of 228 countries for IMR. In 2018, the US IMR was reported at 5.67 infant deaths per 1,000 live births, a rate three times that of the world leader, Slovenia (1.7 deaths per 1,000 live births).[9] The IMR in southern states is substantially higher than the US average. Mississippi has the highest rate (8.41 per 1,000), followed by Louisiana and Arkansas.[9] Compared to other regions of the United States, there are 1.18 excess infant deaths per 1,000 live births in the South, representing 1,600 additional infant deaths each year. (Excess deaths are defined by comparing IMR for southern region states to IMR for other US regions combined.)[10] Congenital malformations are the leading cause of infant mortality in the United States (representing 21% of infant deaths) followed by premature birth/low birth weight (17%), sudden infant death syndrome (SIDS, 6%), maternal complications (6%), and unintentional injuries/accidents (5%).[9] Excess infant mortality in the South is principally driven by higher rates of premature birth and sudden unexpected infant deaths (SUIDs, a term used to describe sudden and unexplained deaths of babies less than 1 year old, which includes SIDS as a cause).[10]

The IMR for Black infants (10.75 per 1,000) remains over twice that of white (4.63 per 1,000), Asian (3.63 per 1,000), and Hispanic infants (4.86 per 1,000).[9] While Black births account for 15.9% of total US births, they represent 29.5% of all US infant deaths.[11] Issues related to premature birth and SUID account for the largest share of excess infant mortality rates for Black infants.[12] Premature birth rates for Black women are 50% higher than for white mothers, and Black infants are four times more likely to die as a result of premature birth than white infants. They are also twice as likely as white infants to die from SIDS and unintentional injuries.[9]

Southern states demonstrate substantial variability in Black infant mortality rates. For example, in the period 2013–2015, Alabama (13.40 per 1,000) reported a rate significantly higher than the national average, while South

Carolina (10.52 per 1,000) reported a rate that was near or below the national average.[13] However, midwestern states currently report the highest Black infant mortality rates: Wisconsin (14.28 per 1,000) and Ohio (13.42 per 1,000) lead the nation in Black infant mortality.[13] Much of this interstate variability in infant mortality rates is driven by rates of extremely premature birth, which are closely related to proportions of Black births.[14]

In recent years, many southern states have reported significant progress in reducing infant mortality for Black infants and decreasing the gap between Black and white infant mortality. Speights et al. found that thirteen states, including Tennessee, Georgia, and South Carolina, achieved statistically significant reductions in overall Black infant mortality in the period 2000 to 2012.[15] Other states, including Alabama and Mississippi, demonstrated statistically significant reductions in the mortality gap between Black and white infants. The study projected that if the current rate of change were to continue, Tennessee could achieve equal infant mortality rates between Black and white infants by 2034 but that mortality gaps would continue for a century or longer in Florida (equity projected by the year 2213) and North Carolina (equity projected by the year 2130).[15]

Elder et al. examined how both explainable factors (e.g. maternal education, age, and marital status and geographic location by state) and unexplainable or unmeasured factors impacted the IMR gap between Black and white infants over a two-decade period (1983–2004).[16] While they found overall declines in the mortality gap between Black and white infants, they reported that socioeconomic and other explainable risk factors became less predictive of IMR over time and that the IMR gap attributable to unexplainable factors was largely unchanged over time. By 2004, unexplainable factors contributed to the majority of the mortality gap in outcomes between Black and white infants and was specifically concentrated among infants who weighed less than 1,000 grams (2.2 pounds) at birth. The authors noted discouragement with these study results because due to the persistent and sizable gap in infant mortality resulting from unexplainable factors, even a complete elimination of the explained gap in Black and white IMRs would reduce the IMR gap by only 25%.[16]

Two-thirds of racial gaps in IMR can be explained by differences in the incidence of and outcomes for Black infants born with very low birth weight (birth weight < 1,500 grams, or 3.3 pounds).[17] A recent publication by Horbar et al. investigated inequities between mortality outcomes for Black infants who weighed less than 1,500 grams at birth and/or were born before 30 weeks gestational age and infants of other racial backgrounds.[18] Using a large database of 743 neonatal intensive care units (NICUs) in the Vermont Oxford Network, that study provided evidence for racial segregation in NICUs across the United States. Horbar and colleagues found that Black infants were most likely to receive medical treatment at lower-quality NICUs after accounting for region of residence. Additionally, there was substantial variability in NICU quality by region; 76% of Black infants were cared for in NICUs in regions with the lowest scores for quality of care. Those regions included all of the southern states.[18]

Survival in the first week of life for infants born extremely premature is significantly impacted by birth hospital. There is substantial variability in approaches to clinical management in birth hospitals that can prejudice morbidity and mortality outcomes for infants at the edges of viability (i.e., 22–24 weeks gestational age).[11,19] Some hospitals and providers choose not to offer neonatal resuscitation for periviable infants or limit interventions that can improve survival and reduce morbidity. Major differences also exist in how parents are counseled antenatally about outcomes for periviable infants that influence their decisions to give consent for interventions (e.g., endotracheal intubation and mechanical ventilation) that may be clinically indicated and beneficial for their baby. A study of 25 leading US academic neonatology centers showed that reductions in racial disparities for certain quality-of-care metrics for Black infants born extremely premature improved over time from 2002 to 2016.[11] Black infants were purported to benefit most from quality improvement initiatives enacted during the study period, as evidenced by increases in practices associated with improved survival, decreases in rates of late-onset sepsis, and lower rates of neurodevelopmental impairments (e.g., using steroids before delivery, performing cesarean sections when indicated).[11] A comparable study by Boghossian et al. reported similar reductions in gaps in quality of care between minority and white infants in the period 2006–2017, again highlighting that quality improvement initiatives in health systems play a crucial role in improving survival rates and reducing complications for Black infants.[19]

Disease-specific racial differences persist among infants born extremely premature, however.[19,20] Black and Hispanic infants in one recent large national database study had higher rates of necrotizing enterocolitis and higher mortality from necrotizing enterocolitis (a significant bowel infection associated with premature birth) after adjusting for both patient and clinical factors.[20] That finding confirmed previous studies showing that Black infants are four times more likely to develop necrotizing enterocolitis than white infants.[21] Black infants have also been shown to have a higher incidence of serious intraventricular hemorrhages, a type of brain bleeding that affects premature infants and can result in severe neurodevelopmental impairments.[19]

In the post-neonatal period (i.e., 29 days of life to 1 year of age), SUIDs and SIDS are the most prevalent cause of infant mortality. Racial disparities in SUID persist; the rate of SUID for Black and American Indian/Alaska Native infants is double that of white infants.[22] SUID rates began to decrease rapidly in 1994 following introduction of the Back to Sleep campaign in the United States, which encouraged a supine sleep position for all infants. Although little has changed at a national level since 1999, SUID rates for Black infants continued to decrease significantly from 1995 to 2013, highlighting the fact that a public health campaign had had substantial and unique benefits for Black infants. Substantial geographic variability exists in rates of SUID. Two regional areas, Alaska and the South (especially Arkansas, Mississippi, and Texas), have significantly higher rates of SUID than the rest of the nation.[23] In addition, SUID rates also remain higher in rural areas of the United States.

Addressing Excess Black Infant Mortality

Structural Inequities

Race is increasingly regarded as a social rather than a genetic construct. Economic and cultural processes have adversely impacted historically disadvantaged populations in multifaceted ways.[17] Societal and systemic racism are believed to contribute to physiological stress for Black women and to lead to higher rates of both maternal and infant mortality.[24] While numerous socioeconomic factors are known to impact women's risk for premature birth, including maternal age, short intervals between pregnancies, and substance abuse, racial disparities for birth outcomes persist for Black women even as socioeconomic and health status improves.[17] One study that examined racial differences in IMR found that compared to college-educated white mothers, college-educated Black mothers had twice the incidence of low-birth-weight deliveries and higher mortality rates for their babies.[25]

A life course conceptual framework that Lu and Halfon proposed to explain disparities in birth outcomes hypothesizes that racial differences re-sult from a combination of the impacts of deleterious early-life (in-utero) epigenetic programming and the cumulative physiological impacts of social inequity on reproduction known as weathering.[26] Weathering drives the pre-mature aging of African American women over time due to a multitude of contextual factors that include challenges in accessing health care, exposures to environmental stress and racism, pollution, high-risk behaviors, and fi-nancial insecurity and negatively impacts their pregnancy outcomes.[17]

Racial concordance between physicians and patients has been suggested as a possible strategy for addressing Black-white infant and maternal mortal-ity gaps. A notable study by Greenwood et al. that examined the outcomes of 1.8 million hospital births in the state of Florida in the period 1992–2015 showed that gaps in Black and white IMRs were reduced by 50% when the infants were cared for by Black providers.[27] The benefit of lower mortality increased as the complexity of medical care required by the infant increased. The authors hypothesized that minority physicians might be more aware of unique challenges Black infants and their parents face and are therefore bet-ter equipped to treat their complex needs. Importantly, 29% of neonatolo-gists in the South are from underrepresented minority backgrounds, a much higher percentage than any other region of the country.[28] Although Green-wood et al.'s study[27] did not show that mortality benefits extended to Black mothers cared for by Black providers, other studies of racially concordant providers for Black mothers have shown substantial reductions in Black-white disparities in premature birth rates and low birth weight when Black women have Black caregivers during pregnancy.[29] It is essential, therefore, to continue to attract and retain a racially, ethnically, and linguistically diverse health care workforce that is best able to meet the needs of all patients.

Disparities in Access to Health Care

In every county of the contiguous United States, the Black IMR is higher than the white IMR.[30] Ninety-three percent of US counties have per-sistent or worsening disparities for low-birth-weight between Black and white infants.[31] Structural racism, which one study characterized as population-level racial inequities in educational attainment, median household income, and rates of jail incarceration, has been shown to have divergent racial im-pacts on IMR; it increases Black IMR by 6% and decreases white IMR by 6%.[32] In an attempt to explain factors that are protective against Black IMR, a 2020 study by Kandasamy et al. looked at the differential impacts of social, economic and health variations by US region.[33] The authors found three specific factors that reduced Black IMR; higher state-level rates of Black-white marriages (which the authors interpreted as an indicator of better interracial integration), higher maternal and child health budgets per capita, and higher values on the index of concentration at the extremes (a variable that measures economic polarization based on household income and unemployment rates).[33]

In the South, almost all counties with a high IMR for Black infants also have a high IMR for white infants. The disparity between Black and white IMRs is greatest in the mid-Atlantic region and parts of Florida.[30] Rossen et al. have shown that the substantial county-by-county variability in Black IMR is driven by unknown factors that are unique to Black infants (which they hypothesized include area-level poverty, access to perinatal care, and social determinants of health) and that Black infants shared only 24% of causal factors for infant mortality with white infants.[30]

In the United States overall, about 7% of infant mortality is attributable to differences in urbanization.[12] The Black IMR in rural areas is nearly 25% higher than the Black IMR in urban areas.[32] The excess mortality rate for Black infants in rural areas is mostly attributable to premature birth/low birth weight and SUID.[12] Vilda et al. have shown that structural racism impacts urban Black IMRs more than rural Black IMRs. They felt that this finding was worthy of addition investigation because rural southern and predominantly Black communities have historically incurred disproportionate impacts of environmental injustices, including exposures to potentially toxic industrial chemicals.[32]

Because rural counties overall have the highest IMR rates in the United States, a better understanding of the disparate impacts of IMR on those communities is needed.[12,34] IMR differences between urban and rural counties are principally driven by higher rates of post-neonatal mortality resulting from higher rates of congenital malformations and SUID.[12,34] Ehrenthal et al. found that urban-rural disparities in overall IMR were linked to socioeconomic disadvantages in rural areas rather than inequities in access to obstetrical services and NICU care, although their study had notable limitations that included the fact that significant data was missing data from Georgia and other states.[34] Further investigation is needed to determine whether those findings reflect successes for perinatal regionalization (e.g., critical access systems in place to ensure that all mothers and infants have access to higher levels of medical care if needed) in rural areas or challenges in data collection for birth outcomes in rural areas.[34]

Because many Black mothers lack health insurance coverage, they may choose to forgo routine prenatal care despite its known health benefits. Improving access to and acceptance of prenatal care is critically important in addressing Black infant mortality, as clinical interventions are available for pregnancies threatened by premature birth.[35] One recent study highlighting decreases in infant mortality potentially attributable to advances in obstetrical care showed that benefits were more substantial for white mothers (who experienced a 48% decrease in infant mortality) than for Black mothers (who experienced only a 31% decrease in infant mortality).[35] Unfortunately, disparities in prenatal care for Black mothers may increase if current trends in access to health care continue. Hospitals in rural areas continue to close at alarming rates; 45% of rural US counties now lack obstetrical services.[36]

The 2010 Patient Protection and Affordable Care Act provided an opportunity for states to expand Medicaid eligibility and close gaps in insurance coverage for pregnant woman and children. Notably, states that adopted Medicaid expansion beginning in 2014 saw reductions in infant mortality, whereas states that did not adopt Medicaid expansion had increases in infant mortality.[37] There is considerable evidence that Black infants benefited most from Medicaid expansion. One study found that states that adopted expansion experienced a 14.5% decrease in Black infant mortality while states that did not adopt expansion experienced only a 6.6% decrease.[37] Another study showed that in states that adopted Medicaid expansion, health disparities between Black and white infants decreased in rates of preterm birth and low birth weight.[38] However, the vast majority of southern states, with the notable exceptions of Arkansas and Louisiana, have not adopted Medicaid expansion. Other government expenditures that have been shown to reduce IMR include increased spending on public health, housing, parks and recreation, and solid waste management.[39]

Addressing Quality

Reductions in the Black-white infant mortality gap will not occur without addressing disparities in the quality of neonatal intensive care. Research to understand how individual provider and institutional attitudes impact NICU care is critically important, as are investigations into technological and staffing disparities (e.g., patient-to-nurse ratio) that may be impacting the quality of care and infant mortality.[18] One nationwide hospital survey of NICU nurses revealed that institutions with higher percentages of Black infants in their units had higher levels of infections, lower levels of maternal breast milk utilization, and more severe nursing staffing shortages.[41] Widespread variability across states exist regarding oversight of levels of NICU care, financial incentives to provide high-quality care, and reimbursement for neonatal intensive care, including financial support for hospitals for neonatal and maternal transportation when a higher level of care is medically necessary.[18]

Interventions to improve the quality of care are also needed to address clinical challenges in the way women's health is optimized in general. Health care for women is separated into reproductive care, which obstetricians and gynecologists provide, and "other" medical care, which internists and family practitioners provide.[40] This lack of comprehensive health care creates gaps in care continuity and fails to address underlying health conditions that can impact pregnancy outcomes for Black mothers, thus increasing the Black IMR.

Conclusions

Racial disparities in Black infant mortality are not inevitable in the United States or in the southern United States specifically. They result from a multitude of complicated factors including state-level variability in public health expenditures, disparities in access to health care, and socioeconomic disadvantages. Much of the Black-white disparity in infant mortality in the southern United States could be impacted by specific efforts to reduce premature birth rates and address differences in quality of care for low-birthweight Black infants and by targeted public health expenditures aimed at further reducing the incidence of SUIDs.

REFERENCES

1. Pearl, Raymond. "Biometric Data on Infant Mortality in the United States Birth Registration Area, 1915–1918." *Am J Epidemiol* 1, no. 4 (1921): 419–439. https://doi.org/10.1093/oxfordjournals.aje.a118046.

2. Brosco, Jeffrey P. "The Early History of the Infant Mortality Rate in America: 'A Reflection upon the Past and Prophecy of the Future.'" *Pediatrics* 103, no. 2 (1999): 478–485. https://doi.org/10.1542/peds.103.2.478.

3. Woodbury, Robert Morse. "Economic Factors in Infant Mortality." *J Am Stat Assoc* 19, no. 146 (1924):137–155. https://doi.org/10.2307/2277226.

4. Newsholme, A. *Thirty-Ninth Annual Report, 1909–1910. Supplement to the Report of the Board's Medical Officer, Containing a Report on Infant and Child Mortality.* London, UK: Local Government Board, 1911.

5. Steckel, Richard H. "A Dreadful Childhood: The Excess Mortality of American Slaves." *Soc Sci Hist* 10, no. 4 (1986):427–465. https://doi.org/10.1017/S0145553200015571.

6. Ewbank, Douglas C. "History of Black Mortality and Health before 1940." *Millbank Q* 65, no. 1 (1987): 100–129. https://doi.org/10.2307/3349953.

7. Newmayer, S. W. "The Warfare against Infant Mortality." *Ann Am Acad of Political Soc Sci* 37, no. 2 (1911): 288–298. https://doi.org/10.1177/000271621103700224.

8. Thakrar, Ashish P., Alexandra D. Forrest, Mitchell G. Maltenfort, and Christopher B. Forrest. "Child Mortality in the US and 19 OECD Comparator Nations: A 50-Year Time-Trend Analysis." *Health Aff (Millwood)* 37, no. 1 (2018): 140–149. https://doi.org/10.1377/hlthaff.2017.0767.

9. Ely, Danielle M., and Anne K. Driscoll. "Infant Mortality in the United States, 2018: Data from the Period Linked Birth / Infant Death File." *Natl Vital Stat Rep* 69, no. 7 (2020): 1–18. Accessed April 5, 2021. https://www.cdc.gov/nchs/data/nvsr/nvsr69/NVSR-69-7-508.pdf.

10. Hirai, Ashley H., William M. Sappenfield, Michael D. Kogan, Wanda D. Barfield, David A. Goodman, Reem M. Ghandour, and Michael C. Lu. "Contributors to Excess Infant Mortality in the U.S. South." *Am J Prev Med* 46, no. 3 (2014): 219–227. https://doi.org/10.1016/j.amepre.2013.12.006.

11. Travers, Colm P., Waldemar A. Carlo, Scott A. McDonald, Abhik Das, Namasivayam Ambalavanan, Edward F. Bell, Pablo J. Sánchez, Barbara J. Stoll, Myra H. Wyckoff, et al. "Racial/Ethnic Disparities among Extremely Preterm Infants in the United States from 2002 to 2016." *JAMA Netw Open* 3, no. 6 (2020): e206757. https://doi.org/10.1001/jamanetworkopen.2020.6757.

12. Womack, Lindsay S., Lauren M. Rossen, and Ashley H. Hirai. "Urban-Rural Infant Mortality Disparities by Race and Ethnicity and Cause of Death." *Am J Prev Med* 58, no. 2 (2020): 254–260. https://doi.org/10.1016/j.amepre.2019.09.010.

13. Matthews, T. J., Danielle M. Ely, and Anne K. Driscoll. "State Variations in Infant Mortality by Race and Hispanic Origin of Mother, 2013–2015." *NCHS Data Brief* 295, nos. 1–6 (2018). Accessed April 6, 2021. https://www.cdc.gov/nchs/data/databriefs/db295.pdf.

14. Travers, Colm P., Luke A. Iannuzzi, Martha S. Wingate, Daniel M. Avery, Namasivayam Ambalavanan, James Leeper, and Waldermar A. Carlo. "Prematurity and Race Account for Much of the Interstate Variation in Infant Mortality Rates in the United States." *J Perinatol* 40, no. 5 (2020): 767–773. https://doi.org/10.1038/s41372-020-0640-2.

15. Speights, Joedrecka S. Brown, Samantha Sittig Goldfarb, Brittny A. Wells, Leslie Beitsch, Robert S. Levine, and George Rust. "State-Level Progress in Reducing the Black-White Infant Mortality Gap, United States, 1999–2013." *Am J Public Health* 107, no. 5 (2017): 775–782. https://doi.org/10.2105/AJPH.2017.303689.

16. Elder, Todd E., John H. Goddeeris, Steven J. Haider, and Nigel Paneth. "The Chang-

ing Character of the Black-White Infant Mortality Gap, 1983–2004." *Am J Public Health* 104, no. S1 (2014): S105–S111. https://doi.org/10.2105/AJPH.2013.301349.

17. Matoba, Nana, and James W. Collins. "Racial Disparity in Infant Mortality." *Semin Perinatol* 41, no. 6 (2017): 354–359. https://doi.org/10.1053/j.semperi.2017.07.003.

18. Horbar, Jeffrey D., Erika M. Edwards, Lucy T. Greenberg, Jochen Profit, David Draper, Daniel Helkey, Scott A. Lorch, Henry C. Lee, Ciaran S. Phibbs, Jeannette Rogowski, Jeffrey B. Gould, and Glenn Firebaugh. "Racial Segregation and Inequality in the Neonatal Intensive Care Unit for Very Low-Birth-Weight and Very Preterm Infants." *JAMA Peds* 173, no. 5 (2019): 455–461. https://doi.org/10.1001/jamapediatrics.2019.0241.

19. Boghossian, Nansi S., Marco Geraci, Scott A. Lorch, Ciaran S. Phibbs, Erika M. Edwards, and Jeffrey D. Horbar. "Racial and Ethics Differences over Time in Outcomes of Infants Born Less than 30 Weeks Gestation." *Pediatrics* 144, no. 3 (2019): e20191106. https://doi.org/10.1542/peds.2019-1106.

20. Jammeh, Momodou L., Obinna O. Abide, Elisabeth T. Tracy, Henry E. Rice, Reese H. Clark, P. Brian Smith, and Rachel G. Greenberg. "Racial/Ethnic Differences in Necrotizing Enterocolitis Incidence and Outcomes in Premature Very Low Birth Weight Infants." *J Perinatol* 38, no. 10 (2018): 1386–1390. https://doi.org/10.1038/s41372-018-0184-x.

21. Llanos, Adofo R., Moss, Mark E., Pinzòn, Timothy Dye, Robert A. Sinkin, and James W. Kendig. "Epidemiology of Neonatal Necrotizing Enterocolitis: A Population-Based Study." *Paediatr Perinat Epidemiol* 16, no. 4 (2002): 342–349. https://doi.org/10.1046/j.1365-3016.2002.00445.X.

22. Parks, Sharyn E., Alexa B. Erck Lambert, and Carrie K. Shapiro-Mendoza. "Racial and Ethnic Trends in Sudden Unexpected Infant Deaths: United States, 1995–2013." *Pediatrics* 139, no. 6 (2017): e20163844. https://doi.org/10.1542/peds.2016-3844.

23. Mitchell, Edwin A., Xiaohan Yan, Shirley You Ren, Tatiana M. Anderson, Jan-Marino Ramirez, Juan M. Lavista Ferres, and Richard Johnston. "Geographic Variation in Sudden Unexpected Infant Death in the United States." *J Pediatr* 220, no. 1 (2020): 49–55. https://doi.org/10.1016/j.jpeds.2020.01.006.

24. Villarosa, Linda. "Why America's Black Mothers and Babies Are in a Life-or-Death Crisis." *New York Times Magazine*, April 11, 2018. Accessed 12/21/2020. https://nyti.ms/2GRP4if.

25. Schoendorf, Kenneth C., Carol J. R. Hogue, Joel C. Kleinman, and Diane Rowley. "Mortality among Infants of Black as Compared with White College-Educated Parents." *NEJM* 326, no. 23 (1992): 1522–1526. https://doi.org/10.1056/NEJM199206043262303.

26. Lu, Michael C., and Neal Halfon. "Racial and Ethnic Disparities in Birth Outcomes: A Life-Course Perspective." *Matern Child Health J* 7, no. 1 (2003): 13–30. https://doi.org/10.1023/A:1022537516969.

27. Greenwood, Brad N., Rachel R. Hardeman, Laura Huang, and Aaron Sojourner. "Physician-Patient Racial Concordance and Disparities in Birth Mortality for Newborns." *Proc Natl Acad Sci USA* 117, no. 35 (2020): 21194–21200. https://doi.org/10.1073/pnas.1913405117.

28. Horowitz, Eric, Mihail Samnaliev, and Renate Savich. "Seeking Racial and Ethnic Equity among Neonatologists." *J Perinatol* 41, no. 3 (2021): 422–434. https://doi.org/10.1038/s41372-021-00915-z.

29. Visionary Vanguard Group, Inc. "The JJ Way®: Community-Based Maternity Center, Final Evaluation Report." Accessed June 29, 2021. [Winter Garden, FL]: Commonsense Childbirth, Inc., 2017. https://perinataltaskforce.com/wp-content/uploads/2021/06/The-JJ-Way%C2%AE-Community-based-Maternity-Center-Evaluation-min.pdf.

30. Rossen, Lauren M., Diba Khan, and Kenneth C. Schoendorf. "Mapping Geographic Variation in Infant Mortality and Related Black-White Disparities in the US." *Epidemiology* 27, no. 5 (2016): 690–696. https://doi.org/10.1097/EDE.0000000000000509.

31. Goldfarb, Samantha S., Kelsey Houser, Brittny A. Wells, Joedrecka S. Brown Speights, Les Beitsch, and George Rust. "Pockets of Progress amidst Persistent Racial Disparities in Low Birthweight Rates." *PLOS One* 13, no. 7 (2018): e0201658. https://doi.org/10.1371/journal.pone.0201658.

32. Vilda, Dovile, Rachel Hardeman, Lauren Dyer, Katherine P. Theall, and Maeve Wallace. "Structural Racism, Racial Inequities and Urban-Rural Differences in Infant Mortality in the US." *J Epidemiol Community Health* 0 (2021): 1–6. https://doi.org/10.1136/jech-2020-214260.

33. Kandasamy, Veni, Ashley H. Hirai, Jay S. Kaufman, Arthur R. James, and Milton Kotelchuck. "Regional Variation in Black Infant Mortality: The Contribution of Contextual Factors." *PLOS One* 15, no. 8 (2020): e0237314. https://doi.org/10.1371/journal.pone.0237314.

34. Ehrenthal, Deborah B., Daphne Kuo Hsiang-Hui, and Russell S. Kirby. "Infant Mortality in Rural and Nonrural Counties in the United States." *Pediatrics* 146, no. 5 (2020): e2020464. https://doi.org/10.1542/peds.2020-0464.

35. Callaghan, William M., Marian F. Macdorman, Carrie K. Shapiro-Mendoza, and Wanda D. Barfield. "Explaining the Recent Decrease in US Infant Mortality Rate, 2007–2013." *Am J Obstet Gynecol* 216, no. 1 (2017): 73.e1–73.e8. https://doi.org/10.1016/j.ajog.2016.09.097.

36. Hung, Peiyin, Carrie E. Henning-Smith, Michelle M. Casey, and Katy B. Kozhimannil. "Access to Obstetric Services in Rural Counties Is Still Declining, with 9 Percent Losing Services, 2000–14." *Health Aff (Millwood)* 36, no. 9 (2017): 1663–1671. https://doi.org/10.1377/hlthaff.2017.0338.

37. Bhatt, Chintan B., and Consuelo Beck-Sagué. "Medicaid Expansion and Infant Mortality in the United States." *Am J Public Health* 108, no. 4 (2018): 565–567. https://doi.org/10.2105/AJPH.2017.304218.

38. Brown, Clare C., Jennifer E. Moore, Holly C. Felix, Kathryn Stewart, T. Mac Bird, Curtis L. Lowery, and J. Mick Tilford. "Association of State Medicaid Expansion Status with Low Birth Weight and Preterm Birth." *JAMA* 321, no. 16 (2019): 1598–1609. https://doi.org/10.1001/jama.2019.3678.

39. Goldstein, Neil D., Aimee J. Palumbo, Scarlett L. Bellamy, Jonathan Purtle, and Robert Locke. "State and Local Government Expenditures and Infant Mortality in the United States." *Pediatrics* 146, no. 5 (2020): e20201134. https://doi.org/10.1542/peds.2020-1134.

40. McCloskey, Lois, Judith Bernstein, and The Bridging the Chasm Collaborative. "Bridging the Chasm between Pregnancy and Health over the Life Course: A National Agenda for Research and Action." *Women's Health Issues* 31, no. 3 (2021): 204–218. https://doi.org/10.1016/j.whi.2021.01.002.

41. Lake, Eileen T., Douglas Staiger, Jeffrey Horbar, Michael J. Kenny, Thelma Patrick, and Jeannette A. Rogowski. "Disparities in Perinatal Quality Outcomes for Very Low Birth Weight Infants in Neonatal Intensive Care." *Health Serv Res* 50, no. 2 (2015):374–397. https://doi.org/10.1111/1475-6773.12225.

19

Maternal Mortality

MARLO VERNON, PhD, MPH,

COLLEEN WALTERS, PhD,

SAMANTHA SOJOURNER, PhD,

and CANDACE BEST, PhD

Across the United States, maternal mortality rates are among the highest of the developed world. In the southern states, rates are typically even higher than national norms. When the Centers for Disease Control and Prevention (CDC) first began tracking maternal deaths in 1986, only 7 out of 100,000 pregnant women died during pregnancy or childbirth or after giving birth. According to the World Health Organization, in the period 2000–2014, the maternal mortality rate doubled from 9.8 to 21.5 maternal deaths per 100,000 live births.[1] In the United States, non-Hispanic Black women have maternal mortality rates of 41.7 deaths per 100,000 live births, compared to 13.4 deaths per 100,000 live births for non-Hispanic white women. Among Hispanic or Latina women, 11.6 die per 100,000 live births nationally, and across the Southeast this rate is much higher. Maternal mortality is defined as death within the first 42 days postpartum (according to the National Vital Statistics System) and pregnancy-related mortality is defined as death up to 365 days postpartum (according to the Pregnancy Mortality Surveillance System).[2,3] These surveillance systems include death for any reason within these time frames, and each state conducts further maternal mortality reviews to determine whether a death is pregnancy related and whether it was preventable. Although both surveillance systems use death certificate data to identify maternal deaths, the information on these certificates is not always complete. The National Vital Statistics System has not published an official maternal mortality rate since 2007; the CDC's Pregnancy Mortality Surveillance System currently tracks US deaths.[4] Maternal mortality is most often reported as a ratio that is calculated by the number of maternal deaths per 100,000 live births.

Data from the CDC's national Pregnancy Mortality Surveillance System for 2011–2015 reports that among the approximately 700 deaths attributed to pregnancy-related complications, 31.3% occurred during pregnancy, 16.9% on the day of delivery, 18.6% 1–6 days postpartum, 21.4% 7–42 days postpartum, and 11.7% 43–365 days postpartum.[5] These numbers highlight the importance of focusing prevention efforts on the first 42 days postpartum. Deaths caused by hypertensive disorders occurred most frequently during days 1–6 postpartum, cerebrovascular accidents (strokes) were most often found in days 1–42 days postpartum, and cardiomyopathy was the most common cause of death in days 43–365 postpartum. Nationally, causes of death included hemorrhage, infection, amniotic fluid embolism or other type of embolism, hypertensive disorders (including preeclampsia), complications from anesthesia, cerebrovascular accidents, cardiomyopathy, other cardiovascular and noncardiovascular medical conditions.[5] Black women's pregnancy-related mortality ratio of 42.8/100,000 live births is 3.3 times higher than the reported rate for white women (13.0/100,000 live births). The most frequently cited causes of death contributing to maternal mortality include heart disease, hemorrhage, and infection.[5] Additionally, the CDC also cited inadequately prepared health systems that are unable to appropriately manage maternal emergencies, missed or delayed diagnoses, and a lack of care coordination as factors influencing maternal mortality.[5] Social determinants of health, including structural barriers to accessing care, systemic barriers, and structural racism contribute to poorer health outcomes and higher maternal mortality rates for Black women. In the United States, African American women access prenatal care less often and at later stages of pregnancy, are more likely to be uninsured, and experience more financial barriers to accessing health care than white women. Additionally, African American women have higher rates of cancer, preventable diseases, diabetes, hypertension, and cardiovascular disease. The history of structural racism in the United States provides some insight into the reasons for the massive health disparities this population experiences, beginning with slavery and continuing to unethical health research practices, lack of inclusion in clinical trials, and unequal treatment by health care providers. African American women fight an uphill battle for equity in health care. They are being failed systemically and geographic, socioeconomic, and racial disparities persist despite efforts to reduce maternal mortality.

When viewed through a socioecological model of health, contributing factors can be found at the individual, family, community, state, and national levels. Barriers to care, lack of access to stable housing, inadequate transportation, low availability of healthy foods, and low health literacy affect maternal health outcomes. Poverty is linked to a higher risk of maternal mortality, but the risk of pregnancy-related death for Black women spans income and education levels.[6] In qualitative work, women reported a lack of confidence when accessing pregnancy and postpartum health information; they were unsure whether online sources were reliable.[7] The combination of low self-efficacy, lack of agency in controlling one's health behaviors due to environmental and structural conditions, and a lack of accountability on the national level contributes to the almost 60% of maternal deaths that the CDC has deemed preventable.

Compared to peer industrialized nations, trends in maternal mortality in the United States have been increasing at a faster rate since 2000 after decades of decreases in maternal mortality rates. A study that compared maternal mortality rates across 27 states and the District of Columbia found a 23% increase between 2008–2009 and 2013–2014 (from 20.6 maternal deaths per 100,000 live births to 25.4).[8] The United States is currently one of only thirteen countries where maternal mortality is worse now than it was fifteen years ago.[1] In fact, most comparable countries in the developed world, including Germany, France, Japan, England, and Canada, are experiencing decreasing maternal mortality and morbidity rates [9] Chronic health conditions (including obesity), increases in cesarean sections, and older maternal age have contributed to this trend.[10] However, these factors are similar across Europe and the developed world and do not adequately explain the recent increases in maternal mortality in the United States. States in the Southern region of the US (as described by the US Census Bureau) have higher rates of maternal mortality compared to other regions.

In a state-by-state evaluation of population-level factors contributing to maternal mortality in the United States, significant associations were found with a higher prevalence of obesity and less than high school education.[11] In addition, fewer prenatal visits (less than 10), diabetes prevalence, and African American ethnicity were also associated with maternal deaths. This is confirmed by state maternal mortality review committees in Virginia and Florida.

Alabama identified 70% of its pregnancy-associated and pregnancy-related deaths as preventable.[12] Key contributors in Alabama included mental health and substance abuse disorders; these were found in almost half of all pregnancy-associated and pregnancy-related deaths. The underlying causes most often found in these deaths were cardiovascular conditions.

Arkansas currently has the fifth highest rate of maternal mortality: 35 maternal deaths per 100,000 births. For African American women in Arkansas, the risk of pregnancy-related deaths is three to four times higher than for white or Hispanic women. Causes of death were attributed to a lack of access to care; chronic conditions such as obesity, diabetes and cardiovascular disease; hypertensive disorders; increased maternal age; and substance abuse and misuse.[13]

In the District of Columbia, closures of obstetrics wards and reduction in labor and delivery services at one hospital in the lowest socioeconomic status areas of the city may be significant factors in the city's maternal mortality rates. These findings point to the importance of access to maternal care. The DC Women's Health Improvement Project reports that for the period 2005–2014, while white women in DC had the lowest maternal mortality rate in the United States (0 deaths per 100,000 live births), African American women in the district carried a burden of 70.6 deaths per 100,000 live births.[14,15] In addition, women who receive Medicaid or who participate in Medicaid's Children's Health Insurance Program tend to have later entry into prenatal care and less than half receive a visit at six weeks postpartum.[15]

In Florida, morbid obesity and late or no prenatal care were significant contributing factors to pregnancy-related mortality rates.[16] Significantly higher rates of pregnancy-related deaths occurred in Florida for African American women compared to white women; their relative risk was 3.3 times higher than that of white women (95% CI, 2.7–4.0). From 2012 to 2018, pregnancy-related maternal ratios for non-Hispanic Black women decreased from a high of 60.5 deaths per 100,000 births to 32.0 deaths per 100,000 births in 2018; among non-Hispanic white women the rate was 12.9 and among Hispanic women it was 10.6.[17] Five leading causes of pregnancy-related death were identified: hypertensive disorders, hemorrhage, infection, cardiomyopathy, and thrombotic embolism. Hernandez et al. report that 42.5% of these were found to be associated with a quality improvement initiative at either the clinical care or health system level.[16]

In Georgia in the period 2012–2016, the cumulative maternal mortality ratio was 66 deaths per 100,000 births. Cardiomyopathy, cardiovascular conditions, hemorrhage, embolism, preeclampsia, and hypertension-related events were identified as significant causes of maternal death. Black non-Hispanic women were 2.7 times more likely to die from pregnancy-related causes than white women. Seventy percent of maternal deaths were found to be from preventable pregnancy-related causes.[71]

According to the America's Health Rankings for 2018, Kentucky dropped from a ranking of 42nd to 45th for overall mortality measures. Maternal mortality rates increased from 80.8 deaths per 100,000 live births in 2013 to 140.9 in 2019. This statistic uses a broader definition of maternal death that is defined as any female between aged 15–55 who was pregnant within one year prior to death or pregnant at death and died from any cause.[72,73]

The Louisiana Pregnancy-Associated Mortality Review for 2017 reported a rate of 106.7 deaths per 100,000 births for pregnancy-associated maternal mortality. The most common causes of pregnancy-related death in Louisiana were cardiovascular and coronary conditions. African American mothers were also found to have a 2.2 higher risk of dying than white mothers. This disparity is even more significant when looking only at pregnancy-related deaths as opposed to all maternal deaths within the first year postpartum. As with other states, older maternal age was a significant risk factor. Eighty percent of pregnancy-related deaths were determined to be "potentially preventable." Provider- and facility-level factors were the most commonly cited factor in pregnancy-related deaths; the review specifically cites a lack of continuity of care.[18]

Maryland has one of the lowest rates of maternal mortality in the southern region. However, the racial disparity widened between 2008–2012 and 2013–2017. In that period, rates decreased 35.4% for white women but increased almost 12% for African American women. The maternal mortality ratio for African American women is approximately four times higher than for white women. Although there was an overall decrease in maternal mortality rate in the state, this improvement was largely driven by white women. In the 2017 report, 80% of the pregnancy-related deaths were deemed to be related to preventable causes.[19]

The Mississippi Health Department also reports a significant racial disparity among maternal mortality deaths: 51.9 deaths per 100,000 live births for African American women and 18.0 for white women. Overall, Mississippi's maternal mortality rate is 1.2 times higher than the national average. In their 2019 report, 86% of pregnancy-related deaths occurred postpartum, almost half before 6 weeks postpartum. The two most common causes of death in Mississippi were related to cardiovascular conditions and hypertensive disorders of pregnancy.[20]

Of all the southern states, North Carolina has the lowest maternal mortality rates, 10.9 per 100,000 live births. A review of maternal deaths in North Carolina identified increased rates of pregnancy-related deaths associated with cardiomyopathy, hemorrhage, and respiratory complications.[21] Black women with a college degree are more likely to die from pregnancy-related causes than white women without a high school diploma. The state considers that 54% of African American maternal deaths were preventable. For white women, the state considered that only 9% were preventable, demonstrating significant racial disparities in risk.

Oklahoma reports similar racial disparities in maternal mortality. African American women are 2.5 more likely to die than white women. The maternal mortality rates for the period 2016–2018 were 54.9 deaths per 100,000 for African American women and 20.4 for white women. Oklahoma found that 85% of maternal deaths due to pregnancy-related causes were preventable with proper and earlier medical intervention. The most frequently cited causes of death included cardiovascular conditions, infections, and noncardiovascular diseases (epilepsy, cirrhosis, asthma, and pneumonia). Three year maternal mortality rates have been trending upward since the trend toward decreasing rates ended in the period 2012–2014.[22]

South Carolina has an overall state mortality rate of 25.5, but for African American women it is 43.3. The state uses the metric of deaths within six weeks postpartum to determine the maternal mortality rate. South Carolina's 2020 Maternal Mortality Review Committee report determined that 55% of the deaths reviewed were preventable. In the period 2016–2019, the highest causes of death were hemorrhage and infections; these two conditions accounted for 50% of all maternal deaths.[23]

A majority of maternal deaths occurred after 42 days postpartum in Tennessee (56%), 22% occurred during the first six weeks postpartum, and the other 22% during pregnancy. Lower education is a significant risk factor in Tennessee. Women with less than a high school degree were two times as likely to die compared to women with at least a high school degree. The state report for 2017 found that approximately 85% of maternal deaths were associated with preventable causes; 96% of the deaths with the contributing factors of substance abuse disorder, mental health challenges, and obesity were considered preventable. Among pregnancy-related deaths, the leading causes were embolism and cardiovascular conditions. Critical factors that contributed to preventable pregnancy-related deaths included lack of coordination of care and delays in seeking treatment. These represent breakdowns in the community systems of care.[24]

The 2020 report of the Texas Maternal Morbidity and Mortality Review Committee provides details on maternal deaths in 2013. Almost 40% of maternal deaths in the first year postpartum were found to be associated with pregnancy-related causes. Eight underlying causes of death were identified: cardiovascular conditions and mental disorders were the two most frequently observed, while hemorrhage, hypertensive disorders, infection, and embolism were the next most frequently cited. Obesity, mental health disorders, and substance use disorders all added significant risks to women. Although race-specific maternal mortality rates were not reported, 31% of deaths were among African American women, who accounted for only 11% of the births.[25]

In Virginia's most recent maternal mortality review team report, chronic conditions affected pregnancy-related deaths differently for white and Black women. Among women with at least one chronic condition, white women died at higher frequencies than Black women. However, Black women had at least one chronic condition at a rate more than twice that of white women (51.4% vs. 25.1%).[26] This report also found that 65% of the women the maternal mortality review team identified were overweight or obese at prepregnancy; a national referent sample was 45% overweight and obese.[27]

In West Virginia, maternal mortality rates were highest among women younger than 20. According to the March of Dimes report *Healthy Moms, Strong Babies* of 2018, 140,000 West Virginians live in a maternity care desert. State-level date for maternal mortality rates were unavailable.

These statewide trends demonstrate significant racial disparities across the southern region of the United States. In many cases, the gap appears to be widening. Causes of death for pregnancy-associated death rates were similar; cardiovascular conditions and hypertensive disorders were the largest contributors to maternal deaths.

African Americans experience higher rates of hypertension than whites outside of pregnancy. The Southeast is known as the Stroke Belt of the United States. During pregnancy, Black women also show signs of preeclampsia earlier in gestation but receive interventions later, often with severe complications and death.[28] The National Partnership for Maternal Safety has identified this as one of the preventable causes of maternal mortality.[29] Shahul et al. found that African American women with preeclampsia were younger and more likely to be in the lowest median income quartile. In this sample, African American women (N = 235,007) had a higher rate of hypertension, diabetes, obesity, and acute renal failure than white women. African American with preeclampsia also had a higher likelihood of severe maternal complications. African American women in this study had an increased unadjusted risk of inpatient maternal mortality (odds ratio 3.70, 95% CI 2.19–6.24); the disparity remained after adjustment for covariates (odds ratio 2.85, 95% CI 1.38–5.53).[28]

Historical Legacies of Slavery

The historical impact of slavery on southern Black women's health outcomes is rooted in social determinants of health that extend to modern times. Slave traders and enslavers prioritized health; they determined the value of enslaved men and women according to their profitability. Insurance companies hired white doctors to examine enslaved persons to evaluate their price and life insurance value in order to protect the investment of the enslavers. The cadavers used in medical schools for teaching purposes were often sourced from dead slaves and pauper graveyards.[30] The ongoing objectification of the Black body in science and medicine has led to what Rana Hogarth refers to as "medicalization of Blackness," the idea that all health outcomes are medical conditions and a search for physiological differences that are the result of race. According to Hogarth, this pathologizing of Blackness has supported the idea that Black bodies are inherently different than white bodies. The differences in how women of different races receive medical care has historical foundations.[31]

Black enslaved women were the subjects of the "father of modern gynecology," Dr. James Marion Sims. They were his patients while he developed surgical techniques and an early understanding of women's health. Unfortunately, he did not provide his subjects with any form of pain management, as he did not believe that Black women felt pain like white women.[32] This belief persists today. Hoff and colleagues report that in a sample of white laypeople, medical students, and residents, over half perceived that Black patients had less pain, resulting in inadequate treatment recommendations. Black and Hispanic patients were also found to be less likely to receive epidurals during labor and delivery than white women.[34] The concept of "obstetrical hardiness," the belief that Black women feel less pain, contributes to how medical providers interact with and treat Black women. At times, they ignore the symptoms Black women experience until it is too late. While the Tuskegee Syphilis Study is often cited as a bellwether for the negligent treatment of African American subjects in medical research, the use of Black women as the earliest patients in the development of women's health care is a significant and all-but-forgotten piece of the narrative.

Exploitation of Black women extended beyond use of their bodies in medical research. Enslavers also required them to serve as their mistresses. The role of mother as a defining characteristic of womanhood was redefined for enslaved women. Enslaved women were often taken from their own children in order to serve as wet nurses for and then to raise the children of the house.[35] Some scholars theorize that this forced role of caretaker and mother has negatively impacted breastfeeding practices among African American women to the present.[36] Women today point to this history when explaining why their mothers and grandmothers did not breastfeed or even discouraged them to breastfeed.[36,37] In addition, high rates of infant mortality during slavery can be connected to this practice, as nutrition deficiencies occurred once mothers were no longer able to breastfeed their own children.

Enslavers saw the fertility of African American women as a financial gain, and their efforts to protect their health was motivated by profitability. Enslaved women preferred midwives and traditional healers to physicians. This cultural preference may still influence African American's women medical-care-seeking behavior today. However, the medicalization of women's health care emphasized a reliance on the physician as best provider of care and slowly eliminated the role of Black midwives. Midwives were framed as ignorant and uneducated about using forceps, and thus physicians and surgeons replaced midwives during birth. The American Medical Association has instituted policies that require doctors to supervise births attended by midwives and set formal requirements for licensure as a midwife. This makes it harder for Black women to receive care from traditional birth attendants and other Black women.[38]

The Impact of Structural Racism on Maternal Mortality

High rates of maternal and infant mortality among African American women in America is partly attributed to wealth and income disparities and to the effects of structural racism, or how social systems, institutions, policies, and practices reinforce and perpetuate inequality.[39] Inequities in the quality of or access to education, quality of and access to health care, and the stress of living in repressive environments contribute to adverse health outcomes, including low birth weight, depression, and heart disease.[40-43] A number of researchers have theorized that the experience of racism produces an underlying state of chronic stress that contributes to increased rates of hypertension, heart disease, and other chronic disease as the body endures a continuous low-grade inflammatory response to the stress state, a concept known as weathering.[44,45] Geronimus et al., who examined allostatic load, a physiological measure of stress burden and one measure of weathering, found that African Americans had higher scores than whites. All African American women regardless of socioeconomic status had the highest probability of high allostatic load scores and the highest scores for excessive stress compared to males and all whites.[45] This study provides physiological evidence of racial differences in health outcomes that are not explained by socioeconomic status and the disproportionate impact of maternal mortality on African American women.

The increased risk of maternal mortality for African American women cannot be explained away by known risk factors, such as advanced maternal age, inadequate prenatal care, low education, or socioeconomic status.[46] Controlling for these known factors has only resulted in a small reduction in odds ratio for pregnancy-related mortality (3.07 to 2.65).[47] These and other data suggest that the negative effects of these recognized health risk factors do not fully explain the disparities seen in maternal mortality among African American women.

African American women are more likely to experience racial discrimination and housing insecurity, to live in disadvantaged neighborhoods, and to experience negative birth outcomes than non-Hispanic white women. This may be the result of structural racism that is built into the fabric of how Black women live and experience an ongoing social culture of discrimination, including historical and current barriers to education, barriers to housing, limits to the generation of intergenerational wealth, and criminal justice disparities.

Jim Crow Laws and the Codification of Racism

Jim Crow laws in the South are an example of how a long history of structural racism relates to accessing care. The Black infant mortality rate in Jim Crow states was 1.19 times higher than non–Jim Crow states in the period 1960–1964. After 1970, this ratio dropped to approximately 1.00, a change that coincides with the abolition of Jim Crow segregation laws.[48] While similar analysis of maternal mortality has not been published, one can surmise that additional burdens were experienced by mothers as well as children.

Structural racism and biases against women of color who access care contribute to health inequities that result in higher maternal and infant mortality rates. Both the American College of Obstetrics and Gynecologists and the American College of Nurse Midwives recognize that these inequities and health disparities affect maternal health.[49] African American women's lack of access to care has its roots in the inability of enslaved persons to access proper medical care and preventive care and their reliance on traditional folklore medicine.[50] Small, Allen and Brown report that countries with a history of enslavement demonstrate comparable disparities in health outcomes.[51] Black women have significantly higher risks of maternal mortality in the UK and Brazil, and the risk remains high for women who self-identify as of African and Afro-Caribbean descent in these countries and in the Netherlands.[52] According to the United Kingdom Obstetric Surveillance System, these risks remained after adjustments for age, socioeconomic status, body mass index, and the number of children born to a woman.[53] The top ten recommendations for addressing the UK maternal mortality crisis include increased and timely access to prenatal care in a welcoming environment and appropriate assessments of family history and chronic conditions. These recommendations that health disparities that are influenced by social determinants of health.

Numerous media stories (such as those reported in the *Atlanta Journal Constitution*, on NPR, and on the ProPublica website) recount stories of women whose health was blamed on issues such as obesity, ignorance, or racist beliefs that negated intervention.[54,55] Examples include a doctor who blamed that fact that woman could not breathe on her obesity; the woman died because her heart failed and her lungs filled with fluid. Another doctor ignored a mother's experienced preeclampsia symptoms; she died because intervention was not done soon enough.[56,57] These and other stories high-light a persistent implicit racial bias that women consistently report in their treatment while pregnant. This bias is thought to prevent women from seek-ing care early enough because of concerns that they will not be heard.[54,58] As Owens and Fett have asked,

> How does a community learn to trust doctors whose forefathers were interested only in repairing and restoring Black women's reproductive health so that slav-ery could be perpetuated? How can doctors learn to be more sensitive to the concerns, both personal and cultural, of Black people who still hold secrets about the forced sterilizations that older southern members of their families endured? How does the medical profession unlearn a pattern of dismissing Black women's self-reported pain when that pattern is rooted in centuries-old soil?[38]

The increased regulation of Black women's fertility through coercive birth control practices is another example of structural racism. The stereo-type of the "welfare queen"—women who received greater benefits with more children—contributes to a negative understanding of Black women and their relationship with motherhood and pregnancy. One editorial in the *Philadel-phia Inquirer* suggested that the Black birth rate could be reduced by implant-ing lower socioeconomic status women with the long-acting contraceptive Norplant. This proposed policy and others like it stemmed from an ideology that economic and social disparities resulted from the higher fertility rates of less intelligent groups.[59] Some federal welfare policies of the 1980s in-cluded a requirement that women receive Norplant in order to be eligible for benefits. While this requirement was for all women, Black women received welfare benefits at a much higher rate and thus the policy discriminated against low-income women of color disproportionately. This policy is remi-niscent of the forced sterilization of Black women in the 1970s.[59]

Similarly, the mandatory prison sentences for drug use during preg-nancy disproportionately affected Black women in the 1980s.[59] Of women who were arrested for using drugs during pregnancy, over 75% were Black. Often women in this group received less-than-optimal prenatal care and were forced to place their children in foster care or with family members until their release, which had negative mental and physical consequences for both the women and their children. These policies and philosophies are rife with racist undertones and provide a lens through which to view the ongoing belief on the part of Black women and their children that they are not valued as highly as their white counterparts.

Ethics of Maternal Health Care for Black Women

The factors associated with maternal mortality in the United States and the disparities noted among non-Hispanic African American women are complex, multifaceted, interrelated, persistent, and far-reaching. But they are largely preventable. To effectively address these factors, a systems approach is needed with interventions that span preconception to the first year postpartum and involves all stakeholder, including federal and state health agencies, primary and acute care facilities, community organizations, and women and their families.

Preconception Care

In 2006, the CDC issued ten recommendations for improving preconception health that are rooted in preventative interventions such as vaccinations, screenings, education, and managing chronic health conditions. The CDC recommends that providers encourage individuals to have a reproductive health plan; increase public awareness of preconception health through culturally appropriate information; improve access to primary care providers for risk assessment visits and early intervention such as folic acid supplements, screenings and treatment for sexually transmitted infections, and smoking and drug use cessation; target high-risk populations with prepregnancy checkups; and create public health programs.[60] At the federal level, expansion of Medicaid to provide coverage for women to access care to identify and manage pre-existing conditions before becoming pregnant is needed. In states that implemented the Medicaid expansion under the Affordable Care Act, improvements in a subset of preconception health measures were noted, including greater preconception health counseling, prepregnancy folic acid intake, and postpartum use of effective birth control methods among low-income women.[61]

Prenatal Care

One of the primary interventions for reducing maternal mortality is early and adequate prenatal care. However, areas of the United States are considered "maternal health deserts"—counties with no obstetrician to provide prenatal care. According to the March of Dimes 2020 report *Nowhere to Go: Maternity Care Deserts across the U.S.*, more than 7 million women of childbearing age live in maternal deserts.[62] In order to provide prenatal care, federal funding needs to be available for training and deployment of obstetricians, nurse practitioners, and certified nurse midwifes to these deserts.

The concept of mother blame, or blaming women for their own ill health and any negative health outcomes of their children, haunts women who seek prenatal care. Social determinants of health play a part in the development of negative health outcomes. For example, women who do not have access to a grocery store because they live in a food desert are told to have healthy diets.[63] Women who have no access to safe places to walk or exercise are instructed to be physically active. Women who do not have reliable transportation or childcare are told to come regularly to prenatal appointments. While women of all ethnicities experience these barriers, they disproportionately affect Black women and their families.[63] Thus, individual health behaviors as the basis for health outcomes cannot be adequately perceived without considering the structural environment. Black women endure "stigmatization, scapegoating, heightened surveillance, and criminalization, all of which disregard the bodily autonomy of pregnant women."[63] Educated and culturally competent medical care provider teams are necessary if the social determinants of health that many Black women endure are to be sufficiently addressed.

Innovative models of prenatal care and education for high-risk patients have demonstrated improvement in health outcomes such as preterm births. These include group prenatal care such as the Becoming a Mom and Centering Pregnancy initiatives of the March of Dimes. The Becoming a Mom program provides group prenatal education for at high-risk women conducted in tandem with routine prenatal care. The 103 women in Kansas who participated in the program had fewer preterm births (5% vs. 10%, $p = 0.4229$).[64] Centering Pregnancy is a full prenatal care experience with a group of women at similar gestation stage and a clinician (a nurse midwife or obstetrician). The women are taught to perform self-assessments such as weight, urine analysis, and blood pressure. Centering Pregnancy has expanded as an evidence-based model of care that has been shown to reduce preterm births, particularly among minority populations.[65–67]

Provider-patient discord is associated with poor outcomes, particularly for non-Hispanic Black women who have a historical basis for mistrust of health care systems. Interventions for addressing this issue during the prenatal period include the CDC's Hear Her campaign, which educates providers to listen to patients and uses nurse-midwives, who non-Hispanic Black women trust more than other medical professionals during pregnancy.[68] Even with the right provider and an innovative prenatal care program, pregnant women need additional assistance in navigating the health care delivery landscape through care coordination by case managers.

Medical providers need a holistic understanding of the cultural and social experiences of the African American women in their care. Community engagement efforts to highlight the bias women of color experience when accessing health care can lead to greater attention to the circumstances, environments, and situations that women must navigate to achieve positive health outcomes. Provider attitudes and practices that fail to recognize or ignore social and structural systems that affect maternal health outcomes do little to improve the disparities in maternal health.

Labor and Delivery

The closure of labor and delivery units in rural hospitals due to high liability and low reimbursement are also significant barriers to access to maternal care. Legislative efforts have been considered to increase reimbursement to hospitals for perinatal care. Some outcomes include agreements on the part of birthing hospitals that they will implement patient safety bundles so that every woman every time receives the same quality of care regardless of preconceived perceptions and provider biases.

Postpartum

The recent expansion of postpartum care coverage to six months was a major step toward access to care and management of women at risk for maternal death. Further recommendations include expanding Medicaid to one year postpartum, as most women die during this time frame. The Post-birth Warning Signs Education Program developed by the Association of Women's Health, Obstetric and Neonatal Nurses provides continued education of nurses and other health care professionals about risk factors for postpartum complications.

Recognizing that there is no "one size fits all" solution for interventions, maternal mortality review committees in California, Florida, Illinois, Kentucky, New Jersey, and North Carolina in 2005–2018 supported multilevel and environmental solutions in their maternal mortality review committee reports, including reducing social inequities, increasing access to quality care, and standardizing hospital approaches to emergencies, such as implementing Alliance for Innovation on Maternal Health bundles. Standardized protocols that are implemented systematically have the greatest chance of reducing the incidence of adverse maternal health outcomes.[16]

Care Coordination

Chronic health conditions that increase the risk of maternal mortality such as obesity, diabetes, hypertension, and cardiovascular disease require particular care and attention during the prenatal and postpartum periods. Preconception care and care coordination are important components of at-risk women's health. Preconception counseling for women who experience these conditions, instruction about how to improve health behaviors and clinical health to best prepare for pregnancy, and medication review are important practices for health care providers and women to address together. This counseling may also address unintended pregnancy or women who have conceived unintentionally. Similarly, a woman's medical history should be taken at each appointment and should include a clinical assessment of her overall health. Women would benefit from a cardiovascular examination by appropriately trained physicians and health care providers on an as-needed basis. These strategies have been correlated with low maternal mortality and greater national mental health.[74]

Several southern states such as Kentucky and Florida stand out in their efforts to address maternal mortality. Kentucky has discussed increasing care coordination across all health care providers and addressing comorbities, among other measures. In Florida, the Pregnancy Associated Mortality Review recommended that the state develop and implement a Maternal Early Warning System protocol based on the National Partnership for Maternal Safety. This protocol uses color-coded metrics to guide health care providers' responses to changes in vital signs so they will know when to escalate care.[69,70] It is the responsibility of all health care providers involved in the care of women to learn from every maternal death, to ensure the quality and safety of maternity care, and to work to improve women's health across the life course.[4]

Conclusion

Women in the United States experience a disproportionate risk of maternal mortality that is greatly increased for African American women in particular. Personal, community, physical, and health care environments all contribute to this risk, and efforts to address this complex issue need to be multifaceted. In the past, little attention has been given to efforts to educate and empower women to increase their self-efficacy when identifying and advocating for timely and appropriate interventions during pregnancy and in the postpartum period. Particularly in the high-risk South, a focus on public health, providers, and health care systems as the usual conduit of health education in combination with improvements in the continuity of care are important interventions for successfully addressing maternal mortality. Prevention strategies that include improving community-level access to adequate health care and patient education may improve maternal mortality outcomes among African American women in the South.

REFERENCES

1. World Health Organization. *Trends in Maternal Mortality: 1990–2015: Estimates from WHO, UNICEF, UNFPA, World Bank Group and the United Nations Population Division*. Geneva: World Health Organization, 2015.

2. Center for Disease Control and Prevention. "Pregnancy Mortality Surveillance System." 2017. https://www.cdc.gov/reproductivehealth/maternal-mortality/pregnancy-mortality-surveillance-system.htm.

3. Hoyert, Donna L. "Maternal Mortality and Related Concepts." *Vital Health Statistics* 3, no. 33 (2007): 1–13. https://www.cdc.gov/nchs/data/series/sr_03/sr03_033.pdf.

4. Lu, M. C. "Reducing Maternal Mortality in the United States." *JAMA* 320, no. 12 (2018): 1237–1238. https://jamanetwork.com/journals/jama/fullarticle/2702413.

5. Petersen, E. E., N. L. Davis, D. Goodman, S. Cox, N. Mayes, E. Johnston, C. Syverson, K. Seed, C. K. Shapiro-Mendoza and W. M. Callaghan. "Vital Signs: Pregnancy-Related Deaths, United States, 2011–2015, and Strategies for Prevention, 13 States, 2013–2017." *Morbidity and Mortality Weekly Report* 68, no. 18 (2019): 423429.

6. Gingrey, J. P. "Maternal Mortality: A US Public Health Crisis." *American Journal of Public Health* 110 (2020): 462–464. https://ajph.aphapublications.org/doi/full/10.2105/AJPH.2019.305552.

7. Vernon, M. "Development of the VidaRPM (Remote Pregnancy and Postpartum Monitoring) App for Women in Georgia to Monitor Blood Pressure, Weight, and Mental Health." Paper presented at the 33rd annual meeting of the Georgia Perinatal Association, St. Simon's Island, GA, September 25, 2019.

8. MacDorman, M. F., E. Declercq, and M. E. Thoma. "Trends in Maternal Mortality by Sociodemographic Characteristics and Cause of Death in 27 States and the District of

Columbia." *Obstetrics and Gynecology* 129, no. 5 (2017): 811–818. https://pubmed.ncbi.nlm
.nih.gov/28383383/.

9. Cox, K. S. "Global Maternal Mortality Rate Declines—Except in America." *American Academy of Nursing* 107, no. 5 (2018): 428–429. https://doi.org/10.1016/j.outlook.2018.08.001.

10. Neggers, Y. H. "Trends in Maternal Mortality in the United States." *Reproductive Toxicology* 64 (September 2016): 72–76. https://www.sciencedirect.com/science/article/pii /S089062381630051X.

11. Daniel B. Nelson, Michelle H. Monez, and Matthew M. Davis. "Population-Level Factors Associated with Maternal Mortality in the United States, 1997–2012." *BMC Public Health* 18 (2018): 1–7. https://bmcpublichealth.biomedcentral.com/articles/10.1186/s12889 -018-5935-2.

12. Mckitt, T. *Review of 2016 Maternal Mortality.* [Montgomery]: Alabama Department of Public Health, [2016].

13. Murtha, M. "Strategies to Improve Maternal Mortality and Morbidity." *Arkansas Physician Newsletter* (March 2018). Accessed June 6, 2022. https://afmc.org/wpfd_file/2018 -03-march-strategies-to-improve-maternal-mortality-and-morbidity/.

14. Moaddab, A., G. A. Dildy, H. L. Brown, Z. H. Bateni, M. A. Belfort, H. Sangi-Hagh-peykar, and S. L. Clark. "Health Care Disparity and State-Specific Pregnancy-Related Mortality in the United States, 2005–2014." *Obstetrics & Gynecology* 128, no. 4 (2016): 869–875. https://journals.lww.com/greenjournal/Fulltext/2016/10000/Health_Care_Disparity _and_State_Specific.25.aspx.

15. Russell, R., C. Rodehau, and P. Quinn. *Human-Centered Solutions to Improve Reproductive and Maternal Health Outcomes in Washington, D.C.* Washington, DC: District of Columbia Primary Care Association, 2018.

16. Hernandez, L. E., W. M. Sappenfield, K. Harris, D. Burch, W. C. Hill, C. L. Clark, and I. Delke. "Pregnancy-Related Deaths, Florida, 1999–2012: Opportunities to Improve Maternal Outcomes." *Maternal and Child Health Journal* 22 (2018): 204–215. https://doi.org/10 .1007/s10995-017-2392-y.

17. Hernandez, Leticia. *Florida's Pregnancy-Associated Mortality Review.* [Tallahassee]: Florida Department of Public Health, 2018. http://www.floridahealth.gov/statistics-and -data/PAMR/_documents/pamr-2018-update.pdf.

18. Benno, J., R. Trichilo, V. Gillispie-Bell, and C. Lake. *Louisiana Pregnancy-Associated Mortality Review, 2017 Report.* [Baton Rouge]: Louisiana Department of Health, 2020.

19. Maryland Department of Health. *Maryland Maternal Mortality Review, 2019.* [Baltimore]: Maryland Department of Health, 2019. https://health.maryland.gov/phpa/mch /Documents/MMR/MMR_2019_AnnualReport.pdf.

20. Mississippi State Department of Health. *Mississippi Maternal Mortality Report, 2013–2016.* Jackson: Mississippi State Department of Health, 2019. https://msdh.ms.gov /msdhsite/index.cfm/31,8127,299,pdf/MS_Maternal_Mortality_Report_2019_Final.pdf.

21. Petersen, E. E., N. L. Davis, D. Goodman, S. Cox, C. Syverson, K. Seed, C. Shapiro-Mendoza, W. M. Callaghan, and W. Barfield. "Racial/Ethnic Disparities in Pregnancy-Related Deaths—United States, 2007–2016." *Morbidity and Mortality Weekly Report* 68, no. 35 (2019): 762–765. https://www.cdc.gov/mmwr/volumes/68/wr/mm6835a3.htm.

22. Oklahoma Maternal Mortality Review Committee. *Maternal Mortality in Oklahoma,*

2004–2018. [Oklahoma City]: [Oklahoma Maternal Mortality Review Committee], [2020]. https://oklahoma.gov/content/dam/ok/en/health/health2/aem-documents/family -health/maternal-and-child-health/maternal-mortality/annual-mmrc-report.pdf.

23. South Carolina Maternal Morbidity and Mortality Review Committee. *South Carolina Maternal Morbidity and Mortality Review Committee Legislative Brief March 2020.* Columbia: South Carolina Maternal Morbidity and Mortality Review Committee, 2020. https:// www.scstatehouse.gov/reports/DHEC/mmmr-2020-Final.pdf.

24. Tennessee Department of Health. *Tennessee Maternal Mortality, Review of 2017 Maternal Deaths.* Nashville: Tennessee Department of Health, 2019.

25. Texas Maternal Mortality and Morbidity Review Committee. *Texas Maternal Mortality and Morbidity Review committee and Department of State Health Services Joint Biennial Report, December 2020.* Austin: Texas Department of Health and Human Services, 2020. https://www.dshs.texas.gov/legislative/2020-Reports/DSHS-MMMRC-2020.pdf.

26. Rouse, M. J., and Virginia Maternal Mortality Review Team. *Chronic Disease in Virginia Pregnancy Associated Deaths, 1999–2012: Need for Coordination of Care.* [Richmond]: Virginia Department of Health, 2019. https://www.vdh.virginia.gov/content/uploads/sites /18/2019/08/MMRT-Chronic-Disease-Report-FINAL-VERSION.pdf.

27. America's Health Rankings. "Maternal Mortality in Georgia, 2018." America's Health Rankings, 2022. https://www.americashealthrankings.org/explore/health-of-women-and -children/measure/maternal_mortality/state/GA?edition-year=2018.

28. Shahul, Sajid, Mohammed Minhaj, Junaid Nizamuddin, Julia Wenger, Eitezaz Mahmood, Ariel Mueller, Shahzad Shaefi, Barbara Scavone, Robb D. Kociol, Daniel Talmor, and Sarosh Rana. "Racial Disparities in Comorbidities, Complications, and Maternal and Fetal Outcomes in Women with Preeclampsia/Eclampsia." *Hypertension in Pregnancy* 34, no. 4 (2015): 506–515. www.ncbi.nlm.nih.gov/pmc/articles/PMC4782921/.

29. Tucker, Myra J., Cynthia J. Berg, William M. Callaghan, and Jason Hsia. "The Black-White Disparity in Pregnancy-Related Mortality from 5 Conditions: Differences in Prevalence and Case-Fatality Rates." *American Journal of Public Health* 97 (February 2007): 247–251. https://ajph.aphapublications.org/doi/10.2105/AJPH.2005.072975.

30. Deirdre Cooper Owens and Sharla M. Fett. "Black Maternal and Infant Health: Historical Legacies of Slavery." *American Journal of Public Health* 109 (October 2019): 1342–1345. https://ajph.aphapublications.org/doi/10.2105/AJPH.2019.305243.

31. Hogarth, R. A. *Medicalizing Blackness: Making Racial Difference in the Atlantic World.* Chapel Hill: University of North Carolina Press, 2017.

32. Cohen, W. "Medical Apartheid: The Dark History of Medical Experimentation on Black Americans from Colonial Times to the Present." *International Journal of Applied Psychoanalytic Studies* 6, no. 4 (2009): 356–630. https://doi.org/10.1002/aps.223.

33. Hoffman, K. M., S. Trawalter, J. R. Axt, and M. N. Oliver. "Racial Bias in Pain Assessment and Treatment Recommendations, and False Beliefs about Biological Differences between Blacks and Whites." *Proceedings of the National Academy of Sciences* 113, no. 16 (2016): 4296–301. https://www.pnas.org/content/pnas/113/16/4296.full.pdf.

34. Glance, Laurent G., R. Wissler, C. Glantz, Turner M. Osler, Dana B. Mukamel, and Andrew W. Dick. "Racial Differences in the Use of Epidural Analgesia for Labor." *Anesthesiology* 106 (2007): 19–25. https://doi.org/10.1097/00000542-200701000-00008.

35. Knight, R. J. "Mistresses, Motherhood, and Maternal Exploitation in the Antebellum South." *Women's History Review* 27, no. 6 (2018): 990–1005. https://doi.org/10.1080/09612025.2017.1336847.

36. DeVane-Johnson, S., C. W. Giscombe, R. Williams II, C. Fogel, and S. Thoyre. "A Qualitative Study of Social, Cultural, and Historical Influences on African American Women's Infant-Feeding Practices." *Journal of Perinatal Education* 27, no. 2 (2018): 71–85. https://www.ncbi.nlm.nih.gov/pmc/articles/PMC6388681/.

37. Green, V. L., N. L. Killings, and C. A. Clare. "The Historical, Psychosocial, and Cultural Context of Breastfeeding in the African American Community." *Breastfeeding Medicine* 16, no. 2 (2021): 116–120. doi: 10.1089/bfm.2020.0316.

38. Owens, D. C., and S. M. Fett. "Black Maternal and Infant Health: Historical Legacies of Slavery." *American Journal of Public Health* 109 (October 2019): 1342–1345. https://doi.org/10.2105/AJPH.2019.305243.

39. Bailey, Z. D., N. Krieger, M. Agénor, J. Graves, N. Linos, and M. T. Bassett. "Structural Racism and Health Inequities in the USA: Evidence and Interventions." *Lancet* 389, no. 10077 (2017): 1453–1463. 10.1016/s0140-6736(17)30569-x.

40. Pabayo, R., A. Ehntholt, K. Davis, S. Y. Liu, P. Muennig, and D. M. Cook. "Structural Racism and Odds for Infant Mortality among Infants Born in the United States 2010." *Journal of Racial and Ethnic Health Disparities* 6, no. 6 (2019): 1095–1106. https://pubmed.ncbi.nlm.nih.gov/31309525.

41. Foster, H. W., L. Wu, M. B. Bracken, K. Semenya, J. Thomas, and J. Thomas. "Intergenerational Effects of High Socioeconomic Status on Low Birthweight and Preterm Birth in African Americans." *Journal of the National Medical Association* 92, no. 5 (2000): 213–221.

42. Mendez, D. D., V. K. Hogan, and J. F. Culhane. "Stress during Pregnancy: The Role of Institutional Racism." *Stress and Health* 29, no. 4 (2013): 266–274.

43. Lukachko, A., M. L. Hatzenbuehler, and K. M. Keyes. "Structural Racism and Myocardial Infarction in the United States." *Social Science & Medicine* 103 (2014): 42–50.

44. Giscombé, C. L., and M. Lobel. "Explaining Disproportionately High Rates of Adverse Birth Outcomes among African Americans: The Impact of Stress, Racism, and Related Factors in Pregnancy." *Psychological Bulletin* 131, no. 5 (2005): 662–683.

45. Geronimus, A. T., M. Hicken, D. Keene, and J. Bound. "'Weathering' and Age Patterns of Allostatic Load Scores among Blacks and Whites in the United States." *American Journal of Public Health* 96 (May 2006): 826–833. https://ajph.aphapublications.org/doi/10.2105/AJPH.2004.060749.

46. Howell, E. A. "Reducing Disparities in Severe Maternal Morbidity and Mortality." *Clinical Obstetrics and Gynecology* 61, no. 2 (2018): 387–399.

47. Harper, M. A., M. A. Espeland, E. Dugan, R. Meyer, K. Lane, and S. Williams. "Racial Disparity in Pregnancy-Related Mortality following a Live Birth Outcome." *Annals of Epidemiology* 14, no. 4 (2004): 274–279.

48. Krieger, N., J. T. Chen, B. Coull, P. D. Waterman, and J. Beckfield. "The Unique Impact of Abolition of Jim Crow Laws on Reducing Inequities in Infant Death Rates and Implications for Choice of Comparison Groups in Analyzing Societal Determinants of Health." *American Journal of Public Health* 103 (December 2013): 2234–2244. https://ajph.aphapublications.org/doi/10.2105/AJPH.2013.301350.

49. Parker, A. M. "Birthing a Slave: Motherhood and Medicine in the Antebellum South (Review)." *Journal of the Early Republic* 26 (2006): 701–704. https://doi.org/10.1353/jer.2006 .0074.

50. Bernice Roberts Kennedy, Christopher Clomus Mathus, and Angela K. Woods. "African Americans and Their Distrust of the Health Care System: Healthcare for Diverse Populations." *Journal of Cultural Diversity* 14, no. 2 (2007): 56–60. https://pubmed.ncbi.nlm.nih .gov/19175244/.

51. Small, M. J., T. K. Allen, and H. L. Brown. "Global Disparities in Maternal Morbidity and Mortality." *Seminars in Perinatology* 41, no. 5 (2017): 318–322. http://www.sciencedirect .com/science/article/pii/S0146000517300514.

52. Bowyer, L. *Saving Mothers' Lives: Reviewing Maternal Deaths to Make Motherhood Safer: 2003–2005. BJOG* 118, Suppl. 1 (2008): 1–203. https://www.oaa-anaes.ac.uk/assets /_managed/editor/File/Reports/2006-2008%20CEMD.pdf.

53. Cantwell, R., T. Clutton-Brock, G. Cooper, A. Dawson, J. Drife, D. Garrod, A. Harper, D. Hulbert, S. Lucas, and J. McClure. *Saving Mothers' Lives: Reviewing Maternal Deaths to Make Motherhood Safer: 2006–2008. BJOG* 118, Suppl. 1 (2011): 1–203.

54. Martin, N., and R. Montagne. "Lost Mothers Nothing Protects Black Women from Dying in Pregnancy and Childbirth." ProPublica, December 7, 2017. https://www.propub lica.org/article/nothing-protects-black-women-from-dying-in-pregnancy-and-childbirth.

55. Hart, A. "Georgia Maternal Death Rate, Once Ranked Worst in U.S., Worse Now." *Atlanta Journal Constitution*, September 30, 2018, https://www.ajc.com/news/state—regional -govt—politics/georgia-maternal-death-rate-once-ranked-worst-worse-now/qG8xWY MufoW2OEiiZNDRmM/.

56. Goode, Keisha, and Barbara Katz Rothman. "African-American Midwifery, a History and a Lament." *American Journal of Economics and Sociology* 76, no. 1 (2017): 65–94. https:// onlinelibrary.wiley.com/doi/full/10.1111/ajes.12173.

57. Bridges, K. *Reproducing Race: An Ethnography of Pregnancy as a Site of Racialization*. Berkeley: University of California Press, 2011.

58. Hoberman, J. *Black and Blue: The Origins and Consequences of Medical Racism*. Berkeley: University of California Press, 2012.

59. Roberts, D. E. *Killing the Black Body: Race, Reproduction and the Meaning of Liberty*. New York: Vintage Books, 1997.

60. Johnson, K., S. F. Posner, J. Biermann, J. F. Cordero, H. K. Atrash, C. S. Parker, S. Boulet, and M. G. Curtis. "Recommendations to Improve Preconception Health and Health Care—United States: Report of the CDC/ATSDR Preconception Care Work Group and the Select Panel on Preconception Care." *Morbidity and Mortality Weekly Report* 55, RR06 (2006): 1–23. https://www.cdc.gov/mmwr/preview/mmwrhtml/rr5506a1.htm.

61. Myerson, R., S. Crawford, and L. Wherry. "Medicaid Expansion Increased Preconception Health Counseling, Folic Acid Intake, and Postpartum Contraception." *Health Affairs* 39, no. 11 (2020): 1883–1890. https://www.healthaffairs.org/doi/abs/10.1377/hlthaff .2020.00106.

62. March of Dimes. *Nowhere to Go: Maternity Care Deserts across the U.S.* [Arlington, VA]: March of Dimes, 2020. https://www.marchofdimes.org/materials/2020-Maternity -Care-Report.pdf.

63. Karen A. Scott, Laura Britton., and Monica R. McLemore. "The Ethics of Perinatal Care for Black Women: Dismantling the Structural Racism in 'Mother Blame' Narratives." *Journal of Perinatal and Neonatal Nursing* 33, no. 2 (2019): 108–115. https://journals.lww .com/jpnnjournal/Fulltext/2019/04000/The_Ethics_of_Perinatal_Care_for_Black_Women _.5.aspx.

64. Woods, N., and A. Chesser. "Becoming a Mom: Improving Birth Outcomes through a Community Collaborative Prenatal Education Model." *Journal of Family Medicine and Disease Prevention* 1 (2015). https://clinmedjournals.org/articles/jfmdp/jfmdp-1-002.pdf.

65. Ickovics, J. R., T. S. Kershaw, C. Westdahl, U. Magriples, Z. Massey, H. Reynolds, and S. S. Rising. "Group Prenatal Care and Perinatal Outcomes: A Randomized Controlled Trial." *Obstetrics and Gynecology* 110 (2007): 330–339. 10.1097/01.A0g.0000275284.24298.23.

66. Picklesimer, A. H., D. Billings, N. Hale, D. Blackhurst, and S. Covington-Kolb. "The Effect of Centering Pregnancy Group Prenatal Care on Preterm Birth in a Low-Income Population." *American Journal of Obstetrics and Gynecology* 206, no. 5 (2012): 415.e1–7. doi: 10 .1016/j.ajog.2012.01.040.

67. Tandon, S. D., L. Colon, P. Vega, J. Murphy, and A. Alonso. "Birth Outcomes Associated with Receipt of Group Prenatal Care among Low-Income Hispanic Women." *Journal of Midwifery & Women's Health* 57, no. 5 (2012): 476–481. https://onlinelibrary.wiley.com/doi /abs/10.1111/j.1542-2011.2012.00184.x.

68. CDC. "Healthcare Professionals." Hear Her Campaign. Last reviewed February 16, 2022. https://www.cdc.gov/hearher/healthcare-providers/index.html.

69. Council on Patient Safety in Women's Health Care. "Maternal Early Warning Signs (MEWS) Protocol." February 24, 2015. https://safehealthcareforeverywoman.org/wp-content /uploads/2017/02/MEWS-Protocol.pdf. April 4, 2021 2021.

70. Mhyre, J. M., R. D'Oria, A. B. Hameed, J. R. Lappen, S. L. Holley, S. K. Hunter, R. L. Jones, J. C. King, and M. E. D'Alton. "The Maternal Early Warning Criteria: A Proposal from the National Partnership for Maternal Safety." *Obstetrics and Gynecology* 124, no. 4 (2014): 782–786. doi: 10.1097/a0g.0000000000000480.

71. Georgia Department of Public Health. *Reducing Maternal Mortality in Georgia: 2013 Case Review Update*. Atlanta: Georgia Department of Health, 2017.

72. United Health Foundation. *America's Health Rankings, 2020 Health of Women and Children Report*. United Health Foundation, 2020. xhttps://assets.americashealthrankings .org/app/uploads/state-summaries-healthofwomenandchildren-2021.pdf

73. Kentucky Department for Public Health and Division of Maternal and Child Health. *Maternal Mortality Review, 2020 Annual Report*. Frankfort: Kentucky Department for Public Health, 2020.

74. Small, M. J., T. K. Allen, and H. L. Brown. "Global Disparities in Maternal Morbidity and Mortality." *Seminars in Perinatology* 41, no. 5 (2017): 318–322. https://doi.org/10.1053/j .semperi.2017.04.009.

IV FUTURE DIRECTIONS

20

Ameliorating Health Inequities

STEVEN S. COUGHLIN, PhD, MPH,

LOVORIA B. WILLIAMS, PhD, FNP-BC, FAAN,

and TABIA HENRY AKINTOBI, PhD, MPH

The chapters in this book detail the unacceptably higher morbidity and mortality rates related to health conditions among African Americans, particularly those who reside in the southern United States. This disproportionate burden results in noteworthy health disparities when comparing this group to others. The chapters explore the root causes of the persistent health inequities in this population subgroup. In this concluding chapter, we consider measures that can ameliorate health disparities among African Americans in the South.

Increase Access to Quality, Affordable Health Care

Studies indicate that racial/ethnic minorities are less likely to receive routine medical care and that when they access care they often experience a lower quality of health care than whites.[1] For example, research indicates that when accessing health care, African Americans wait longer than whites to be seen, receive a less thorough clinical workup, and are often viewed by white providers as less intelligent and less likely to follow medical advice.[2] These negative interactions contribute to dissatisfaction and make African American less likely to access health care when needed. Disparities in health and health care not only affect the groups facing disparities but also limit overall improvements in quality of care and health for the broader population, thereby resulting in unnecessary health care costs.[3] To address health disparities among African Americans in the South and elsewhere in the United States, concerted cross-sector efforts are necessary.

One intervention that will advance health equity is improving the Affordable Care Act (ACA) and expanding Medicaid. The ACA created new coverage options, including health insurance marketplaces and Medicaid expansion. Following enactment of the ACA in 2010, there were large gains in coverage, particularly among low-income persons and racial/ethnic minorities.[3-5] The ACA also included protections for people with preexisting conditions, thereby increasing access to health care for populations that were previously denied coverage.[5] The online marketplace HealthCare.gov, which was launched in 2014, enabled qualified individuals to purchase health insurance from private insurers that offered plans that met federal criteria.[6] Qualified individuals included self-employed individuals and people who could not obtain affordable insurance coverage through their employers.[6] However, as of 2018, African Americans and other racial/ethnic minority groups remained more likely than whites to be uninsured.[3]

One component of the ACA that is likely to have the greatest impact on health outcomes is the increased funding it provides for public health and prevention capacity, which has improved access to preventive services and encouraged private employers and insurers to incorporate prevention and wellness in workplaces and coverage policies.[7]

Federal initiatives such as increased support for community health centers are critical for ameliorating health disparities, particularly among African Americans. The ACA's coverage expansions and funding for community health centers have both increased access to coverage and care for African Americans and other groups facing disproportionately higher disparities.[3] States, local communities, private organizations, and health care providers are also engaged in efforts to reduce health disparities.[3]

Criticisms of the ACA include concern about the high and increasing insurance premiums. As Ho has noted, a relatively healthy single person earning a salary of $50,000 will likely find the cost of health insurance in the Marketplace unacceptable, partly because these plans require a significant deductible and copayments.[6] Effective steps are needed to lower premiums through a variety of strategies that affect potential enrollees, insurers, and health care providers.[6] In addition, continued efforts are needed to improve the health care delivery system and the quality of health care.

Increase Access to Culturally Appropriate Health Care

In order to address health disparities among African Americans in the southern United States, increasing access to affordable health care is necessary but not sufficient. There is also a need to ensure that health care is culturally appropriate and that measures are taken to eliminate race bias in health care.

Addressing Racism and Race Bias in Medicine

The Institute of Medicine's landmark report titled *Unequal Treatment: Confronting Racial and Ethnic Disparities in Health Care* compiled a convincing body of evidence that minority populations receive less care than whites.[8] The report, which assessed differences in the kinds and quality of health care racial/ethnic minorities and non-minorities receive in the United States, found that that the disparities that exist health care exist are associated with worse health outcomes. Health care disparities occur in the context of broader inequality and social determinants of health, such as neighborhood environment, unemployment, lack of access to healthy foods, and poor education. Upstream sustained approaches are necessary to address the deeply rooted social determinants that contribute to the poor health of African Americans.

While most of the studies reviewed in the report focused on comparisons between African Americans and whites, disparities exist across all race and ethnic groups and span a wide spectrum of health conditions.[9] Several steps have been taken to address these inequities, including increasing the number of practicing Black physicians, providing cultural competency training in medical education and in the health care workforce, and addressing medical distrust among African Americans and other minority populations.

The report recommended numerous interventions to eliminate racial/ethnic disparities in health care. They include the following:

— Defragmenting health care financing and delivery
— Strengthening doctor-patient relationships
— Strengthening the stability of patient-provider relationships in publicly funded health care plans
— Increasing the proportion of underrepresented US racial and ethnic minorities among health professionals
— Applying the same managed care protections to publicly funded enrollees in health maintenance organizations that apply to enrollees in private health insurance
— Providing more resources to the Office for Civil Rights of the United

States Department of Health and Human Services for enforcing civil rights laws
— Promoting the consistency and equity of care through the use of evidence-based guidelines
— Enhancing patient-provider communication and trust by providing financial incentives for practices that reduce barriers and encourage evidence-based practice
— Supporting the use of community health care workers
— Implementing multidisciplinary treatment and preventive care teams; providing cross-cultural education in the health professions
— Integrating cross-cultural education into the training of all current and future health professionals.[8]

Increase the Number of Practicing Black Physicians

African Americans are persistently underrepresented in the health care professions. Lack of diversity is well documented within both nursing and medicine. For instance, Black physicians account for only 5% of all physicians even though African Americans make up 13% of the United States population.[10] The situation is especially concerning for Black males. Research indicates that demographic representation improves access to health care for underserved populations and improves the cultural effectiveness of the physician workforce as a whole.[11-14] Despite efforts to address the lack of diversity among the medical profession, the underrepresentation of Black physicians has not significantly changed since the Liaison Committee on Medical Education issued diversity accreditation guidelines in 2009.[11] In fact, according to a report by the Association of American Medical Colleges, the number of African American men who applied to medical school between 1978 and 2014 decreased slightly.[10] There is a need for robust policies and programs designed to create a physician workforce that is demographically representative of the United States population. Underrepresented minority medical students tend to go into primary care more often and choose to serve Black, Latino, or Native American populations more often than students of other races or ethnicities.[15] Historically Black colleges and universities have played a significant role in the education of Black physicians. Although these institutions represent 2.4% of medical colleges, they house 31% of Black chairs, 10% of Black faculty, and 14% of Black medical students.[14]

To increase the diversity of physicians and other health professions, efforts must begin early, such as exposing minority populations to the STEM programs related to the health professions, funding pipeline programs, and providing mentoring for underrepresented students.

Cultural Competency Training in Medical Education and in the Health Care Workforce

Efforts to eliminate racial/ethnic disparities are strengthened by cultural competency training in medical education and in the health care workforce. Cultural competency influences how health messages are transmitted and perceived, how illness is defined, when and where care is obtained, and how treatment options are considered.[15] However, cultural competency must begin with cultural humility; individuals who seek to become culturally competent must engage in self-reflection and become aware of their personal biases. Cultural competency can be taught as part of medical education and continuing professional education programs and includes the acquisition and integration of knowledge about culture and cultural differences that enables health care professionals to provide optimal care to patients from different racial, ethnic, socioeconomic, and cultural backgrounds.[16–18] When cultural competence is balanced with cultural humility, individuals acknowledge their personal limitations about acquiring complete knowledge of every culture and make a lifelong commitment to understanding the complexity of identities. They know that they will never be fully competent about the evolving and dynamic nature of a population's experiences.[18]

The American Medical Association developed the Health Disparities Toolkit, which focused on the theme of "Working Together to End Racial and Ethnic Disparities: One Physician at a Time."[1] The toolkit included DVD interviews with physicians, nurses and patients and a CD of information on topics such as cultural competence and health literacy.

Addressing Medical Distrust among African Americans

Medical distrust among African Americans stems from historical medical mistreatment and unethical medical research by medical professionals that dates as far back as chattel slavery. It also stems from contemporary experiences of discrimination when African Americans access health care and when they interact socially. African Americans are more likely to report that they believe their physician will expose them to unnecessary risk, prescribe them experimental medications, not provide them with the best care available, and be motivated by profit.[19-21] The literature on medical distrust has documented how distrust of health care systems and providers among African Americans and other minorities contributes to poor patient outcomes and decreased access to health care.[8] Contrarily, research indicates that greater interpersonal trust between a physician and patient is a significant predicator of acceptance of recommended care and self-reported improvement in health.[22] Expert reports and individual research studies have identified several measures that decrease medical trust.[8] These include ensuring that the health care workforce is diverse, increasing the number of practicing Black physicians, addressing racial bias in medicine, and strengthening cultural competency training for the health care workforce. Important trends such as patient-centered care and shared decision-making between patients and providers also help alleviate medical distrust and improve health outcomes.

Enhance Surveillance Activities to Monitor Health Disparities among African Americans

At the federal level, the United States Department of Health and Human Services is engaged in a range of activities to monitor the health of African Americans and other important population subgroups. This includes surveillance systems maintained by the Centers for Disease Control and Prevention (CDC), the National Center for Health Statistics, the National Institutes of Health, the Centers for Medicare and Medicaid Services, and the Health Resources Services Administration. Two such systems are the National Health Interview Survey and the Behavioral Risk Factor Surveillance System, both of which are maintained by the CDC. Additionally, the Agency for Healthcare Research and Quality maintains the *National Quality and Disparities Report*, which features data on the quality of and access to health care with a particular focus on racial and ethnic disparities.[23] In 2013, the CDC released its second *Health Disparities and Inequalities Report*.[24]

To monitor progress toward eliminating health care disparities among African Americans, particularly those who live in the southern United States, public health professionals must leverage these national surveillance activities to identify regional and state-specific disparities and develop targeted strategies to address them.

Designing and Implementing Culturally Tailored Interventions to Address Health Disparities

As Coughlin et al. noted in chapter 1, efforts to address health disparities among African Americans are furthered by evidence-based interventions to improve the health of diverse communities. This includes information provided by the Guide to Community Preventive Services and by leading health advocacy organizations and professional associations.[25] Interventions the Community Guide has identified as evidence-based effective practices based on systematic literature reviews can be recommended to local and state health departments and to other stakeholders for routine use in public health. Instances where the Community Guide has concluded that there is insufficient evidence that an intervention is effective in improving health suggest opportunities for further research.

The Department of Health and Human Services supports noteworthy federal infrastructures designed to advance community-engaged research, related infrastructures, and related translation. The National Institute on Minority Health and Health Disparities conducts and supports research in minority health and health disparities and promotes and supports the training of a diverse research workforce.[26] For example, the institute supports community-based participatory research aimed at addressing health disparities in racial and ethnic communities. The CDC also supports community-based participatory research in diverse communities, including African Americans in the South.

Programs described in the *Strategies for Reducing Health Disparities— Selected CDC-Sponsored Interventions, United States, 2016*, a supplement to the *Morbidity and Mortality Weekly Report*, are examples of CDC-sponsored initiatives that address health disparities with the goal of advancing health equity.[27] The 2016 supplement includes interventions to address disparities by race and ethnicity, socioeconomic status, geographic location, disability, and sexual orientation across a range of conditions.

Disseminating Effective, Evidence-Based Programs

Health disparities and inequities are best addressed at the individual, neighborhood, group, community, social, and policy levels.[28] Several community-based research studies have used the socio-ecological model to plan multilevel health interventions.[29] According to this model, health interventions can be aimed at the individual, the social, or interpersonal level (e.g., friends, family, coworkers); the organizational level (e.g., health care providers and employers); and the structural or environmental level (e.g., the built environment). Health interventions can also be aimed at the level of the community or public policy. In practice, health intervention research (e.g., community context, organizational setting, policy environment) is often multilevel and crosses socioecological levels, even when it is not conducted or reported as such.[30]

In order to address health disparities among African Americans in the southern United States, evidence-based interventions that have been found to be effective need to be disseminated and implemented more broadly. Dissemination refers to the active promotion or support of a health program to encourage its widespread adoption.[31] This includes the adaptation, evaluation, implementation, and maintenance of an intervention that has been shown to be effective. In contrast, diffusion is the passive process by which a health program becomes routine practice. Even when research findings are published, successful evidence-based programs rarely diffuse passively to become routine practice. Instead, active efforts are needed to disseminate research-tested health interventions to other communities.[31] Dissemination requires foresight, long-term planning, and support. The potential for dissemination should be a consideration throughout the planning, implementation, evaluation, and reporting stages of health intervention research.[31] The dissemination and translation of community-based research findings to address public health concerns helps ensure that the research has practical results that lead to the greatest possible benefit.

Partnerships at the Local, State, and National Levels

Effective partnerships are essential for addressing health disparities among African Americans and other important population subgroups. This includes partnerships at the local level such as community advisory boards and local health coalitions. For example, in order for community-based research projects to be successful, a community advisory board or committee that consists of community residents and representatives of group organizations should be established. When implemented successfully, such groups function to advance equity in the planning and conduct of the research. The experiences of exploitation in research or other social systems (economic, political, racial/ethnic) of community members can be channeled through community advisory boards, where they can inform research development and implementation plans that demonstrate the trustworthiness of the researcher or clinician.[32]

Many community advisory boards include patient representatives and other community residents, representatives from local nonprofit organizations and faith-based institutions, teachers, business owners, primary care providers, and representatives from local hospitals or clinics. Community advisory board members and academic researchers work together to identify priority health concerns, identify community resources, undertake health needs assessments, and plan and monitor community-based research studies. Academic researchers who engage a community advisory board in order to plan and conduct community-based research projects must foster communication and seek to develop trust within the partnership. The focus should be on encouraging equitable participation and establishing norms for working together.[32] To build a partnership, academic researchers can confer with people in their institution who have existing community partnerships for guidance and can provide introductions to community leaders and key informants. Local public health departments, agencies, nonprofit organizations, and coalitions are also likely to be helpful. Potential partners may differ in the extent to which they focus on research versus delivery of health services, acquiring new scientific knowledge versus building infrastructure, or publishing versus informing policy change. Building and sustaining a community-based research partnership requires a long-term commitment of time and effort on the part of the partners.[28]

Examples of successful partnerships at the state and national levels include the National Black Leadership Initiative on Cancer (NBLIC), which was funded by the National Cancer Institute, and the National Comprehensive Cancer Control Program of the CDC.[33] In 1986, the National Cancer Advisory Board, recognizing the significant disparity in cancer incidence and mortality between Blacks and whites, approved a special initiative to reach African Americans. NBLIC was launched as the first minority outreach project of the National Cancer Institute. Under the leadership of Dr. Louis W. Sullivan, president emeritus of the Morehouse School of Medicine and former secretary of the United States Department of Health and Human Services, NBLIC elicited interest in, support for, and participation in dissemination of information about smoking cessation, dietary modification, cancer screening, and early detection across the nation. These efforts improved access to care and advocacy. The National Comprehensive Cancer Control Program, which was established in 1998, provides funding, guidance, and technical assistance that programs use to design and implement impactful, strategic, and sustainable plans to prevent and control cancer.[34]

Conclusions

Addressing health disparities among African Americans in the southern United States involves an array of challenges, including limited capacity to address social determinants of health, declines in funding for prevention and for public health and health care workforce initiatives, and gaps in surveillance data for measuring and understanding disparities.[3] Although the breadth and depth of health disparities among African Americans may seem daunting, several important measures can be taken to address them, as summarized in this chapter and throughout this book, and such measures should be strengthened and continued. To improve the situation, we recommend that public health officials routinely collect surveillance data that includes data on race, ethnicity and geographic locality and make concerted efforts to monitor health disparities among African Americans living in the southern United States. In addition, we recommend that additional centers of excellence and research networks on minority health be established in southern states to further identify and disseminate effective, evidence-based interventions to improve the health of African Americans and other socioeconomically disadvantaged population subgroups.

It is essential that efforts to ensure quality, affordable, and culturally appropriate health care be strengthened and continued, such as improving and revitalizing the ACA and continuing the expansion of Medicaid in southern states. Still, we recognize that ensuring access to affordable health care is not enough and that in order to ameliorate health disparities among African Americans in the southern United States and other socioeconomically disadvantaged populations, it is necessary to address social determinants of health such as poverty, unemployment, lack of education, inadequate housing, and structural racism. Evidence-based interventions that are likely to improve the health of African Americans in the South and elsewhere in the United States include policy interventions targeted at education and early childhood, urban planning and community development, housing, employment, and income enhancements and supplements.[35,36]

REFERENCES

1. American Medical Association. "Reducing Disparities in Health Care." https://www
.ama-assn.org/delivering-care/patient-support-advocacy/reducing-disparities-health-care.

2. Hall, W. J., M. V. Chapman, K. M. Lee, Y. M. Merino, T. W. Thomas, B. K. Payne,
E. Eng, S. H. Day, and T. Coyne-Beasley. "Implicit Racial/Ethnic Bias among Health Care
Professionals and Its Influence on Health Care Outcomes: A Systematic Review." *American
Journal of Public Health* 105, no. 12 (2015): e60–e76.

3. Ndugga, N., and S. Artiga. "Disparities in Health and Health Care: Five Key Questions
and Answers." Kaiser Family Foundation, May 11, 2021. https://www.kff.org/racial-equity
-and-health-policy/issue-brief/disparities-in-health-and-health-care-five-key-questions
-and-answers/.

4. Renna, F., V. D. Kosteas, and K. Dinkar. "Inequality in Health Insurance Coverage
before and after the Affordable Care Act." *Health Economics* 30, no. 2 (2021): 384–402.

5. Blumenthal, D., S. R. Collins, and E. J. Fowler. "The Affordable Care Act at 10 Years—
Its Coverage and Access Provisions." *New England Journal of Medicine* 382 (2020): 963–969.

6. Ho, V. "Refinement of the Affordable Care Act." *Annual Review of Medicine* 69 (2018):
19–28.

7. Chait, N., and S. Glied. "Promoting Prevention under the Affordable Care Act." *Annual Review of Public Health* 39 (2018): 507–524.

8. Smedley, B. D., A. Y. Stith, and A. R. Nelson, eds. 2003. *Unequal Treatment: Confronting Racial and Ethnic Disparities in Health Care*. Washington, DC: National Academies Press.

9. Lurie, N. "Addressing Health Disparities: Where Should We Start?" *Health Services
Research* 37, no. 5 (2002): 1125–1127.

10. American Association of Medical Colleges. *Altering the Course: Black Males in Medicine*. [Washington, DC: American Association of Medical Colleges, 2015.

11. Lett, L. A., H. M. Murdock, W. U. Orji, J. Aysola, and R. Sebrol. "Trends in Racial/
Ethnic Representation among US Medical Students." *JAMA Network Open* 2, no. 9 (2019):
e1910490.

12. Cohen, J. J., B. A. Gabriel, and C. Terrell. "The Case for Diversity in the Health Care
Workforce." *Health Affairs (Millwood)* 21, no. 5 (2002): 90–102.

13. Moy, E., Bartman, B. A. 'Physician Race and Care of Minority and Medically Indigent Patients." *Journal of the American Medical Association* 273 (1995): 1515–20.

14. Komaromy, M., K. Grumbach, M. Drake, K. Vranizan, N. Lurie, D. Keane, and A. B.
Bindman. "The Role of Black and Hispanic Physicians in Providing Health Care for Underserved Populations." *New England Journal of Medicine* 334, no. 20 (1996): 1305–1310.

15. Rodriguez, J. E., I. A. Lopez, K. M. Campbell, and M. Dutton. "The Role of Historically Black College and University Medical Schools in Academic Medicine." *Journal of Health
Care for the Poor and Underserved* 28, no. 1 (2017): 266–278.

16. Coughlin, S. S., P. Matthews-Juarez, P. D. Juarez, C. E. Melton, and M. King. "Opportunities to Address Lung Cancer Disparities among African Americans." *Cancer Medicine*
3, no. 6 (2014): 1467–1776.

17. Agner, J. "Moving From Cultural Competence to Cultural Humility in Occupational
Therapy: A Paradigm Shift." *American Journal of Occupational Therapy* 2020 74 (2020): 18.

18. Masters, C., D. Robinson, S. Faulkner, E. Patterson, T. McIlraith, and A. Ansari. "Addressing Biases in Patient Care with The 5Rs of Cultural Humility, a Clinician Coaching Tool." *Journal of General Internal Medicine* 34, no. 4 (2019): 627–630.

19. Whetten, K., J. Leserman, R. Whetten, J. Ostermann, N. Thielman, M. Swartz, and D. Stangl. "Exploring Lack of Trust in Care Providers and the Government as a Barrier to Health Service Use." *American Journal of Public Health* 96, no. 4 (2006): 716–721.

20. Corbie-Smith, G., S. B. Thomas, and M. M. St. George. "Distrust, Race, and Research." *Archives of Intern Medicine* 162 (2002): 2458–63.

21. Miller, S. T., H. M. Seib, and S. P. Dennie. "African American Perspectives on Health Care: The Voice of the Community." *Journal of Ambulatory Care Management* 24 (2001): 37–44.

22. Jacobs, E. A., I. Rolle, C. E. Ferrans, E. Whittaker, and R. B. Warnecke. "Understanding African Americans' Views of the Trustworthiness of Physicians." *Journal of General Internal Medicine* 21, no. 6 (2006): 642–647.

23. Agency for Healthcare Research and Quality. *2018 National Healthcare Quality and Disparities Report.* Rockville, MD: AHRQ, 2019. https://www.ahrq.gov/research/findings /nhqrdr/nhqdr18/index.html.

24. CDC. "CDC Health Disparities and Inequalities Report—United States, 2013." *Morbidity and Mortality Weekly Report* 63, no. 2 (Suppl.) (2013): 1–186.

25. CDC. "The Guide to Community Preventive Services." www.thecommunityguide .org.

26. National Institute on Minority Health and Health Disparities. "About NIMHD." Last reviewed February 21, 2022. https://www.nimhd.nih.gov/about/.

27. Centers for Disease Prevention and Control. "Strategies for Reducing Health Disparities. Selected CDC-Sponsored Interventions, United States, 2016." Last reviewed October 3, 2016. https://www.cdc.gov/minorityhealth/strategies2016/index.html.

28. Rhodes, S. D., R. M. Malow, and C. Jolly. "Community-Based Participatory Research (CBPR): A New and Not-So-New Approach to HIV/AIDS Prevention, Care, and Treatment." *AIDS Education and Prevention* 22, no. 3 (2010): 173–183.

29. Breslow, L. "Social Ecological Strategies for Promoting Healthy Lifestyles." *American Journal of Health Promotion* 10, no. 4 (1996): 253–257.

30. Neta, G., R. E. Glasgow, C. R. Carpenter, J. M. Grimshaw, B. A. Rabin, M. E. Fernandez, and R. C. Brownson. "A Framework for Enhancing the Value of Research for Dissemination and Implementation." *American Journal of Public Health* 105, no. 1 (2015): 49–57.

31. Glasgow, R. E., A. C. Marcus, S. S. Bull, and K. M. Wilson. "Disseminating Effective Cancer Screening Interventions." *Cancer* 101, Suppl. 5 (2004): 1239–1250.

32. Baldwin, J. A., J. L. Johnson, and C. C. Benally. "Building Partnerships between Indigenous Communities and Universities: Lessons Learned in HIV/AIDS and Substance Abuse Prevention Research." *American Journal of Public Health* 99, Suppl. 1 (2009): S77–S82.

33. National Black Leadership Initiative on Cancer. http://nblicfoundation.org/.

34. CDC. "About the National Comprehensive Cancer Control Program." Last reviewed July 30, 2021. https://www.cdc.gov/cancer/ncccp/about.htm.

35. Thornton, R. L. J., C. M. Glover, C. W. Cene, D. C. Glik, J. A. Henderson, and D. R.

Williams. "Evaluating Strategies for Reducing Health Disparities by Addressing the Social Determinants of Health." *Health Affairs (Millwood)* 35, no. 8 (2016): 1416–1423.

36. U.S. Dept. of Health and Human Services, Office of the Secretary, Office of the Assistant Secretary for Planning and Evaluation and Office of Minority Health. "HHS Action Plan to Reduce Racial and Ethnic Health Disparities Implementation Progress Report." November 2015. https://aspe.hhs.gov/reports/hhs-action-plan-reduce-racial-ethnic-health -disparities-implementation-progress-report-2011-2014-0.

Index

abortion, 345–46, 347, 359

access to health care: and colorectal cancer, 309, 314, 318, 322; and diabetes, 183, 190, 192–93; and infant mortality, 372, 377–79; and kidney disease, 164–66; and maternal mortality, 386, 388–90, 394, 397–98; and mental health, 254; in overview, 8, 9, 10; and prostate cancer, 271–72, 294; and recruiting physicians, 39–42, 44; and reproductive justice, 346; and residential segregation, 9, 22; and rurality, 248; and socioeconomic status, 184; as systemic problem, 9, 10, 31–45

acculturation and prostate cancer, 282, 283, 285, 286–87, 294

Active and Healthy Brotherhood, 72–73

acute myocardial infarction, 137, 140–41

ADHD (attention deficit hyperactivity disorder), 240

adherence to treatment, 126, 144, 169–70, 183, 193, 314, 338, 339

adiponectin, 211

Advancing American Kidney Health Initiative, 160, 170

adverse birth outcomes: and discrimination, 25; and doula care, 359; genetic factors in, 11; and interpersonal violence, 225; and life course perspective, 10; and residential segregation, 9; and rurality, 378–79. *See also* low birth weight; preterm birth

adverse childhood experiences, 8, 23, 225, 227–28, 234, 247–48

Affordable Care Act: and colorectal cancer, 319–20, 322–23; improvement suggestions, 409–10; and infant mortality, 379; and kidney disease, 165–66, 170; and Medicaid expansion, 41–42, 163, 165–66, 319–20, 322, 379, 397, 409–10

African sleeping sickness, 153

age: and diabetes, 187; maternal, 349, 376, 387; and mental health, 240; and prostate cancer, 272–73; and weathering, 377, 394

agency, patient, 59–60, 346–47, 387

Agency for Healthcare Research and Quality, 97, 98, 220, 414

AIDS/HIV. *See* HIV/AIDS

albuminuria, 156

alcohol use: and adverse childhood experiences, 247; and colorectal cancer, 312–13; and depression, 252; and discrimination, 23, 25; and gender, 25; and interpersonal racism, 10; and mental health, 252; and prostate cancer, 273, 274; rates of, 250

allostatic load, 11, 23, 168–69, 182, 209, 252, 394

Ambulatory Sentinel Practice Network, 97

American Cancer Society, 274, 318, 321, 335

American College of Cardiology, 117–18, 143

American College of Gastroenterology, 317

American Diabetes Association, 181, 185, 195

American Gastroenterological Association, 319

American Heart Association, 117–18, 120, 121–22, 142, 143, 144, 219–20

American Medical Association, 20, 36–37, 393, 413

American Stoke Association, 210, 212, 219, 220

amputations, 190, 191

androgen receptors, 275–76

anger, 26, 252

angina, 135

angiography, 216

anxiety, 26, 182, 225, 232, 247, 249, 252, 287

APOL1 (apolipoprotein L1 gene), 152–54, 158–59, 161–62

asbestos, 337

aspirin, 143, 280

asthma, 11, 357

Atherosclerosis Risk in Communities Study (ARIC), 119, 136–37, 139, 141

atherosclerotic cardiovascular disease. *See* coronary heart disease

attention deficit hyperactivity disorder (ADHD), 240

Milton Keynes UK
Ingram Content Group UK Ltd.
UKHW041852150224
437889UK00007B/146/J

9 781421 445465